Neuropharmacotherapy in Critical Illness

Updates in Neurocritical Care

Updates in Neurocritical Care
Edited by Romergryko G. Geocadin

Neuropharmacotherapy in Critical Illness
Edited by Gretchen M. Brophy

Cerebral Herniation Syndromes and Intracranial Hypertension
Edited by Matthew Koenig

Neuropharmacotherapy in Critical Illness

Updates in Neurocritical Care

Edited by **Gretchen M. Brophy**

Series Editor
Romergryko G. Geocadin

MEDICINE

New Brunswick, Camden, and Newark, New Jersey, and London

Library of Congress Cataloging-in-Publication Data

Names: Brophy, Gretchen M., editor.
Title: Neuropharmacotherapy in critical illness / edited by Gretchen M. Brophy.
Description: New Brunswick, New Jersey : Rutgers University Press Medicine, 2017. | Series: Updates in neurocritical care | Includes bibliographical references and index.
Identifiers: LCCN 2017017718 (print) | LCCN 2017018903 (ebook) | ISBN 9780813584690 (E-pub) | ISBN 9780813584706 (Web PDF) | ISBN 9780813590356 (paperback : alk. paper) | ISBN 9780813584690 (epub) | ISBN 9780813590585 (mobi) | ISBN 9780813584706 (PDF)
Subjects: | MESH: Trauma, Nervous System—drug therapy | Brain Injuries, Traumatic—drug therapy | Cerebrovascular Disorders—drug therapy
Classification: LCC RC387.5 (ebook) | LCC RC387.5 (print) | NLM WL 140 | DDC 617.4/81061—dc23
LC record available at https://lccn.loc.gov/2017017718

A British Cataloging-in-Publication record for this book is available from the British Library.

This publication was supported in part by the Eleanor J. and Jason F. Dreibelbis Fund

Executive Editor: Kel McGowan
Design and composition: Westchester Publishing Services

♾ The paper used in this publication meets the requirements of the American National Standard for Information Sciences—Permanence of Paper for Printed Library Materials, ANSI Z39.48-1992.

www.rutgersuniversitypress.org

Manufactured in the United States of America

CONTENTS

FOREWORD

Welcome to the second volume in the Updates in Neurocritical Care series, *Neuropharmacotherapy in Critical Illness.*

Updates in Neurocritical Care was developed in response to clinical demands for expertise in neurocritical care. This series bring state-of-the-art knowledge and best practices to the health care providers in the field of neurocritical care. We are excited to bring together leading experts to provide clinicians with the various relevant and practical factors for treating patients with neurocritical illnesses.

We are privileged to have Gretchen M. Brophy serve as the editor of this volume. Dr. Brophy is Professor of Pharmacotherapy and Outcomes Science and Neurosurgery at Virginia Commonwealth University. She is also vice-president of the Neurocritical Care Society (NCS) and the overall chair of the NCS 2017 Annual Meeting.

Dr. Brophy has put together for this book a team of clinical pharmacy specialists that are experts in the field of neurocritical care, and have years of experience in teaching, research and clinical practice.

The clinical practice of neurocritical care addresses neurological illness with the predominant issues not only centered within the nervous system, but also involving complex direct and indirect systemic factors. Management of these complex illnesses requires both understanding the pathophysiology and mastering the neuropharmacology. In this book, Dr. Brophy has assembled pharmacy experts that are in active practice at top medical institutions in the United States. They have extensive knowledge and real-world experience in utilizing the medications relevant to neuerocritical care. These pharmacists practice in a multidisciplinary setting; they are also active in teaching health care professionals, residents, and students about therapeutic entities and management in neurocritical care.

I extend my sincerest appreciation to Dr. Brophy and to the contributors of this volume. I also extend my deep appreciation for the dedication and professionalism of Kel McGowan, Executive Editor for Clinical Health and Medicine, and her team at Rutgers University Press. The development of this series is made possible by the collaboration of the editors, authors, and Rutgers University Press.

Romergryko G. Geocadin, MD FNCS, FANA, FAAN

PREFACE

Neurocritical care patients often pose significant management challenges, which are often commonly complicated by concomitant drug therapies. To avoid unwanted adverse drug effects and drug-drug interactions, it is important to choose the right drug for the right patient. *Updates in Neurocritical Care: Neuropharmacotherapy in Critical Illness* focuses on pharmacotherapeutic strategies in critically ill patients with neurological injuries.

This book is written by a team of clinical pharmacy specialists who are experts in the field of neurocritical care and have years of experience in teaching, research, and clinical practice. These pharmacy experts provide care for neurocritical care patients in institutions all across the United States and have extensive knowledge and experience using the medications that are discussed. In addition, these pharmacists practice in a multidisciplinary setting, teaching health care professionals, residents, and students about neurocritical care therapeutic entities and management strategies at the bedside, as well as in the didactic setting. Each author has contributed a chapter focusing on neurocritical care pharmacotherapies that are clinically relevant, comprehensive, and highly specific to the care of neurologically injured patients.

Therapeutic strategies for the treatment of neurocritical care patients can be variable around the globe but are also similar in regards to the drug class being used for treatment. These common drug classes are discussed in this book and include hyperosmolar therapies for traumatic brain injury, sedation and neuromuscular blockade, antithrombotic therapies for ischemic stroke, coagulopathy reversal strategies for intracranial hemorrhage, pharmacotherapy for vasospasm prophylaxis and treatment in subarachnoid hemorrhage, pharmacotherapy of acute spinal cord injury, hemodynamic management strategies for hypertensive emergencies and shock, antiepileptic agents for seizure prophylaxis and treatment, neurostimulants for acute brain injury, and intraventricular and intrathecal drug therapies. Evidence-based, clinically significant neuropharmacotherapy pearls on medication mechanisms of action, pharmacokinetics, pharmacodynamics, drug-drug interactions, and adverse drug reactions are provided to assist in optimizing treatment strategies for neurocritical care patients.

GRETCHEN M. BROPHY

CONTRIBUTING AUTHORS

Teresa A. Allison, PharmD, BCPS, BCCCP
Clinical Pharmacist Specialist, Neurosciences
Program Director, PGY2 Critical Care Residency
Memorial Hermann Texas Medical Center
Department of Pharmacy Services
Houston, TX

Karen Berger, PharmD, BCPS, BCCCP
Clinical Pharmacy Manager
Neurosciences Intensive Care Unit
New York Presbyterian Hospital
Weill Cornell Medical Center
New York, NY

Kathleen A. Bledsoe, PharmD, BCPS
Pharmacy Clinical Coordinator of Neurosciences
University of Virginia Health System
Charlottesville, VA

Jennifer Bushwitz, PharmD
BJC Healthcare
Washington University in St Louis
St Louis, MO

Amber Castle, PharmD, BCPS, BCCCP
Pharmacy Supervisor, Education & Residencies
PGY-1 Residency Program Coordinator
Yale New Haven Hospital
Yale University
New Haven, CT

Katleen Chester, PharmD, BCCCP
Clinical Pharmacist Specialist, Neurocritical Care
Director, PGY-2 Critical Care Specialty Residency Program
Director, PGY-2 Neuroscience Specialty Residency Program
Adjunct Assistant Professor, Emory University School of Nursing
Grady Health System
Atlanta, GA

Aaron M. Cook, PharmD, BCPS
Clinical Coordinator-Neuroscience-Pulmonary/Critical Care
Associate Adjunct Professor, Pharmacy
Director, PGY1 Pharmacy Residency Program
University of Kentucky
Lexington, KY

Emily Durr, PharmD, BCCCP
Critical Care Clinical Specialist
Grady Medical Center
Atlanta, GA

Olabisi Falana, PharmD, BCPS, BCCCP
Clinical Pharmacy Specialist—Neurocritical Care
The University of Chicago Medicine
Chicago, IL

Jose Guzman Garcia, PharmD, BCCCP
Clinical Pharmacy Specialist
Dignity Health
Mercy General Hospital
Sacramento, CA

Haley Goodwin Gibbs, PharmD, MPH
Medication Strategy Specialist
Wake Forest Baptist Health
Winston-Salem, NC

Kristy N. Greene, PharmD, BCPS, BCCCP
Clinical Pharmacist Specialist, Neuroscience Critical Care Medicine
Emory University Hospital Midtown
Atlanta, GA

Jimmi Hatton-Kolpek, PharmD, FCCP, FCCM
Professor
Department of Pharmacy Practice and Science
University of Kentucky College of Pharmacy
Lexington, KY

Theresa Human, PharmD, BCPS, FNCS
Neuroscience Clinical Specialist
Washington University
Barnes-Jewish Hospital
St Louis, MO

Lisa Kurczewski, PharmD, BCPS, BCCCP
Clinical Pharmacy Specialist, Neurocritical Care
Virginia Commonwealth University Health System
Clinical Assistant Professor
Virginia Commonwealth University School of Pharmacy
Richmond, VA

John J. Lewin III, PharmD, MBA, FASHP, FCCM, FNCS, BCCCP
Division Director—Critical Care and Surgery Pharmacy
The Johns Hopkins Hospital
Associate Professor
Anesthesiology & Critical Care Medicine, Johns Hopkins University
    School of Medicine
Clinical Professor
University of Maryland School of Pharmacy
The Johns Hopkins Hospital
Baltimore, MD

Norah Liang, PharmD, BCPS
Clinical Pharmacist—Neurocritical Care/Neurology
Hartford Hospital
Hartford, CT

Kathryn Morbitzer, PharmD
Business Intelligence and Data Analytics Pharmacist
UNC Health Care
Assistant Professor of Clinical Education
Division of Practice Advancement and Clinical Education
UNC Eshelman School of Pharmacy
Chapel Hill, NC

Christopher Morrison, PharmD, BCCCP
Clinical Specialist—Critical Care
Memorial Hospital West
Pembroke Pines, FL

Ron Neyens, PharmD
Neurocritical Care Clinical Pharmacy Specialist
Medical University of South Carolina
Charleston, SC

Viet Nguyen, PharmD, MPH, MS, BCPS
Assistant Professor
Chapman University School of Pharmacy
Orange, CA

Nicholas G. Panos, PharmD, BCPS
Clinical Pharmacy Specialist, Neuroscience Intensive Care
Department of Pharmacy
Rush University Medical Center
Chicago, IL

Denise H. Rhoney, PharmD, FCCP, FCCM, FNCS
Ron and Nancy McFarlane Distinguished Professor and Chair
Division of Practice Advancement and Clinical Education
UNC Eshelman School of Pharmacy
Chapel Hill, NC

A. Shaun Rowe, PharmD, BCPS, BCCCP, FNCS
Associate Professor of Clinical Pharmacy
University of Tennessee Health Science Center
College of Pharmacy–Knoxville Campus
Pharmacist Specialist, Neurocritical Care
University of Tennessee Medical Center
Knoxville, TN

Ted Sindlinger, PharmD
Neurology Clinical Pharmacist
University of Virginia
Charlottesville, VA

Eljim P. Tesoro, PharmD, BCPS
Clinical Associate Professor
University of Illinois at Chicago
Chicago, IL

Neuropharmacotherapy in Critical Illness

Hyperosmolar Therapy in Traumatic Brain Injury

Haley Goodwin Gibbs, Jose Guzman Garcia, and Ron Neyens

INTRODUCTION

Severe brain injury results in a complex secondary injury cascade, with ensuing cerebral edema and elevated intracranial pressure (ICP). This process is a common contributor to permanent neurological sequelae and death. Cerebral edema is primarily manifested as 2 distinct physiological processes: vasogenic (eg, capillary permeability) and/or cytotoxic (eg, cellular apoptosis).[1] Osmotherapy is designed to create an osmotic gradient across the blood-brain barrier (BBB), resulting in an intended reduction of brain water content.

Osmotherapy has a long-standing history, with concentrated electrolyte solutions shown to decrease ICP and brain bulk in the early 1900s. It was not until the 1950s before osmotic formulations were routinely used clinically as a therapeutic tool in the management of intracranial hypertension. Initially, formulations of urea were standard therapy, but adverse effects and observations of intracranial pressure rebound limited its use, driving a transition to glycerol and sorbitol in the 1960s, followed by mannitol in the late 1960s and hypertonic saline in the 1990s.[2] The latter 2 osmotic agents now stand as guideline-based recommendations and a major component of neurocritical care treatment strategies for cerebral edema and intracranial hypertension.

1

MECHANISM

The exact mechanism of ICP reduction with osmotherapy remains ill-defined yet potentially involves several characteristics. The major therapeutic impact is felt to be a complex and dynamic result of osmotic dehydration and rheologically induced cerebrovascular vasoconstriction with reduced cerebral blood volume (CBV).

Osmotic Dehydration

The BBB is a highly selective permeability barrier separating the brain extracellular fluid from the circulating blood. It is composed of endothelial cells, connected by high-density cellular tight junctions. It serves as a self-protective mechanism allowing passive transport of water and small lipid-soluble molecules, as well as active transport of molecules necessary for optimal neuronal function.[3] It relies on the osmotic principle that the BBB allows transport of water from compartments with low osmolality to those with higher osmolality. An induced high-osmole concentration gradient mobilizes water from the interstitial and intracellular compartments of the brain into the intravascular compartment, therefore reducing brain water content, mass effect, and ICP. Clinical practice has evolved to using mannitol and hypertonic sodium solutions as they are more effective osmoles than urea, glycerol, and sorbitol. Therefore, they display low permeability across the BBB, referred to as its reflection coefficient (σ), which is an index of the effectiveness of a solute in generating an osmotic driving force ($\sigma = 1$ for hypertonic sodium solutions and $\sigma = 0.9$ for mannitol on a scale of $0-1$, with the most effective being 1). The osmotic model assumes an intact BBB, expressing low hydraulic conductivity.[4] The degree of BBB disruption is not readily determined clinically in the neurologically injured patient. Therefore, the osmotic dehydration effect may occur more effectively in normal rather than injured or impaired brain tissue; however, the clinical relevance remains debatable and ill-defined.[5]

Rheology and Vascular Reactivity

The brain has little capacity to store oxygen, with its survivability dependent on an adequate cerebral blood flow (CBF) and cerebral oxygen delivery (CDO_2). In normal physiological conditions, homeostatic cerebral autoregulation is in place to ensure that supply (ie, CBF and CDO_2) is coupled to meet demand (ie, cerebral metabolic rate for oxygen consumption), despite variations in cerebral perfusion pressure (CPP). This occurs via a tight regulation of cerebral vascular resistance, stimulated by various interrelated processes involving pressure, chemical, and electrical gradients.[6] The rheological principle of osmotherapy relies on its ability to increase red blood cell deformity resulting in reduced blood viscosity, independent of changes in hematocrit.[2] It is proposed that this promotes compensatory vasoconstriction of both arterioles and venules on the surface of the brain to maintain homeostatic CBF and thus reduces CBV and resultant ICP.[7] This model assumes intact vascular reactivity and has been challenged in the pathology of acute brain injury.[8]

Pleotropic

Several other proposed mechanisms exist, including immunomodulatory, free radical scavenging, and neuroendocrine effects.[9–11] With unclear clinical relevance, hypertonic sodium solutions may assist in preserving the BBB by restoring normal resting membrane potential, which is not observed with mannitol.[12]

HYPEROSMOLAR AGENTS

There are several different concentrations of mannitol and hypertonic sodium solutions used in clinical practice. The agents and doses used display variable osmolarities but are believed to yield a therapeutic response via similar principles. For osmotic agents routinely used in clinical practice, see Table 1.1.

Pharmacokinetics and Pharmacodynamics

An optimal dose-response relationship has not been clearly defined, and many of the relevant comparative studies have not used equiosmolar dosing strategies. Based on initial clinical observations, an osmotic gradient of 5 to 10 mOsmol/kg was considered necessary for therapeutic efficacy.[13,14] However, it remains incompletely understood as it is clear that hypertonic sodium solutions effectively reduce ICP, with relatively small total osmole doses (eg, 23.4% 30 mL = 240 mOsm), even in the face of high serum osmolarity (eg, >320 mOsm/L).[15] In addition, it is a common clinical practice that doses of mannitol 20% and hypertonic sodium solutions are often not equiosmolar, yet both are effective at reducing elevated ICPs. An equiosmolar dose of 1 g/kg 20% mannitol is approximately 5.3 mL/kg 3% saline, 3.2 mL/kg 5% saline, 2.1 mL/kg 7.5% saline, 1.6 mL/kg 10% saline, 1.1 mL/kg 14.6%, and 0.69 mL/kg 23.4% saline.

For both mannitol and hypertonic sodium solutions, the effect on ICP tends to be biphasic. The initial rapid ICP reduction, occurring within minutes, is possibly related to the previously mentioned rheological and cerebral vascular

TABLE 1.1 Hyperosmolar Agents

Agent	Osmolarity, mOsm/L	Dosing	Osmole Dose (70-kg Patient)	Commercial Availability
Mannitol				
20%	1098	Crisis: 0.25 to 1 g/kg over 5 to 15 min	1 g/kg = 384 mOsm	250 mL, 500 mL
25%	1372	Repeat dosing: 0.5 g/kg, can be redosed every 4 to 6 hours	1 g/kg = 384 mOsm	50 mL
Hypertonic saline				
2%	684	Continuous infusion: 0.5 to 2 mL/kg/h	—	—
3%	1027	Crisis: 250 to 300 mL or 2.5 to 5 mL/kg over 5 to 20 min	250 mL = 257 mOsm	500 mL
		Continuous infusion: 0.5 to 2 mL/kg/h		
5%	1711	Crisis: 150 to 200 mL/min or 2.5 to 5 mL/kg over 5 to 20 min	150 mL = 257 mOsm	500 mL
7.5%	2566	Crisis: 1.5 to 2.5 mL/kg over 20 min	1.5 mL/kg = 269 mOsm	—
10%	3422	Crisis: 75 to 100 mL over 20 min	75 mL = 257 mOsm	—
14.6%	4996	Crisis: 40 to 60 mL over 20 min	40 mL = 200 mOsm	20 mL, 40 mL
23.4%	8008	Crisis: 30 mL over 10 to 20 min	30 L = 240 mOsm	30 L

Sources: Adapted from Hinson HE. *J Intensive Care Med.* 2013;28:3–11; Eskandari R. *J Neurosurg.* 2013;119:338–46; and Brophy GM. *Neurocrit Care.* 2015;23(suppl 2):48–68.

reactivity principles. However, the intensity of effect may be dependent on the mean arterial blood pressure (MAP). It has been shown that in the face of elevated blood pressure, an impressive rise in CBF occurred, particularly in the noninjured regions of the brain. However, the CBV was not significantly reduced. Therefore, it has been proposed that osmotherapy-reduced viscosity and reflexive vasoconstriction may be lost at high perfusion pressures (eg, MAPs ≥ 120–130 mm Hg), exceeding the upper limits of autoregulation and reactivity of cerebral resistance arterioles. In effect, they may be maximally vasoconstricted and unable to further respond to reduced viscosity.[8] Although unproven, compensatory vasoconstriction may remain intact at moderate perfusion pressures, assuming autoregulation remains intact.

The later phase, which is delayed 15 to 30 minutes after drug administration, is related to osmotic principles and cellular dehydration. Pharmacokinetic data specifically with hypertonic saline are lacking, but it is observed to be similar to mannitol, with initial effects within minutes, a peak between 15 and 120 minutes, and a duration of response up to 4 to 6 hours.[16] The hydration of brain tissue with osmotherapy persists longer than one would expect given the relatively short serum half-life of the osmotically active agents.

ADMINISTRATION AND STORAGE

Access and Infusion Considerations

Mannitol doses for the treatment of elevated ICP can be infused over 5 to 30 minutes through a peripheral or central line.[17,18] The ability to infuse peripherally makes mannitol an ideal agent in the emergency department or in patients without central access. Rapid infusion over a few minutes produces maximal effects to decrease ICP. Mannitol solutions with concentrations greater than 15% have a tendency to crystallize and therefore require administration through an in-line filter.[17,18]

Hypertonic saline solutions with concentrations greater than 3% are to be administered via a central venous catheter, although the infusion of 3% saline solutions through peripheral venous access at infusion rates of up to 50 mL/h has been associated with a low risk of infusion-related complications.[19] Because rapid infusions of 23.4% can cause hypotension, 30- to 60-mL doses can be administered over 20 minutes or via slow intravenous push as tolerated by the patient. Doses and infusion rates for boluses of lesser concentrated hypertonic saline solutions are patient specific but are generally between 250 and 500 mL and can be infused rapidly via an infusion pump.

As the intraosseous route of administration has been promoted for emergency settings, such as in advanced cardiac life support, it begs the question of whether there is a role to play in neurological emergencies, especially when laying the patient flat for line placement is not possible due to the patient's clinical condition. The effective administration of 7.5% sodium chloride/6% dextran 70 via the intraosseous route has been established in military medicine studies. In addition, Chavez–Negrete et al[20] showed that intraosseous administration of 250 mL of 7.5% sodium chloride/6% dextran 60 was an effective initial treatment for hemorrhagic shock secondary to upper gastrointestinal bleeding. Soft tissue and bone necrosis has been observed following hypertonic saline administration via the intraosseous route in swine models of uncontrolled hemorrhagic shock. As a result, it is recommended to limit hypertonic saline infusions via the intraosseous route to a single 250-mL bolus dose.[20] Mannitol can be administered via intraosseous access safely and effectively.

Bolus vs Continuous Infusions

As suggested by the literature and highlighted in clinical practice, there is no consensus on the optimal mode of administration for hypertonic saline— namely, bolus dosing vs continuous infusions for maintenance therapy. Theoretically, bolus dosing targeting goal serum sodium level would maximize the osmolar gradient after administration and minimize the opportunity for osmotic equilibrium to be established in the setting of a disrupted BBB. Conversely, others believe that the establishment and maintenance of the gradient through reaching a target sodium concentration are responsible for the therapeutic benefit and thus can be done via continuous infusion without diminishing the therapeutic effects, although this has not been studied directly.[21]

Storage

The Joint Commission classifies concentrated electrolytes as high-alert medications. High-alert medications bear increased potential of causing significant patient harm. As a result, The Joint Commission mandates that concentrated electrolyte solutions be obtained from pharmacy services and not be available in patient care areas, unless their unavailability compromises patient care.[22] Because of this, institutions may be reluctant to store hypertonic saline in neurocritical care units; however, mediations given as a standard for the treatment of neurological emergencies should be readily available in areas where these events are likely to occur.[23] This includes hypertonic saline preparations such as 23.4%. The Joint Commission requires health care systems to implement policies and procedures to prevent the inadvertent administration of concentrated electrolytes when stored in patient care areas.[22] Minimum safeguards outlined in policy and procedures should include limiting access, placing warning labels highlighting concentrated electrolyte status as a high-alert medication, and storing separately from other medications.[22] Automatic dispensing machines can aid health systems in preventing inadvertent administration of hypertonic saline when stored in patient care areas. Concentrated saline solutions do not carry the same risk as other concentrated electrolytes (ie, potassium), and because of hypertonic saline's low potential for patient harm, we believe the benefits of having hypertonic saline readily available for the treatment of neurological emergencies in patient care areas outweigh the risk of patient harm.

Mannitol solutions are prone to crystallization, especially at temperatures below 20°C.[18] Crystallization is concentration dependent and more likely to occur with concentrations of greater than 15%. Crystallized mannitol solutions can be warmed using dry heat for 20% mannitol in flexible bags and warm water baths for 25% glass vials. Crystallized solutions should be dissolved into solution prior to administration.[18]

ADVERSE EFFECTS

Rebound Intracranial Hypertension

One of the most concerning adverse effects of osmotic therapy is rebound cerebral edema with subsequent intracranial hypertension and/or herniation syndromes. This is typically thought to occur after a rapid discontinuation of prolonged osmotic therapy, in which a new transcellular equilibrium has been achieved following a relatively high osmolar state.[2,23] The exact mechanism is not well understood but may involve the generation of intracellular osmotically active particles, which then results in a reverse osmotic gradient upon a rapid decline in serum sodium.[23,24] A reverse gradient, with a higher intracellular osmolarity, would then promote an increase in brain water content, which is unintended and of particular importance in patients with low brain compliance.[23] Consequently, when osmotherapy has been employed and a prolonged state of high osmolarity has been maintained, for the ongoing management of intracranial hypertension or cerebral edema, reversal of the hyperosmolar state should be done carefully, regardless of which agent is used. Specifically for hypertonic saline, it is reasonable to continue to frequently monitor sodium levels upon therapy discontinuation to ensure that they do not decline too rapidly. In conjunction, the patient's clinical exam and ICP should be monitored for signs of potential rebound to understand if the rate of decrease is clinically appropriate for that individual patient. A stepwise weaning approach may be required in some patients. For those on continuous infusions, the concentration of hypertonic solution is decreased (eg, 3% to 2% sodium solution) and/or the rate of infusion is slowly decreased to provide a controlled strategy for normalizing serum osmolarity. For those receiving intermittent boluses, the size or concentration of the bolus could be decreased or the interval between boluses could be lengthened.

The other concern for rebound revolves around the potential for intracellular accumulation of osmotically active substances in relation to the principle of hydraulic conductivity and the reflection coefficient. With a reflection coefficient of 0.9, mannitol is more likely to penetrate the intact BBB and accumulate in the transcellular environment.[23,25] This is largely theoretical, but studies have demonstrated the accumulation of mannitol into the central nervous system, as well as captured rebound effects after mannitol administration.[26,27] The accumulation of mannitol seems more likely with repeated dosing and in the presence of impaired renal function; however, it is not likely to occur after single doses used for the treatment of emergent intracranial hypertension or pending herniation syndromes. For this particular reason, it is logical to avoid scheduled dosing of mannitol if other therapies can be used in its place. Continuous infusions of mannitol should never be used. Hypertonic saline, with a reflection coefficient of 1, is not likely to result in accumulation in the setting of an intact BBB, providing a theoretical advantage over mannitol.[2] However, it is unlikely that the integrity of this barrier is completely maintained in the setting of a brain injury; therefore, the reflection coefficient may not entirely explain the pharmacological profile and concerns of accumulation with osmotherapy.

Osmotic Demyelination

Osmotic demyelination is a feared complication that can result from a rapid rise in serum sodium. It is described in individuals with chronic severe hyponatremia, most commonly having a serum sodium concentration of 120 mEq/L or less. The exact mechanism of injury of osmotic demyelination has not been well characterized. However, it is believed that in the setting of chronic hyponatremia, brain cells adapt by decreasing the level of intracellular sodium, potassium, and organic solutes.[28] This adaptive process seems to occur within 24 to 48 hours following severe hyponatremia.[28] After this time, if serum sodium is corrected too rapidly, the brain cells are unable to adapt to the new homeostatic tonicity.[28] Regions of compact interdigitation of white and gray matter (eg, mid-brain, pons, basal ganglia, and cerebellum) are sensitive to fluctuating osmotic forces, resulting in compromised BBB, interstitial edema, and compression of fiber tracts that seems to trigger demyelination and apoptosis.[28] Most neurocritical care patients have a normal or near-normal serum sodium, which is often quickly induced to a hypernatremic state using hypertonic sodium solutions. In this patient subset, very limited data exist, but postherniation magnetic resonance imaging following boluses of hypertonic solutions did not suggest the presence of demyelination.[29,30] The neurocritical care patient may not be completely void of the risk, but it seems that the most important risk factor, baseline serum sodium (<120 mEq/L), is often not present in most of these patients. Anecdotally, expert opinion is that the risk of osmotic demyelination is exceptionally low during induced hypernatremia in the normonatremic neurocritical care patient. In those patients who may have chronic severe hyponatermia, the increase of sodium concentration should generally be limited to 8 to 12 mEq/L over 24 hours or 0.5 to 1 mEq/L/h.[28] Although more caution should be employed, osmotherapy may still be used, particularly in cases of acute intracranial hypertension or herniation syndromes.

Changes in Volume Status

The impact of the 2 osmolar agents on volume status is perhaps one of the most distinguishing characteristics. Mannitol is an osmotic diuretic, which by nature leads to volume depletion and dehydration if adequate measures are not taken for fluid replacement.[17] Conversely, hypertonic saline is a volume expander and has been used as an agent for fluid resuscitation in multiple populations.[17] In most patients with traumatic brain injury (TBI), volume expansion is thought to give the advantage to hypertonic saline as dehydration should be avoided to promote optimal cerebral perfusion. However, in certain patient populations, the diuretic effects might benefit other organ systems. Patients with acute heart failure and pulmonary edema might worsen in the setting of volume expansion and may benefit from diuresis. Conversely, patients with preexisting renal impairment may retain mannitol for an extended period of time and are unable to regulate fluid balance, making them more susceptible to volume overload in the setting of mannitol.[31] In general, patients receiving hyperosmolar agents should be monitored closely with regard to fluid balance and plans should be developed to maintain clinical euvolemia.

Electrolyte Imbalances

Electrolyte imbalances can result from both mannitol and hypertonic saline administration. Initially, mannitol causes osmotic movement of water from cells into the extracellular fluid, causing solvent drag, which may result in transient hyperkalemia and dilutional hyponatremia.[32] Following this initial phenomenon, osmotic diuresis induced by mannitol leads to excretion of potassium and free water, contributing to hypokalemia and hypernatremia.[32] This was observed in a study following repeated doses of mannitol, in which 52% of patients developed hypokalemia and 10% hypernatremia.[32]

Hypertonic saline, although an initial volume expander, promotes natriuresis and renal potassium loss, contributing to hypokalemia. In addition, hypertonic sodium solutions may lead to hyperchloremia with associated non–anion gap metabolic acidosis. Buffered sodium chloride/sodium acetate solutions can be used to reduce the chloride load of hypertonic saline administration, especially when using continuous infusions.[23,31] It remains unknown if this strategy should be empiric in efforts to avoid any complications or reactionary when hyperchloremia develops. The serum pH, chloride, and HCO_3- concentration at which buffered sodium solutions should be considered have not been established. Unfortunately, buffered hypertonic solutions are not commercially available. Therefore, it is reasonable to consider initiation with a nonbuffered commercially available formulation (eg, 3%) to avoid administration delays with plans to switch to a buffered solution when compounded and available from pharmacy services. Overall, the goal should be to maintain a normal pH without excessive compensation.

Renal Dysfunction

Mannitol can cause acute renal failure via several mechanisms, including vasoconstrictor effects on the afferent renal artery, vacuolization of the renal tubular epithelial cells, and depletion of intravascular volume as a result of osmotic diuresis.[31] Patients with preexisting renal impairment and those being administered nephrotoxic drugs are at greater risk of developing acute renal failure. To minimize adverse effects on the kidney, mannitol should not be administered if the serum osmolar gap is greater than 55 mOsm/L, although some clinicians use a more conservative target of 20 mOsm/L.[31,33] Mannitol-induced acute renal failure may be treated by discontinuing mannitol and restoring extracellular fluid volume.[31] If discontinuation of mannitol and volume repletion is not effective, hemodialysis may be required.

Hypertonic sodium solutions may contribute to acute injury as well. Although not well understood, excessive serum chloride induces afferent renal artery vasoconstriction, leading to increased arteriolar resistance and a subsequent decrease in renal blood flow. Multiple general critical care studies have been conducted evaluating the adverse effects of chloride-rich solutions. These studies detail mixed results depending on the volume and type of chloride-rich fluid administered.[34–36] A recent randomized study resulted in a similar incidence of clinically significant acute kidney injury between rather small volumes (~2 L) of a buffered vs chloride-rich solution.[36] Studies specifically with hypertonic saline, carrying a much higher chloride exposure, have not definitively shown a correlation between hyperchloremia and acute kidney injury.[37] In the absence of conclusive data, it is reasonable to minimize hyperchloremia, especially when using continuous infusions of hypertonic sodium solutions.

Impaired Coagulation

Hypertonic saline has been shown to impair coagulation in both animal and in vitro studies.[38,39] Reed et al[38] showed that significant alterations in prothrombin time, activated partial thromboplastin time, and platelet aggregation occur when 10% of plasma was replaced with 7.5% hypertonic saline. Possible mechanisms include impaired enzymatic function in the clotting cascade as a result of increased sodium load and dilution of clotting factors and platelets secondary to transcellular fluid movement. Other research suggests this effect may be minimal.[40,41] Further research is needed to evaluate the clinical implications of hypertonic saline administration on coagulation in humans.

Extravasation and Phlebitis

Hyperosmolar agents pose a major risk for the development of phlebitis and extravasation injuries. Osmotic movement of fluid into the fixed tissue compartment around an infiltration of a hyperosmolar agent produces hypoperfusion, ischemia, and edema, which can progress to tissue necrosis. After extravasation of hyperosmolar agents, patients should be monitored for compartment syndrome. In the event of extravasation, the offending agent should be stopped immediately, the affected limb should be elevated, and attempts to aspirate as much of the infiltrated drug as possible should be made. Cold or hot dry compresses may be applied to the affected area.[42,43] Hyaluronidase has been successfully used in the treatment of extravasated mannitol, and animal data have found tissue-sparing effects during hypertonic saline infiltrations.[44] Hyaluronidase for the treatment of extravasation is administered via multiple 0.5- to 1-mL injections of a 15-U/mL solution injected intradermally or subcutaneously around the periphery of the extravasation. Hyaluronidase must be administered within 1 hour of extravasation.[43]

Hypotension

Rapid infusion of 23.4% can induce transient hypotension.[30] This can be avoided if administered slowly over 20 minutes. Hypotension in the setting of herniation is significant as it can impair cerebral perfusion pressure. Systolic blood pressure must be monitored and maintained to keep cerebral perfusion pressure between 50 and 70 mm Hg.[45,46]

MONITORING PARAMETERS

Normal serum osmolality is 285 to 295 mOsm/L.[25] An osmotic gradient is created when serum osmolality reaches 300 to 320 mOsm/L, and thus the latter range has historically been used as a target for hyperosmolar therapy; however, the osmolar gap is a better estimate of mannitol plasma levels and should be used in place of absolute serum osmolarity thresholds.[24,25,47] An osmolar gap greater than 55 indicates excess accumulation of mannitol in the plasma, and patients with an osmolar gap greater than 55 are at an increased risk of renal complications. However, many clinicians, including the authors of this chapter, prefer a more conservative threshold of 20 mOsm/L for when alternative therapies should be considered, although this practice is not well supported by data.[31,33] A serum osmolality of greater than 320 mOsm/L should not limit the use of mannitol if the osmolar gap is less than the threshold. This is particularly relevant in patients receiving frequent repeated or scheduled doses of mannitol. In the case of emergent therapy for herniation events or ICP crises, the administration of hyperosmolar therapy should not be delayed for this calculation.

The administration of hypertonic saline requires serum sodium concentrations to be monitored initially every 4 to 6 hours and less frequently after sodium levels are consistently within the therapeutic range on a single regimen.[25] No goal serum sodium concentration for the management of TBI has been firmly established in the literature but should generally target sodium levels that correlate with an improvement in exam for each specific patient. Serum sodium concentrations of greater than 160 mEq/L should not limit the use of hypertonic saline for the emergent treatment of sustained ICP greater than 20 or herniation syndromes. In addition to monitoring serum sodium concentrations, it is also important to monitor serum potassium and chloride concentrations for potential development of hypokalemia and hyperchloremic metabolic acidosis.[17,23,25]

While monitoring serum markers of osmolarity and electrolytes is important, it is equally important to monitor the patient's ICPs and neurological status to track the success of the therapies. Normal ICP is 5 to 15 mm Hg. An ICP of 20 to 25 mm Hg is considered the upper threshold at which treatment to lower ICP should generally be initiated.[47,48] The most frequently used methods used to measure ICP are intraventricular and intraparenchymal catheters. Other less common catheters include the extradural and subdural catheters, but they are more prone to concerns regarding accuracy and reliability. Regardless of the ICP catheter used, it is imperative to understand the functionality and associated limitations to best apply to the clinical scenario.[47-49]

Locally measured pressures do not always correlate with herniation events and clinical status, and thus clinical signs and symptoms of elevated ICP should be assessed regularly.[25,45,50] These include progressive deterioration in conscious level, headache, papilledema, and vomiting, but there is no consistent relation between the severity of symptoms and degree of ICP elevation. Fundal hemorrhage is indicative of an acute and severe rise in ICP. Cushing's triad (hypertension, bradycardia, and apnea) in addition to pupillary dilatation, bilateral ptosis, impaired upgaze, extension to pain, and respiratory irregularity are associated with cerebral herniation syndrome. Neurological examination should be performed at least hourly in the acute phase of injury. Post-acute phase neurological examination frequency should be guided by patient condition.

Computed tomography signs that are indicative of cerebral edema and raised ICP include effacement of the sulci, slit-like or obliterated ventricles, loss of gray-white matter differentiation, effacement of the cisterns, and midline shift.[25] The absence of these signs, however, does not indicate normal ICP.

EVIDENCE BASE

Although many publications have attempted to evaluate differences between mannitol and hypertonic saline, there have been very few randomized, controlled studies performed in the human TBI population. Interpreting that body of literature can be challenging given the number of different dosing regimens and the fact that some studies have not evaluated equiosmolar doses of the 2 agents. Given that the hyperosmolar nature of these therapies is thought to in large part drive the efficacy of these agents, this is a significant limitation. This chapter reviews select human studies with randomized controlled designs that studied equiosmolar doses of these therapies.

Comparative Studies

One of the earlier studies, published in 2005, evaluated the effect of a short infusion of either 7.2% hypertonic saline hydroxyethyl starch or 15% mannitol for ICP exceeding 20 mm Hg for longer than 5 minutes in 32 patients with TBI.[51] The infusion ran until the ICP was less than 15 mm Hg, rather than to a prespecified dose. Although the investigators do not report the rate of the infusion, the average doses of each medication were 1.4 and 1.8 mL/kg for the hypertonic saline and mannitol, respectively. The mean starting ICP was 22 for the hypertonic saline group and 23 for the mannitol group. Although the investigators found that both were successful in reducing ICP, the hypertonic saline took less time by several minutes (8.7 vs 6) and required lower total doses. The maximum increase in CPP was also greater in the hypertonic saline group. Overall, there were no differences in outcomes between the 2 groups.[51] The design of the study was strong and the investigators did have a standard algorithm for treating elevated ICP with other therapies, including sedation and hyperventilation, which makes it easier to evaluate the response to hyperosmolar therapies.

They also approached the treatment dose in a unique way, giving each patient the amount required based on response, rather than a flat dose, and thus this study is included despite not giving equiosmolar doses. However, the study did have limitations, most notably the small size. In addition, the starting rate for the infusion is not clear, making it difficult to replicate their process. Finally, one could argue that the difference in time to ICP less than 15 was not clinically significant; however, this difference could be greater for patients with a higher starting ICP, and therefore it is difficult to truly assess the clinical significance of these findings.

Another study, also published in 2005, described the results of a 9-patient, randomized, crossover study.[52] Six patients had had a TBI, and the others had subarachnoid hemorrhage. The investigators compared the effects of 200 mL 20% mannitol (249 mOsm/dose) to 100 mL of 7.5% saline/6% dextran solution (250 mOsm/dose). Each treatment was administered over 5 minutes in response to ICPs exceeding a predetermined threshold sustained for a predetermined time (which for most patients was >20 mm Hg for >5 minutes), and each patient received each treatment twice for 4 different episodes. This study found that the absolute decrease in ICP was greater for those episodes treated with the hypertonic saline/dextran solution compared with mannitol (−5 mm Hg; 95% confidence interval [CI], −10.8 to −3; $P = .041$). In addition, the duration of the effect was significantly longer for hypertonic saline/dextran (−46 minutes; 95% CI, −182 to −6; $P = .044$). In addition, the investigators found that MAP decreased after hypertonic saline/dextran by 7 mm Hg, and no differences was found for mannitol; despite this decrease in MAP, patients had higher cerebral perfusion pressures after administration of hypertonic saline/dextran due to the greater drop in the ICP after this treatment compared with mannitol.[52] A crossover design seems reasonable for the treatment of transient events (elevated ICP) and can increase power, allowing for small populations, but it does not allow for the evaluation of long-term outcomes and can make it difficult to evaluate the use of one therapy in isolation if there are carryover effects from previous treatments. It is therefore difficult to say if the difference of 5 mm Hg produces improved outcomes and clinically may be viewed as a small difference since both of the medians after treatment ICPs were well below the clinically accepted treatment threshold of 20 mm Hg.

Francony and colleagues[53] published a report in 2008 describing the results of a randomized controlled trial comparing the effects of 20% mannitol to 7.45% saline in patients with TBI, both at doses of 255 mOsm/treatment and delivered over 20 minutes in response to a sustained ICP greater than 20 mm Hg. The investigators found that in the 20 patients who were randomized, both hypertonic saline and mannitol reduced ICP by 37% and 41%, respectively, but the difference in reduction was not significantly different between the 2 therapies. There were no changes in the MAP in either group. There were differential effects on certain cerebral hemodynamic parameters, primarily diastolic blood flow velocities and pulsatility index, reflecting potential changes in brain compliance after treatment in the mannitol group.[53] Like the previous studies, the randomized design was strong; however, the sample was very small, which is especially noteworthy in negative studies, given that it was only powered to detect large differences between treatments. Interestingly, this study evaluated whether the autoregulatory response was preserved prior to treatment. Only 1 patient in the study did not have preservation of autoregulation; thus, results from this study might not apply to a patient without autoregulation. This is also the first study that evaluated hypertonic saline in isolation of other components (dextran and hydroxyethyl starch), which could potentially explain the differences in findings from previous studies.

In 2009, another study was published comparing similar interventions.[54] This group evaluated 1.5-mL/kg infusions of 20% mannitol vs an equiosmolar sodium lactate solution infused over 15 minutes in 34 patients with TBI. Treatments were infused in response to a sustained ICP greater than 25 mm Hg. In this study, the sodium lactate solution was more often successful at reaching goal ICP (90.4% vs 70.4%, $P = .053$) and had a more pronounced decrease in ICP at 4 hours (5.9 vs 3.2 mm Hg, $P = .009$). In addition, the hypertonic saline group had more persistent positive effects on the cerebral perfusion pressure compared with mannitol. This study concluded that hypertonic saline lactate solution was more effective than mannitol.[54] Like the other studies, the randomized design was high quality, but the sample was quite small. The results described above are from the intention-to-treat analysis. The authors did allow for patients to cross over to the other therapy after treatment failure. This occurred more often in the mannitol group. Although the authors did analyze the data using "as administered" groups, this technique removes the benefits of randomization, and results from that analysis should be interpreted carefully and are thus not described here.

More recently, in 2011, Cottenceau and colleagues[55] compared the effects of equiosmolar infusions of 20% mannitol (4 mL/kg) or 7.5% hypertonic saline (2 mL/kg). Forty-seven patients with TBI were randomized at 2 different centers. The treatment threshold used in this study was lower than others at 15 mm Hg. The authors found that both treatments reduced ICP but did not differ significantly from one another, although in a sensitivity analysis, the absolute magnitude of ICP decrease was greater in the hypertonic saline group. Both therapies exhibited a durable response at 2 hours as well.[55] Cerebral blood flow was also significantly increased in both groups at 30 minutes, but the increase was higher in patients receiving hypertonic saline. Because rheology is thought to play an important role in the mechanism of these agents, the investigators also evaluated markers of rheology, hematocrit, and ICA shear rate. While in the hypertonic saline group, the hematocrit was found to decrease slightly and had a higher shear rate, the mannitol patients were found to have a significantly elevated hematocrit at 30 minutes and no evidence of increased shear rate. There were no differences in neurological outcomes between the groups.[55] As with the other studies discussed, randomization is a high-quality feature of this study, but the sample size is quite small; despite the small size of this study, it is actually the largest that has examined these 2 therapies in the TBI population to date.

Again in 2011, Sakellaridis et al[56] randomized 29 patients with TBI (a total of 199 events) to receive either 2 mL/kg of 20% mannitol or 0.42 mL/kg of 15% hypertonic saline. Mannitol was infused over 20 minutes, and the hypertonic saline was administered as a bolus over an unspecified duration. Each treatment was given in response to an ICP greater than 20 mm Hg. Patients were randomized to one of the therapies on their first episode of intracranial hypertension, but treatment between agents alternated on the same patient for subsequent episodes. Osmotic therapy was only used until serum osmolarity reached 320 mOsm/L. Both were found to decrease ICP, but one was not significantly better than the other. The duration of effect was similar for the treatments as well.[56] Although patients were randomized to the order in which treatments were received, all patients received both therapies, making it difficult to understand the success of each therapy in isolation of the other. Although outcomes were reported, the design also limits the ability to comment on long-term outcomes of individual therapies.

Meta-analyses

Two meta-analyses have been published on the comparison of the 2 agents in the context of randomized trials, mostly including the literature summarized above. The earlier one, published in 2011, included 5 studies comparing the 2 treatments for elevated ICP but was not specific to TBI.[23] Two of the studies did not include any patients with TBI and were thus not reviewed. This meta-analysis ultimately included a total of 112 patients and 184 episodes of intracranial hypertension and found that hypertonic saline was more effective in achieving ICP control (relative risk, 1.16; 95% CI, 1.00 to 1.33; $P=.046$), but the mean difference in ICP reduction was only 2 mm Hg (95% CI, −1.6 to 5.7; P = .276), which is not clinically or statistically significant.[57]

A second meta-analysis published in 2014 limited the studies to those done in TBI comparing mannitol to hypertonic saline.[58] This meta-analysis included a total of 171 patients and 599 episodes of intracranial hypertension. Hypertonic saline was found to decrease ICP by 1.39 mm Hg (95% CI, −0.74 to 3.53) compared with mannitol, but this difference was not statistically significant.

Other meta-analyses that included nonrandomized and retrospective data have been published.[59–61] The conclusion of all 3 studies was that hypertonic saline was superior to mannitol; however, the inclusion of noncontrolled data leaves significant room for selection bias and thus should be interpreted with caution.

This body of literature suffers from significant limitations. The drug regimens, especially those in the hypertonic saline arms, differed dramatically. Some of the trials used only sodium chloride solutions, whereas others used sodium chloride in combination with dextran or hydroxyethyl starch. In addition, differing doses and administration rates were used across trials. This heterogeneity in clinical trials is mirrored in clinical practice with widely varying practices between institutions, making this a very complex treatment to study. Interestingly, standard dosing for mannitol is considered from 0.25 to 1 g/kg. Most of these studies evaluated doses in the lower to middle portion of this range, although in practice, many use the upper limit of the range. Second, all of the trials evaluated ICP lowering rather than reversal of clinical herniation. All of the trials discussed are very small. And while some trials did find significant differences in certain end points, the randomization process does not always hold up well to small samples. None of the studies were large enough to evaluate outcomes, so even if we knew that one therapy is better than the other at lowering ICP, the question still remains if it affects outcomes. Despite these limitations, both therapies appear to effectively lower ICP and thus seem like reasonable options, although there may be a modest benefit of using hypertonic saline in terms of the magnitude of ICP lowering.

23.4% Sodium Chloride

Hypertonic saline is commercially available in various concentrations. One available product containing 120 mEq Na/30 mL (23.4%) is significantly more hyperosmolar than the most concentrated commercial mannitol (25%) product (8008 vs 1375 mOsm/L). A number of publications have described experience with this product. One retrospective cohort study evaluated the use of 23.4%

on the reversal of transtentorial herniation.[30] Unlike the comparative studies above, this group of investigators used a clinical end point for their primary outcome. In this study, 68 patients received treatment for 76 events with 30 mL of 23.4%. No patients with TBI were included in this study, and most had either had an intracranial hemorrhage or SAH. In 75% of the events, clinical reversal of transtentorial herniation was achieved. Adverse events were limited to transient episodes of hypotension. While interesting, interpretation of these results is complicated by the lack of a control group and simultaneous use of other therapies for herniation. There were also no patients with TBI included in this study. Another group retrospectively evaluated the use of 23.4% in patients with elevated serum osmolality (>320 mOsm/L) at baseline to see if there was an additional ICP-lowering benefit with osmotic therapy.[15] They found no correlation between the magnitude of ICP decrease and starting serum or cerebrospinal fluid osmolality. This would indicate that 23.4% has the potential to benefit patients, even when they have already received hyperosmolar therapy and have achieved serum osmolality greater than 320 mOsm/L, which has been used as a historical cutoff. Kerwin and colleagues[62] conducted a nonrandomized pilot study including 22 patients with TBI who had received both mannitol and hypertonic saline (23.4%). For all patients, hypertonic saline was dosed at 30 mL, and the mannitol dose was at the discretion of the providers, ranging from 15 to 75 g. The investigators found that the mean reduction in ICP from hypertonic saline was greater than that from mannitol (9.3 vs 6.4 mm Hg, $P<.01$). Although these data suggest that 23.4% is safe and effective, all studies described in this section were observational in nature rather than randomized controlled evaluations.

Usefulness of ICP Monitoring

The most recent guidelines on the management of TBI were written by the Brain Trauma Foundation in 2007.[45] Its recommendation on hyperosmolar therapy at that time was mannitol was effective in managing intracranial hypertension; however, the evidence was not strong enough to make a recommendation regarding hypertonic saline. Since that time, more data have been published. To complicate matters, the 2012 BEST-TRIP trial study compared therapy directed at maintaining an ICP less than 20 mm Hg to therapy targeting clinical and radiological findings.[63] This study found that there were not significant benefits of treating ICP in isolation of the clinical exam. This highlights the limitations of the available literature given that most of it focuses solely on ICP reduction rather than clinical end points. Despite the limitations of the current literature, both therapies are reasonable, and the choice should be driven by type of intravenous access, the differences in known adverse effects across the 2 agents, and their implications on patient-specific factors.

CHOICE OF AGENT

Clinical trials have shown both hypertonic saline and mannitol to be effective in lowering ICP. The literature, however, does not clearly support the superiority of one agent over the other. The choice of hyperosmolar agent for the treatment of intracranial hypertension thus should be influenced by specific patient characteristics, side effect profiles, ease of administration, and availability. Mannitol would be the preferred agent in the settings of chronic hyponatremia, lack of central line access, fluid overload state, and severe chronic or acute decompensated heart failure. Hypertonic saline is preferred in patients with renal impairment, negative fluid balance, an osmolar gap greater than 20, or in patients in whom mannitol has become ineffective after repeated doses. Patients who are experiencing herniation syndrome require emergent hyperosmolar therapy, and the agent of choice should be most readily available for administration barring any contraindications.

CONCLUSION

Despite limited data, hyperosmolar therapies remain a standard of care for patients with TBI and elevated ICP. Given the lack of clear direction provided by the evidence, a robust understanding of the potential adverse effects and the practical pearls associated with each osmolar agent is essential for optimizing clinical practice. The agent of choice may certainly vary depending on institution-specific barriers as well as patient-specific factors and their individual relationship to the associated adverse effects. It is important for institutions to have policies and procedures in place to facilitate their rapid use, given the emergent nature of their indications.

References

1. Nau R. Osmotherapy for elevated intracranial pressure: a critical reappraisal. *Clin Pharmacokinet*. 2000;38:23–40.
2. Hinson HE, Stein D, Sheth KN. Hypertonic saline and mannitol therapy in critical care neurology. *J Intensive Care Med*. 2013;28:3–11.
3. Selmaj K. Pathophysiology of the blood-brain barrier. *Semin Immunopathol*. 1996; 18:57–73.

4. Ziai WC, Toung TJ, Bhardwaj A. Hypertonic saline: first-line therapy for cerebral edema? *J Neurol Sci.* 2007;261:157–166.
5. Videen TO, Zazulia AR, Manno EM, et al. Mannitol bolus preferentially shrinks non-infarcted brain in patients with ischemic stroke. *Neurology.* 2001;57:2120–2122.
6. Dunn IF, Ellegala DB, Fox JF, Kim DH. Principles of cerebral oxygenation and blood flow in the neurological critical care unit. *Neurocrit Care.* 2006;4:77–82.
7. Muizelaar JP, Wei EP, Kontos HA, and Becker DP. Mannitol causes compensatory cerebral vasoconstriction and vasodilation in response to blood viscosity changes. *J Neurosurg.* 1983;59:822–828.
8. Diringer MN, Scalfani MT, Zazulia AR, et al. Cerebral hemodynamic and metabolic effects of equi-osmolar doses mannitol and 23.4% saline in patients with edema following large ischemic stroke. *Neurocrit Care.* 2011;14:11–17.
9. Marko FN. Hyperosmolar therapy for intracranial hypertension: time to dispel antiquated myths. *Am J Respir Crit Care Med.* 2012;185(5):467–478.
10. Qureshi AI, Suarez JI. Use of hypertonic saline solutions in treatment of cerebral edema and intracranial hypertension. *Crit Care Med.* 2000;28:3301–3313.
11. Torre-Healy A, Marko NF, Weil RJ. Hyperosmolar therapy for intracranial hypertension. *Neurocrit Care.* 2012;17(1):117–130.
12. Nakayama S, Kramer GC, Carlsen RC, Holcroft JW. Infusion of very hypertonic saline to bled rats: membrane potentials and fluid shifts. *J Surg Res.* 1985;38:180–186.
13. Rottenberg DA, Hurwitz BJ, Posner JB. The effect of oral glycerol on intraventricular pressure in man. *Neurology.* 1977;27:600–608.
14. Nath F, Galbraith S. The effect of mannitol on cerebral white matter water content. *J Neurosurg.* 1986;65:41–43.
15. Paredes-Andrade E, Solid CA, Rockswold SB, et al. Hypertonic saline reduces intracranial hypertension in the presence of high serum and cerebrospinal fluid osmolalities. *Neurocrit Care.* 2012;17:204–210.
16. Sorani MD, Manley GT. Dose-response relationship of mannitol and intracranial pressure: a metaanalysis. *J Neurosurg.* 2008;108:80–87.
17. Papangelou A, Lewin JJ, Mirski MA, Stevens RD. Pharmacologic management of brain edema. *Curr Treat Options Neurol.* 2009;11:64–73.
18. Mannitol [package insert]. Lake Forest, IL: Hospira; 2009.
19. Perez C, Coffie P, Kacir C, et al. Complications rates of 3% hypertonic saline infusion through peripheral intravenous access. *Neurology.* 2015;84(14)(suppl P6.020).
20. Chavez-Negrete A, Majluf Cruz S, Frati Munari A, et al. Treatment of hemorrhagic shock with intraosseous or intravenous infusion of hypertonic saline dextran solution. *Eur Surg Res.* 1991;23(2):123–129.
21. Kalanuria AA, Geocadin RG, Puttgen HA. Brain code and coma recovery: aggressive management of cerebral herniation. *Semin Neurol.* 2013;133:1410.
22. Rich D. New JACHO medication management standards for 2004. *Am J Health Syst Pharm.* 2004;61(13):1349–1358.
23. Forsyth LL, Liu-DeRyke X, Parker DP, Rhoney DH. Role of hypertonic saline for the management of intracranial hypertension after stroke and traumatic brain injury. *Pharmacotherapy.* 2008;28(4):469–484.
24. Diringer MN, Zazulia AR. Osmotic therapy fact and fiction. *Neurocrit Care.* 2004;1:219–234.
25. Raslan A, Bhardwaj A. Medical management of cerebral Edema. *Neurosurg Focus.* 2007;22(5):E12.

26. Rudehill A, Gordon E, Ohman G, et al. Pharmacokinetics and effects of mannitol on hemodynamics, blood and cerebrospinal fluid electrolytes, and osmolarity during intracranial surgery. *J Neurosurg Anesthesiol.* 1993;5:4–12.

27. Node Y, Yajima K, Nakazawa S. Rebound phenomenon of mannitol and glycerol: clinical studies [in Japanese]. *No To Shinkei.* 1983;35(12):1241–1246.

28. King JD, Rosner MH. Osmotic demyelination syndrome. *Am J Med Sci.* 2010;339(6): 561–567.

29. Saltarini M, Massarutti D, Baldassarre M, et al. Determination of cerebral water content by magnetic resonance imaging after small volume infusion of 18% hypertonic saline solution in a patient with refractory intracranial hypertension. *Eur J Emerg Med.* 2002;9(3):262–265.

30. Koenig MA, Bryan M, Lewin JL, et al. Reversal of transtentorial herniation with hypertonic saline. *Neurology.* 2008;70:1023–1029.

31. Visweswaran P, Massin EK, Dubose TD. Mannitol-induced acute renal failure. *J Am Soc Nephrol.* 1997;8:1028–1033.

32. Seo W, Oh H. Alterations in serum osmolality, sodium and potassium levels after repeated mannitol administration. *J Neurosci Nurs.* 2010;24(4):201–207.

33. Fink ME. Osmotherapy for intracranial hypertension: mannitol versus hypertonic saline. *Continuum Lifelong Learning Neurol.* 2012;18(3):640–654.

34. Yunos NM, Bellomo R, Glassford N, et al. Chloride-liberal vs. chloride restrictive intravenous fluid administration and acute kidney injury: an extended analysis. *Intensive Care Med.* 2015;4(2):257–269.

35. Lobo DM, Awad S. Should chloride rich crystalloids remain the mainstay of fluid resuscitation to prevent 'pre-renal' acute kidney injury? *Kidney Int.* 2014;86:1096–1105.

36. Young P, Bailey R, Henderson S, et al. Effect of a buffered crystalloid solution vs saline on acute kidney injury among patients in the intensive care unit: the SPLIT randomized clinical trial. *JAMA.* 2015;314(16):1701–1710.

37. Corry JJ, Varelas P, Abdelhak T, et al. Variable change in renal function by hypertonic saline. *World J Crit Care Med.* 2014;3(2):61–67.

38. Reed RL II, Johnston, TD, Chen Y, Fischer RP. Hypertonic saline alters plasma clotting times and platelet aggregation. *J Trauma.* 1991;31(1):8–14.

39. Wilder DM1, Reid TJ, Bakaltcheva IB. Hypertonic resuscitation and blood coagulation: in vitro comparison of several hypertonic solutions for their action on platelets and plasma coagulation. *Thromb Res.* 2002;107(5):255–261.

40. Hess JR, Dubick MA, Summary JJ, et al. The effects of 7.5% NaCl/6% dextran 70 on coagulation and platelet aggregation in humans. *J Trauma.* 1992;32(1):40–44.

41. Dubick MA, Kilani AF, Summary JJ, et al. Further evaluation of the effects of 7.5% sodium chloride/6% Dextran-70 (HSD) administration on coagulation and platelet aggregation in hemorrhaged and euvolemic swine. *Circ Shock.* 1993;40(3):200–205.

42. Rosenthal K. Reducing the risks of infiltration and extravasation. *Nursing.* 2007;37(suppl): 4–8.

43. Dougherty L. Extravasation: prevention, recognition, and management. *Nurs Stand.* 2010;52:48–55.

44. Zimmet SE. The prevention of cutaneous necrosis following extravasation of hypertonic saline and sodium tetradecyl sulfate. *J Dermatol Surg Oncol.* 1993;19(7):641–646.

45. Brain Trauma Foundation. Guidelines for the management of severe traumatic brain injury. *J Neurotrauma.* 2007;24(suppl 1):S1–S106.

46. Haddad S, Arabi YM. Critical care management of severe traumatic brain injury in adults. *Scan J Trauma Resusc Emerg Med.* 2012;20:12.

47. Rangel-Castillo L, Gopinath S, Robertson CS. Management of intracranial hypertension. *Neurol Clin.* 2008;26:521–541.
48. Czosnyka M, Picard JD. Monitoring and interpretation of intracranial pressure. *J Neurol Neurosurg Psychiatry.* 2004;75:813–821.
49. Bhatia A, Gupta AK. Neuromonitoring in the intensive care unit, I: intracranial pressure and cerebral blood flow monitoring. *Intensive Care Med.* 2007;33:1263–1271.
50. Dahlqvist MB, Andres RH, Raabe A, et al. Brain herniation in a patient with apparently normal intracranial pressure: a case report. *J Med Case Rep.* 2010;4:297–300.
51. Harutijunyan L, Holz C, Rieger A, et al. Efficiency of 7.2% hypertonic saline hydroxyethyl starch 200/0.5 versus mannitol 15% in the treatment of increased intracranial pressure in neurosurgical patients—a randomized clinical trial. *Crit Care.* 2005;9:R530–R540.
52. Battison C, Hons BA, Andrews PJD, et al. Randomized, controlled trial on the effect of a 20% mannitol solution and a 7.5% saline/6% dextran solution on increased intracranial pressure after brain injury. *Crit Care Med.* 2005;33:196–202.
53. Francony G, Fauvage B, Falcon D, et al. Equimolar doses of mannitol and hypertonic saline in the treatment of increased intracranial pressure. *Crit Care Med.* 2008; 36:795–800.
54. Ichai C, Armadno G, Orban JC, et al. Sodium lactate versus mannitol in the treatment of intracranial hypertensive episodes in severe traumatic brain-injured patients. *Int Care Med.* 2009;356:471–479.
55. Cottenceau V, Masson F, Mahamid E, et al. Comparison of effects of equiosmolar doses of mannitol and hypertonic saline on cerebral blood flow and metabolism in traumatic brain injury. *J Neurotrauma.* 2011;28:2003–2012.
56. Sakellaridis N, Pavlou E, Karatzas S, et al. Comparison of mannitol and hypertonic saline in the treatment of severe brain injuries. *J Neurosurg.* 2011;114:545–548.
57. Kamel H, Navi BB, Nakagawa K, et al. Hypertonic saline versus mannitol for the treatment of the elevated intracranial pressure: a meta-analysis of randomized clinical trials. *Crit Care Med.* 2011;39:554–559.
58. Rickard AC, Smith JE, Newell P, et al. Salt of sugar for your injured brain? A meta-analysis of randomized controlled trials of mannitol versus hypertonic sodium solutions to manage raised intracranial pressure in traumatic brain injury. *Emerg Med J.* 2014; 31:679–683.
59. Mortazavi MM, Romeo AK, Deep A, et al. Hypertonic saline for treating raised intracranial pressure: literature review with meta-analysis. *J Neurosurg.* 2012;116:210–221.
60. Li M, Chen T, Chen S, et al. Comparison of Equimolar doses of mannitol and hypertonic saline for the treatment of elevated intracranial pressure after traumatic brain injury. *Medicine.* 2015;94(17):e736.
61. Lazarides C, Neyens R, Bodle J, DeSantis SM. High-osmolarity saline in neurocritical care: systematic review and meta-analysis. *Crit Care Med.* 2013;41:1353–1360.
62. Kerwin AJ, Schinco MA, Tepas JJ, et al. The use of 23.4% hypertonic saline for the management of elevated intracranial pressure in patients with severe traumatic brain injury: a pilot study. *J Trauma.* 2009;67:277–282.
63. Chestnut RM, Temkin N, Carney N, et al. A trial of intracranial pressure monitoring in traumatic brain injury. *N Engl J Med.* 2012;367:2471–2481.

Sedation and Neuromuscular Blockade for Neurocritical Care Patients

2

Katleen Chester
and Kristy N. Greene

SEDATION

Introduction

Intensive care unit (ICU) sedation is a foundational principle in the management of the critically ill patient, routinely being used for indications, including cardiorespiratory stabilization, endotracheal intubations, invasive procedures, withdrawal syndromes, metabolic derangements, and more. Most patients are exposed to numerous noxious stimuli and experience both emotional and physical stressors while in the ICU. Providing patient comfort with analgesics and sedatives has remained at the forefront of ICU patient care for the management and prevention of pain, anxiety, and agitation.

Further complications necessitating sedative therapy are introduced when considering the neurologically injured patient. Specifically, patients with intracranial pathologies have unique requirements for sedative therapy related to cerebral ischemia or hemorrhage, cerebral edema, diffuse axonal injury, and elevated intracranial pressure (ICP). Maintenance of sedation may be employed as part of overall management in patients who cannot protect their airway. From a respiratory perspective, sedation permits manipulation of ventilation to optimize cerebral metabolic rates, cerebral blood flow, and ICPs. Sedatives also prove useful for brain–injured patients whose underlying condition is exacerbated by alcohol or illicit drug intoxication and in patients with refractory status epilepticus[1] or refractory shivering during therapeutic hypothermia or

TABLE 2.1 Indications for Sedation for Neurocritically Ill Patients

1. Patient discomfort
2. Anxiety and agitation
3. Facilitation of procedures
4. Adjunctive therapy with ventilatory support
5. Blunt central hyperventilation
6. Status epilepticus
7. Reduction of increased intracranial pressure
8. Shivering during therapeutic hypothermia
9. Withdrawal from alcohol and other agents
10. Stroke
11. Metabolic encephalopathies
12. Neurodegenerative disorders
13. Central infections
14. Neoplastic pathologies

Source: Adapted from references 49, 156, 157, and 158.

normothermia.[2] For a comprehensive list of sedation indications in the neuro-critically ill patient, see Table 2.1.

While sedation is often paramount in neurologic illness, it frequently contradicts the general rules of ICU sedation. The renaissance of critical care sedation management strongly criticizes a deep state of sedation since this level of sedation is known to reduce ventilator-free days, increase nosocomial infections, lengthen ICU stay, and increase the incidence of delirium.[3] Meanwhile, there has been increasing focus on achieving a comfortable yet arousable patient under the least amount of sedation. This concept mirrors a longstanding doctrine in neurointensive care in which the least amount of sedatives and analgesics is used to maintain patient comfort while preserving the neurologic examination; however, the goals of care may not always align with this doctrine when sedation is necessary for certain acute, neurologic indications. Such indications often call for extreme amounts of sedation to manage particular intracranial pathologies. This chapter will primarily focus on routine sedative and analgosedative strategies in the neurocritically ill population.

Analgesia

It is estimated that more than 50% of patients experience pain within the ICU.[4–6] Neurocritically ill patients are inherently at risk for experiencing pain due to the neuro-pathophysiology of their conditions. Pain in this patient population may exist as a consequence of neurosurgical procedures such as external ventricular drain placement, craniotomies, spinal surgeries, and tumor resections or as a result of conditions such as neuropathies, subarachnoid hemorrhage, tumors, meningitis, cerebral venous thrombosis, and elevated ICP as examples.

Pain and discomfort should always be considered a cause of ICU agitation.[7] This theory, along with supporting evidence, prompted the recommendation for analgesics as first-line therapy (analgosedation) prior to institution of a traditional sedative for agitation and anxiety. Analgesia to control agitation and anxiety has been associated with a reduction or even omission of doses of sedative agents, an increase in ventilator-free days, and decreased length of ICU stay.[3,4,8,9] Contrary to supporting data and practices supporting analgesia-based sedation in the general ICU population, total reliance on analgesics for initial management of neurocritical care patients is essentially impossible depending on the acuity of the intracranial pathology. For example, a patient experiencing increased ICP after severe head trauma would likely benefit from hypnotic-like, sedative therapy with an agent such as propofol in addition to fentanyl due to the lack of profound ICP-reducing properties associated with analgesic therapy alone.

Opioids

Opioids bind to μ_1 receptors (suprapsinal) and κ receptors (sedation, spinal analgesia) in the central nervous system (CNS) to produce analgesic and sedative properties. Opioids are routinely used in combination with hypnotic agents for their pain-relieving properties and to augment sedation. They are devoid of amnestic properties but are useful due to ease of titration and reversible nature. For commonly used opioids for analgosedation in the ICU, see Table 2.2.

Studies regarding opioid effects on ICP have been inconsistent. Some literature indicates that bolus dosing may transiently increase ICP secondary to decreases in mean arterial pressures resulting in a decline in cerebral blood.[10–12] Decreased sympathetic tone and release of histamine are 2 mechanisms by which opioids have been shown to cause hypotension. Opioids indirectly alter ICP secondary to hypercarbic effects that occur as a result of respiratory depression. Narcotic-associated seizures have been much debated with the consensus being that high doses cause muscle rigidity rather than true clinical seizures, with the exception of meperidine, whose active metabolite has epileptogenic properties.[13] The side effects associated with meperidine administration preclude its use for analgosedation in the neurointensive care unit; however, it has been shown to be effective for the management of shivering in this population.[2]

Fentanyl is most popular among opioids for its high lipid solubility and rapid distribution. Its reputation for use in the hemodynamically unstable patient is largely due to the absence of vasodilatory hypotension and active metabolites

TABLE 2.2 Common Analgosedation and Traditional Sedatives in the Neurocritically Ill Population

Class/Drug	Sedation/Analgesia	MOA	ICP Effects	Adverse Events	Pearls
Opioid					
Morphine	+/+++	μ receptor agonist	Indirect elevation (hypercarbia); may lower MAP, which could decrease CPP	Respiratory depression, gastric dysmotility, hypotension, hallucinations	Avoid in renal failure (morphine-3-glucuronide and morphine-6-glucuronide) Accumulation and prolonged sedation in obese and elderly
Fentanyl	+/+++	μ receptor agonist	Indirect elevation (hypercarbia)	Respiratory depression, chest wall rigidity, gastric dysmotility, hypotension	Rapid onset Preferred for hemodynamically unstable
Remifentanil	+/+++	μ receptor agonist	Indirect elevation (hypercarbia)	Respiratory depression, chest wall rigidity, gastric dysmotility, hypotension	Mostly reserved for perioperative use by anesthesiology; ultra-short acting; limited data on postoperative recovery time after craniotomy show little benefit over fentanyl
Benzodiazepine					
Diazepam	+++/+	GABA$_A$ receptor agonist	Indirect elevation (hypercarbia)	Respiratory depression, hypotension, confusion	Active metabolites causing prolonged half-life; contains propylene glycol
Lorazepam	+++/+	GABA$_A$ receptor agonist	Indirect elevation (hypercarbia)	Respiratory depression, hypotension, confusion	Contains propylene glycol Osmolal gap of 10–12 may identify those at risk for propylene glycol toxicity IV infusion not recommended for status epilepticus
Midazolam	+++/+	GABA$_A$ receptor agonist	Indirect elevation (hypercarbia and hypotension)	Respiratory depression, hypotension, confusion	Active metabolite causing prolonged half-life in renal dysfunction

TABLE 2.2 *Continued*

Class/Drug	Sedation/Analgesia	MOA	ICP Effects	Adverse Events	Pearls
Barbiturate					
Pentobarbital	+++/−	$GABA_A$ receptor agonist	Reduction	Respiratory depression, hypotension, gastric dysmotility, bronchospasm, angioedema	Half-life: (phenobarbital > **pentobarbital** > thiopental)
Phenobarbital	+++/−	$GABA_A$ receptor agonist	Reduction (with large doses)	Respiratory depression, hypotension, gastric dysmotility, bronchospasm, angioedema	Half-life: (**phenobarbital** > pentobarbital > thiopental) Contains propylene glycol
Thiopental	+++/−	$GABA_A$ receptor agonist	Reduction	Respiratory depression, hypotension, gastric dysmotility, bronchospasm, angioedema	Redistribution of drug from the brain, resulting in short half-life Half-life: (phenobarbital > pentobarbital > **thiopental**)
Neuroleptic					
Droperidol	+++/−	Blocks dopamine, adrenergic, serotonin, acetylcholine, and histamine receptors	Not studied	Extrapyramidal signs, may lower seizure threshold, QT prolongation	Lacks respiratory depressant effects Maintain $K^+ \geq 4$ and $Mg^{+2} \geq 2$ to prevent QT prolongation
Haloperidol	+++/−	Blocks dopamine, adrenergic, serotonin, acetylcholine, and histamine receptors	None	Extrapyramidal signs, may lower seizure threshold, QT prolongation	Lacks respiratory depressant effects Maintain $K^+ \geq 4$ and $Mg^{+2} \geq 2$ to prevent QT prolongation
α_2 Agonist					
Clonidine	++/+	α_2 receptor agonist (pre- and postsynaptic)	None	Dry mouth, bradycardia, hypotension, rebound hypotension	$\alpha_2 : \alpha_1$ activity 220:1

(continued)

TABLE 2.2 *Continued*

Class/Drug	Sedation/Analgesia	MOA	ICP Effects	Adverse Events	Pearls
Dexmedetomidine	++/+	α_2 receptor agonist (pre- and postsynaptic)	None	Dry mouth, bradycardia, hypotension, adrenal suppression, atrial fibrillation, rebound hypotension with prolonged administration	Greater specificity for α_2-receptor (α_2 : α_1 activity 1620:1) ~50% reduction in hepatic metabolism in elderly and those with liver failure Has moderate analgesic properties but should not be used as a primary analgesic AE: hypotension and bradycardia Does not suppress respiratory drive
Other					
Propofol	+++/−	Poorly understood; $GABA_A$ receptor agonist and sodium channel blocker	Reduction	Hypotension, respiratory depression, metabolic acidosis, rhabdomyolysis, anaphylaxis, pain on injection	Rapid onset and offset Easily titrated; short duration of action PRIS (rare)—higher risk with higher doses > 70 mcg/kg/min in adults PK of drug not affected by metabolism but can accumulate in adipose tissue with prolonged use Contains 1.1 kcal/mL of lipid content
Ketamine	+++/+++	Dissociative agent; noncompetitive NMDA receptor antagonist	Conflicting evidence; newer data suggest possible reduction in ICP (limited data)	Hypertension, emergence reactions, injection site pain; tachycardia, excessive salivation, hypertension, laryngospasm,	Extensively hepatically metabolized—consider dose reductions with liver dysfunction No adjustments necessary with renal insufficiency

Source: Compiled from references 3, 117, 157, 159, and 160.

Note: AE, adverse effect; CPP, cerebral perfusion pressure; GABA, gamma-aminobutyric acid; ICP, intracranial pressure; IV, intravenous; MOA, mechanism of action; MAP, mean arterial pressure; NMDA, N-methyl D aspartate; PK, pharmacokinetics; PRIS, propofol-related infusion syndrome.

commonly associated with morphine use. Fentanyl boasts nonspecific clearance by nonspecific esterases, allowing for usage in patients with both renal and hepatic dysfunction. Overall, it has a quick onset and short duration of action, but use may be limited by accumulation within fatty tissues with prolonged administration, making awakening times less predictable.[14–16] For additional details about analgesics that may be used in the neurointensive care unit, see Table 2.3.

Sedation

Prior to choosing a sedative, special consideration should be given to identifying underlying etiologies of agitation and anxiety with initial management focused on nonpharmacologic strategies (eg, reducing noise, promoting normal sleep-wake cycles, attention to patients' general care). Routine, mundane aspects of care such as tracheal suctioning, repositioning, and catheter removals can become the culprit of ICU pain and agitation and can often be managed with analgesics vs sedation.[3, 17] Concomitant administrations of psychoactive therapies that can adversely affect behavior should be noted and discontinued if necessary. These agents may include corticosteroids, anticonvulsants, agents increasing gastric motility, antivirals, antibiotics, antidepressants, and so on.[18–23]

Sedation acts through CNS depressant mechanisms, contributing to decreased cognitive abilities, which can ultimately result in deterioration of neurologic status. Consequently, this interferes with neurologic monitoring, the most critical determinant for providing care of the brain-injured patient. Unfortunately, no sedative in the ICU completely circumvents this process. An optimal sedative is one that has a rapid onset, short duration of action, and a predictable dose-response relationship so that prolonged sedation after discontinuation of therapy could be avoided. An agent that lacks drug accumulation and has minimal risk of adverse effects is also desired.[24,25] The process for selecting and titrating a sedative agent for the neurocritically ill patient becomes manifold, taking into consideration the indication for therapy, neurologic therapeutic goals, pharmacokinetic and pharmacodynamic properties of the drug, and knowledge of the potential toxicity profile along with advantages and disadvantages of each agent. For additional details about sedative characteristics and dosing, see Table 2.2 and Table 2.3.

Commonly Used Sedatives

Benzodiazepines. Benzodiazepines (BZDs) and propofol are commonly used sedatives in the neurocritically ill population.[6,26] Despite recent clinical data

TABLE 2.3 Pharmacokinetics and Dosing Suggestions for Sedation in the Neurointensive Care Unit

Drug	Half-Life	Initial Dose	Titration	Protein Binding, %	Metabolism	Active Metabolite(s)
Opioids						
Morphine	1.5–4.5 h IV, IM, SQ	IV: 2–10 mg every 4 hours IM: 5–20 mg every 4 hours	Postoperative pain (PCAP): 0.2–3 mg every 5–20 minutes	20–30	Hepatic	Morphine-3-glucoronide, morphine-6-glucoronide
Fentanyl	30–60 minutes (single IV dose). Repeated doses significantly increase half-life	12.5–100 µg IV every 20 minutes	Infusion .01–0.03 µg/kg/h	80–86	Hepatic	None
Remifentanil	3–10 minutes after single dose	0.5–1 µg/kg IV bolus	Infusion 0.05–2 µg/kg/min	92	Plasma esterases	None
Benzodiazepines						
Diazepam	30–60 hours	2 mg IV every 0–60 minutes	None	99	Hepatic	Desmethyl-diazepam, oxazepam, hydroxydiazepam
Lorazepam	10–20 hours	0.25–2 mg IV every 1–2 hours	Infusion 0.01–0.1 mg/kg/h IV	91–93	Hepatic	None
Midazolam	1–2.5 hours	0.5–2 mg IV every 5–30 minutes	Infusion 0.25–1.0 µg/kg/min	97	Hepatic	1-hyroxymethylmidazolam
Barbiturates						
Pentobarbital	15–50 hours	3–30 mg/kg	Infusion 1–2 mg/kg/h to burst suppression EEG	35–45	Mostly hepatic	None
Phenobarbital	53–120 hours	Sedation: 1–3 mg/kg/IV or IM; status epilepticus: 15–20 mg/kg IV	None	20–40	Mostly hepatic	None

TABLE 2.3 *Continued*

Drug	Half-Life	Initial Dose	Titration	Protein Binding, %	Metabolism	Active Metabolite(s)
Thiopental	5–10 minutes after single dose; infusion 8–12 hours	1–5 mg/kg IV	None	30–40	Mostly hepatic; also renal and brain	None
Neuroleptics						
Haloperidol	12–36	0.5–5 mg IV	None	92	Hepatic	None
Droperidol	4–12	0.625–2.50 mg IV	None	92	Hepatic	None
α₂ Agonist						
Clonidine	12–16 hours	0.1 mg PO every 8–24 hours; increase 0.1 mg/d every 1–2 days up to 0.6 mg/d	None	20–40	Hepatic (50%), unchanged in urine (50%)	None
Dexmedetomidine	2 hours	1 µg/kg IV over 10 minutes	Infusion 0.2–1.4 µg/kg/h	94	Hepatic	None
Other						
Propofol	4–10 minutes	Anesthesia induction: 1–2.5 mg/kg IV	Infusion 5–125 µg/kg/min	Not found	Hepatic and extrahepatic	None
Ketamine	2–3 hours	Sedation: 0.2–0.5 mg/kg over 2 minutes Intermittent bolus (pain, agitation, procedure): 0.1–0.2 mg/kg IV over 2 minutes	Infusion 0.1–0.5 mg/kg/h	12	Hepatic	Nor-ketamine

Source: Compiled from references 156, 157, and 160.

Note: EEG, electroencephalogram; IM, intramuscular; IV, intravenous; PCAP, patient-controlled analgesia pump; PO, by mouth; SQ, subcutaneous.

suggesting increased prevalence of delirium with BZDs compared with other sedatives such as dexmedetomidine, BZDs continue to be mainstay treatments in neurocritically ill patients due to their versatility in managing refractory intracranial hypertension, refractory status epilepticus, and withdrawal syndromes related to ethanol or previous BZD usage.[3,27–29]

BZDs exert their pharmacologic effects by enhancing the effects of the neurotransmitter gamma-aminobutyric acid (GABA) at the GABA$_A$ receptor, resulting in sedative, anxiolysis, hypnotic, and muscle-relaxing properties.[30] Anterograde amnesia, the inability to recall recent events and create new ones after the amnestic event, is a particularly unique feature of BZD therapy.[31] BZDs are opioid-sparing agents due to their ability to modulate the pain anticipatory response. BZDs have been shown to lower ICP[1]; however, they may adversely affect cerebral perfusion pressure if the BZD infusion reduces the mean arterial pressure (MAP), particularly with higher infusion rates.[32–34] In cases where large amounts of BZDs are needed for burst suppression, vasopressor therapy may be needed to mitigate any adverse effects from sedative-related hypotension.

Disadvantages of BZDs are dose-related respiratory depression and inhibition of the cough reflex, limiting use in nonventilated patients. Patients receiving prolonged, continuous infusions can also develop tolerance and, more important, experience significant withdrawal effects, including but not limited to tremors, seizures, hypertension, and insomnia.[35] In such instances, resuming the BZD may be required while determining appropriate weaning strategies.

BZD-induced cognitive decline and withdrawal symptoms as a result of long-term use (>1 month) continue to emerge as a controversial issue. While short-term memory is least affected negatively and often a desired effect with anterograde-like characteristics in the acute setting, long-term memory can be hampered, affecting several domains such as visuospatial abilities, verbal learning, and speed of processing.[31] A recent meta-analysis investigating withdrawal affects found a correlation between prolonged cognitive dysfunction after daily administration of 17 mg/d of diazepam. Three months after diazepam discontinuation, this cognitive dysfunction failed to resolve.[36] Non-anxiety-related withdrawal symptoms following prolonged exposure include tinnitus, involuntary movements and perceptual changes.[37]

Midazolam. Midazolam is a staple therapy in neurological patients owing to its lipophilic nature. Midazolam's lipophilicity results in a quick onset of 2 to 5 minutes and relatively short half-life of 3 to 11 hours.[3] Midazolam metabolism produces an active metabolite, α-hydroxy midazolam, that accumulates in the elderly and renally impaired, resulting in prolonged sedation. Midazolam possesses anticonvulsant properties, and in contrast to lorazepam, it can be used in excessively high doses via continuous infusion for sedation and treatment of refractory status epilepticus or elevated ICP without concern for propylene glycol toxicity. Relating to cerebral hemodynamics, midazolam reduces cerebral blood flow and blood volume; however, it blunts effects against the response to hypoxia and hypercarbia, making it suboptimal for nonventilated patients who may be at risk for intracranial hypertension.[38,39]

Lorazepam. Contrary to lorazepam's class effects as a BZD, its usage has grown unpopular over the past decade and a rarity in neurocritically ill patients. Its ability to cause propylene glycol toxicity with higher doses precludes its use for indications where high infusion rates are needed, such as with burst suppression. This toxicity manifests as a metabolic acidosis with concomitant acute kidney failure and can be identified by an osmolar gap in the range of 10 to 12 mOsm/kg H_2O. More recent literature reports reduced thresholds for toxicity appearing at minimum doses of 1 mg/kg[3,40] compared with previous dose thresholds of 25 mg/h administered for several hours to days.[41–43] Lorazepam has a similar elimination half-life as midazolam; however, this agent has a delayed peak effect of 15 to 20 minutes. It undergoes glucuronidation without cytochrome P450 metabolism, making it suitable for patients with renal and hepatic dysfunction.[30]

Diazepam. The myorelaxant properties mediated through α_2 receptors in the spinal cord make diazepam useful in postoperative management of neurological spinal surgery patients; however, its use as a general sedative is limited in the ICU setting. Diazepam's sedative properties are α_1-mediated and are present with higher doses of this medication. Intramuscular (IM), intravenous (IV), oral, and rectal dosage forms are available, but it is not recommended to administer diazepam as a continuous infusion due to its long half-life and duration of action. Previous IV formulations were compounded with propylene glycol; however, sterile fat preparations now permit ease of administration, thereby reducing injection site pain and thrombophlebitis.

As with the lipophilic nature of BZDs as a class, it has a rapid onset of 2 to 5 minutes intravenously. Nonetheless, its long distribution half-life (20–120 hours) and multiple active metabolites (oxazepam, hydroxydiazepam, desmethyldiazepam) that rely on renal excretion prohibit its routine use as a sedative in neurological patients. Advanced age and renal dysfunction further prolong the duration of action, making this agent a less than ideal sedative, especially for continuous sedation in the neurointensive care unit.[30]

Propofol. As a general anesthetic agent, propofol administration has been used with much success in brain-injured patients due to its ability to reduce cerebral blood flow and metabolism as well as its ICP-lowering properties. Therapy should not be withheld in an attempt to provide analgosedation first when intracranial pathologies are present that could increase ICPs. Instead, a combination of analgesia and propofol can be initiated simultaneously. Propofol provides sedative and amnestic properties through a degree of GABA mediation. Propofol's high lipid solubility and rapid distribution with hepatic and extrahepatic clearance contribute to its quick onset and short duration of action, thus making it beneficial to perform neurologic assessments in a timely manner. While previously recommended as a short-term sedative, prolonged usage (greater than 3 days) with careful monitoring for adverse effects is not uncommon in neurological patients. Wakeup times have been reported to be less predictable in these circumstances, partly due to drug accumulation.[44,45]

Propofol-related infusion syndrome (PRIS) presents as a constellation of symptoms, including metabolic acidosis, cardiac and renal failure, elevated creatinine kinase, and arrhythmias. The development of PRIS is thought to be a result of the accumulation of free fatty acids from the inhibition of mitochondrial fatty acid oxidation process. Manifestations of this syndrome have been reported to occur at less than 1% incidence with approximately 33% mortality. PRIS more commonly manifests at doses greater than 70 mcg/kg/min but has also been shown to occur at lower doses.[26,46–48] When higher sedative doses are necessary, propofol may be abandoned for an agent such as midazolam that can be uptitrated without less risk of severe adverse effects. Propofol is manufactured as a 10% lipid emulsion, which can infrequently cause pancreatitis as a result of hypertriglyceridemia with higher doses or prolonged utilization. While hypertriglyceridemia itself does not appear to cause PRIS, if present, it may be a harbinger for this fatal adverse effect. In general, serum triglycerides should be checked routinely, particularly with higher doses, and hypertriglyceridemia should prompt reevaluation of sedative therapy.

Hypotension, usually associated with volume depletion, is also an adverse effect that can be mitigated with adequate volume repletion. Bradycardia is another adverse effect of propofol, seen more commonly with bolus dosing and higher infusion rates. Dose-related respiratory depression is predictable with higher doses and often not an issue in an ICU setting, as administration requires a controlled airway; however, every attempt should be made to wean patients from the propofol infusion prior to extubation.[49]

A nontoxic adverse effect of propofol is green discoloration of urine that occurs when the clearance exceeds metabolism, which promotes metabolism by extrahepatic mechanisms. This alternative pathway can be augmented during parenchymal liver damage evidenced by the presence of urobilinogen. Dosage and duration of propofol infusion are not related to discoloration, and there is subsequent resolution after medication discontinuation.[50–52] Green discoloration of the urine is not a harbinger for PRIS.

α_2-*Agonists.* Dexmedetomidine's unique effects on pre-and postcentral α_2-adrenoreceptors, inhibiting the release of norepinephrine and central sympathetic activity, makes it suitable for analgesic, sedative, and anxiolytic properties. Even at higher doses, it sedates in a manner similar to the normal sleep cycle, which allows for rapid arousal upon stimulation without severely impairing the ability to obtain a neurologic examination.[53] Dexmedetomidine has gained favor over BZDs as an ICU sedative in mechanically ventilated patients. There is evidence supporting less time spent in deeply sedated states compared with BZD therapy. Consequently, this translates into shorter durations of mechanical ventilation days and lower incidences of delirium.[27,29]

Dexmedetomidine is lipophilic and possesses a short half-life, allowing for rapid titrations. It is available IV and is 8 times more potent for α_2-receptors than its counterpart clonidine, which enhances its sedative properties and reduces the incidence of less desirable sympatholytic effects, including hypotension and bradycardia. IV loading doses have been associated with both hypo- and hypertension.

Dexmedetomidine's mechanism of action allows for a calm patient who can be easily aroused and interactive upon stimulation but returning to a tranquil state when undisturbed. This type of sedative necessitates an ideal environment to be most effective. Unlike other sedatives, dexmedetomidine can be administered to nonintubated patients as it lacks any significant respiratory depressive effects[54,55]; however, concern for loss of oropharyngeal tone and reflexes still exists. Originally approved in 1999 for mechanically ventilated patients and in short-term (24 hours) procedural sedation, dexmedetomidine is clinically used for longer periods of time in the ICU setting. Although rebound effects have been associated with clonidine's abrupt discontinuation, this phenomenon has not been evidenced with prolonged dexmedetomidine infusions up to 7 days.[56]

Dexmedetomidine may be advantageous for facilitation of procedures or for agitated patients not requiring deep sedation. Examples of such scenarios include prevention of intubation in severely agitated patients who are candidates for light sedation, initial management of paroxysmal sympathetic hyperactivity, and adjunctive therapy in the management of alcohol withdrawal syndrome (AWS). To date, no evidence supports the use of dexmedetomidine for AWS. Theoretically having similar properties to clonidine, it may be desirable to control hypersympathetic output and prevent intubation from respiratory depression associated with BZD therapy, although most patients with AWS should have high tolerances to the respiratory depression of BZD unless the effects of the BZD are enhanced by the underlying brain injury. From a favorable standpoint, a few case series have demonstrated reduced BZD requirements and the avoidance of intubation.[57,58] On the other hand, there are reports of dexmedetomidine failing to control agitation when used as a single agent and increased BZD doses after initiation.[59,60]

In general, dexmedetomidine utilization is limited by the cost of the agent. When cost is a concern, many institutional protocols prefer the use of propofol as an initial ICU sedative and reserve dexmedetomidine for ventilator weaning or as an antishivering agent.

Ketamine. Ketamine, a phencyclidine derivative, produces potent analgesic, hypnotic, and amnestic effects by actions on μ, κ, and δ opioid receptors as well as antagonism at N-methyl D aspartate (NMDA) receptors. There is also evidence of muscarinic activity contributing to additional analgesic effects.[61,62] Different from the traditional stages of sedation continuum, ketamine offers dissociative sedative effects in which patients enter a fugue state and are completely unresponsive to any stimuli. During this sedated state, there is no respiratory depression, and patients maintain some degree of muscle tone. The latter would indicate that it might not be an ideal agent in brain-injured patients in whom complete immobility is desired unless combined with other sedatives or used in higher doses that promote burst suppression.[63,64]

Ketamine is gaining popularity in the ICU setting for its high lipid solubility resulting in a rapid onset of action (30 seconds). Equally favorable is ketamine's short duration of action of 5 to 10 minutes and elimination half-life of 2 to 3 hours with single IV bolus dosing. Ketamine also boasts the ability to maintain airway integrity without loss of protective pharyngeal reflexes unlike other IV sedatives and analgesics. Ketamine maintains MAP and pulmonary vascular resistance. This agent may yield negative inotropic effects; however, they are counteracted by CNS stimulation and inhibition of catecholamine uptake. Metabolically, ketamine undergoes hepatic metabolism via microsomal enzymes (CYP3A4, CY2B6, and CYP2C9), producing an active metabolite, nor-ketamine, which has 33% greater potency than the parent compound.[65]

Perhaps the most notable concerns with ketamine utilization are emergence delirium and psychotropic effects. The incidence of hallucinations is 7.4% vs 3.7% in controls.[66] Additional adverse effects include hypersalivation, hypertension, and supraventricular tachycardia, particularly in patients receiving thyroid replacement therapies; however, these adverse effects could occur in any patient. Ketamine should be used cautiously in patients on thyroid replacement therapies, those with significant histories for coronary artery disease, or patients with uncontrolled hypertension.

The benefits of ketamine in the neurologically injured patient remain inconclusive due to the lack of controlled data to validate its neuroprotective effects. There is also question of ketamine's negative effects on ICP and cerebral perfusion pressures in spontaneously breathing patients. Recent reviews actually negate these effects when patients are receiving mechanical ventilation.[67,68] On the other hand, ketamine does allow for preservation of responses to hypercarbia during administration.[64] Other than its negative behavioral side effects, it remains an attractive, safe, and relatively efficacious agent with growing use for the management of refractory status epilepticus through its antagonism at NMDA receptors.[69]

Barbiturates. Barbiturates produce dose-dependent CNS depressant activity through chloride conductance at inhibitory $GABA_A$ ion channels, exhibiting sedation at lower doses and hypnosis at higher concentrations. Barbiturates' lipophilic nature allows rapid penetration of the blood-brain barrier, producing a quick onset of action. Barbiturates also undergo hepatic metabolism and function as notorious enzyme inducers, necessitating awareness of the potential for significant drug interactions with these agents. Historically, thiopental, phenobarbital, and pentobarbital have played a central role in the ICU setting for sedation, anticonvulsant activity, and burst suppression for treatment of elevated ICP. Their effects on ICP are believed to occur via suppression of cerebral metabolism, thus reducing metabolic demands and cerebral blood volume.

Overall, the use of barbiturates as a continuous infusion for sedation is rare due to their long half-lives (range, 8–120 hours) and nontitratable nature. When administered in supra-anesthetic doses, they are commonly associated with hypotension (with vasopressor requirements), which has led to a decline in their routine use for management of intracranial pressures. A recent Cochrane Review on traumatic brain-injured patients advised against this class of agents, concluding that the blood pressure–lowering adverse effect (occurring in 1 of every 4 patients) refuted any benefits with ICP lowering and improvements in cerebral blood flow.[70]

Methohexital is a barbiturate that is rarely used except in the procedural setting of Wada testing, a process by which hemispheric language dominance and single-hemisphere capability of memory support is determined in patients prior to intracranial surgeries. It is also useful during cerebral angiography in patients being evaluated for tumor or vascular anomaly resection. In these instances, methohexital is administered intra-arterially, targeted at a single hemisphere, and may require multiple injections. Although sodium amobarbital has been a standard, methohexital is favored due to its greater lipophilicity and shorter half-life.[71,72]

Butyrophenones. Butyrophenones, also known as neuroleptics, include haloperidol and droperidol. Both have sedative, anxiolytic, and antipsychotic potential. Mechanistically, they antagonize a combination of dopamine, adrenergic, serotonin, acetylcholine, and histamine receptors, creating a multitude of effects. Neuroleptics are frequently criticized and commonly avoided in the neurocritically ill populations secondary to their ability to lower the seizure threshold, although this property is controversial. On the contrary, they are beneficial when seeking control of the combative, agitated, demented, or even delirious patient. Butyrophenones fall low in the sedative hierarchy owing to their inability to lightly sedate, making them least attractive for general sedative use in the ICU aside from the aforementioned indications. More important, they have a rapid onset, lack the common respiratory depressant effects associated with many other sedatives, and are titratable (although tolerance as well as accumulation may occur with repeated dosing). Haloperidol can be given by various routes of administration, including oral, IM, and IV, while droperidol lacks an oral formulation. Overall metabolism of these agents occurs hepatically and may be reduced in the elderly population, necessitating lower starting doses.

An additional concern with neuroleptics is extrapyramidal side effects (Parkinsonism, acute and tardive dystonias, tardive dyskinesia, akathisia, and perioral tremor), systemic hypotension with IV dosing, neuroleptic malignant syndrome, and QT prolongation. The latter is more pronounced with droperidol, which gained a black box warning for the adverse effect and consequently prohibited its usage in patients exhibiting a prolonged QT at baseline. QT interval thresholds for avoiding use are commonly physician dependent, and patients should have an initial 12-lead electrocardiogram (EKG) performed along with additional monitoring for the duration of use, especially in the setting of repeated cumulative dosing. Due to the heightened concern with droperidol, continuous serial EKG monitoring is warranted during the initial hours after its administration with preparation of necessary medications to treat arrhythmias/dysrhythmias and hypotension should they occur. Maintaining electrolytes (K^+ and Mg^{+2}) within goal range prior to and during administration of the neuroleptic is recommended. It is recommended to avoid the use of concomitant QT-prolonging medications if possible, and it is an absolute contraindication to administer droperidol when a patient is already receiving a QT-prolonging agent.[73]

The effects of haloperidol on ICP have not been studied, although some data indicate a reduction in cerebral blood flow secondary to hypotension in a limited clinical study with droperidol usage.[74]

Monitoring

There is a plethora of subjective scales available for monitoring sedation in the ICU environment[15,75-78]: (1) Observer's Assessment of Alertness/Sedation Scale, (2) Ramsay Sedation Scale, (3) New Sheffield Sedation Scale, (4) Sedation Intensive Care Score, (5) Motor Activity Assessment Scale, (6) Adaptation to the Intensive Care Environment, (7) Minnesota Sedation Assessment Tool, (8) Vancouver Interaction and Calmness Scale, (9) The Richmond-Agitation Scale (SAS), and (10) Richmond Agitation-Sedation Scale (RASS). Latest recommendations support RASS and SAS to adequately measure depth of sedation and agitation with emphasis on achieving lighter sedation in critically ill patients.[79] Validation studies for the RASS included neurologically ill patients in the validity and reliability analyses.

Both scales have high interrater reliability. Validation of these scales is attributed to their ability to differentiate various levels of sedation in correlation with electroencephalogram (EEG) and bispectral index values (BIS).[75,80,81] The Nursing Instrument for Communication of Sedation and the RASS scales have direct significance to the neurological population—historically, being the only scales that included this population in validity and reliability assessments. Hence, of the two, the RASS specifically allows for goal-directed administration of sedatives with consecutive detection of sedative changes.[53,82] Despite the relevance with sedation titration, its utility diminishes in indications where the goal of sedative therapy is to burst suppress rather than achieving a particular target RASS score. In other words, it is appropriate to allow a RASS of −5 if this is the level of sedation that promotes termination of seizure activity. Furthermore, it is important to note that in patients requiring burst suppression, sedation holidays may lead to deleterious consequences and should be avoided.

Neurological monitors including EEG and BIS continue to have utility in specific situations. EEG monitoring is a necessary for detecting nonconvulsive seizures in at-risk patients with neurologic injury. Furthermore, it is a beneficial measure when titrating sedatives and anticonvulsant medications to burst suppression for termination of refractory seizures and possibly in patients experiencing increased ICP.[83]

BIS monitoring is historically favorable in the setting of assessing brain function during general anesthesia; however, it has not been sufficiently validated for use in the neurocritically ill patient. BIS is not programmed to interpret changes with nonbarbiturate therapies (eg, BZDs, narcotics). Furthermore, being affected by numerous factors such as targeted temperature management, shock states, and even metabolic disturbances, it lacks reliability as an objective scoring system. The BIS monitor may produce artifacts, rendering it an unacceptable mode of sedation monitoring in noncomatose, nonparalyzed patients since these artifacts could further complicate interpretation of the results.[84-86] Anecdotally, BIS monitors are used as part of neuromuscular blocking agent protocols to monitor and titrate sedation during induced paralysis for indications such as elevated intracranial pressures and shivering. The goal in these scenarios may be to achieve burst suppression with BIS monitoring in the setting of intracranial hypertension and to prevent patient awareness when used during shivering protocols.

Conclusions

Overall goals of sedative care with neurological patients are to safely produce comfort while avoiding anxiety and agitation along with the least amount of medication necessary while ensuring that neurophysiologic needs are met. These endeavors also align with the latest recommendations to achieve light levels of sedation to decrease mechanical ventilation days. Particularly, maintaining the ability to perform neurological assessments is of utmost importance; however, acute neurologic conditions often obviate the need for high doses of sedative and analgesic combinations. When used for routine ICU sedation, RASS is the most validated sedation scoring tool for mechanically ventilated, neurologically ill patients. When burst suppression is necessary, other modalities of sedative and neurologic monitoring should be used.

NEUROMUSCULAR BLOCKING AGENTS

Introduction

Neuromuscular blocking agents (NMBAs) are used sparingly in neurocritically ill patients but are a crucial consideration in patient care when other measures have been exhausted for neurologic indications such as malignant ICP, refractory shivering, and supportive care in the management of muscle spasms associated with tetanus, drug overdose, or status epilepticus.[87] Some nonneurologic indications for NMBAs that may arise in any ICU setting include the need for rapid sequence intubation (RSI), acute respiratory distress syndrome (ARDS), and ventilator dyssynchrony.[87–89] Regardless of the indication, when used in the neurocritically ill patient population, proper consideration of the pharmacology of NMBAs is prudent in selecting the optimal agent and recovering the neurologic examination as soon as clinically possible.

There are several characteristics that make an ideal paralytic agent for neurologically ill patients. First, the ideal paralytic agent should be fast acting, particularly when used during RSI but also when used for other indications such as refractory malignant ICP when the threat of significant morbidity and mortality is imminent. Second, the ideal NMBA should have a short duration of action, which would allow for a timely neurologic examination soon after termination of the paralytic infusion or after bolus administration of the paralytic agent. An ideal paralytic agent should also be cost-effective, quickly and easily reversed if necessary, and free from adverse drug reactions. The next section reviews the pharmacology of the most common paralytic agents used in neurocritically ill patients.

General Pharmacology of Neuromuscular Blocking Agents

All NMBAs exert their effects on nicotinic acetylcholine receptors (nAChRs) on the motor endplate by reversibly blocking impulse transmission. Most of these agents have minimal to no effects on muscarinic receptors.[87] Each motor endplate holds up to 10 million nAChRs, and each receptor comprises 5 subunits that form a glycoprotein complex, ligand-gated ion channel.[89] During normal receptor function, the channel's 2 α subunits attract the positive quaternary nitrogen group on acetylcholine (ACh). When 1 ACh substrate binds each of these subunits, conformational changes of the receptor occur, resulting in channel opening, depolarization of the muscle membrane, and subsequent muscle contraction. ACh is hydrolyzed in the synaptic cleft by acetylcholinesterase (AChE).

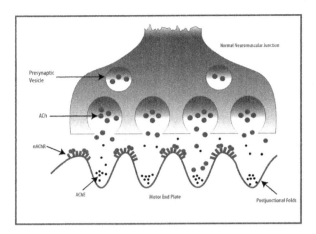

FIGURE 2.1. Normal neuromuscular junction.

Normal cholinergic activity is critical for maintaining a high concentration of mature nAChRs at the motor endplate (Figure 2.1).[90] In neurologic conditions that promote loss of nerve function, the skeletal muscle upregulates the production of short-lived, immature, fetal-variant nAChRs that have longer channel "open times" and that are distributed on the extra-junctional membrane in addition to usual placement of mature nAChRs on the motor endplate crests (Figure 2.2). Upregulation and suboptimal placement of these immature receptors is a plausible explanation for some of the adverse effects seen with NMBA use in patients with underlying disorders of neuromuscular junctional transmission.[88] Alterations in the anticipated response to NMBAs may also be seen with elderly patients. These changes may be a result of reduced organ function such as heart failure or renal insufficiency, but they may also be due to morphological changes in the neuromuscular junction (NMJ) that happen over time. Such changes that reduce the functional capacity of the postsynaptic response include a reduced number and depth of postjunctional folds that lead to spatial uncoupling of presynaptic ACh release near locations with greatest receptor density.[91,92] Similar morphologic changes have been seen with varying extremes in disorders of neuromuscular transmission such as myasthenia gravis (see Figure 2.2).[93]

The NMBAs can be classified as depolarizing or nondepolarizing agents. Depolarizing agents exert their actions by first activating nAChRs and then deactivating the receptors. Nondepolarizing agents do not cause the nACh receptor to be activated prior to inhibition and can be further divided based on chemical structure into benzylisoquinoliniums and aminosteroidal agents.

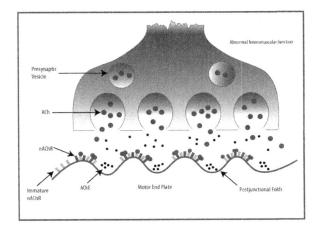

FIGURE 2.2. Abnormal neuromuscular junction.

As a result of the chemical structures, each paralytic agent has a unique pharmacokinetic and pharmacodynamic profile. This section will focus on paralytics that may be considered for use in neurocritically ill patients. See Table 2.4 for a list of undesirable NMBAs for neurocritically ill patients.

Depolarizing Agent—Succinylcholine

Pharmacology. Succinylcholine was approved by the US Food and Drug Administration (FDA) in 1952 and is the only *depolarizing* NMBA in clinical use. It comprises 2 ACh molecules joined together. Each of these bound molecules binds one of the α subunits on the nACH receptor, leading initially to a depolarization followed by closure of the ion channel and inactivation. Unlike ACh, succinylcholine is not degraded by AChE in the synaptic cleft but rather diffuses through a concentration gradient out of the synaptic area and is degraded by plasma cholinesterases. Initial depolarization may cause muscle fasiculations prior to the muscle becoming flaccid.[94]

Succinylcholine at a dose of 1 to 1.5 mg/kg IV push can produce profound paralysis within 60 seconds of administration and is the fastest acting NMBA currently on the US market. With a duration of action of approximately 8 to 10 minutes, the use of succinylcholine is primarily limited to the setting of RSI due to its favorable pharmacokinetic profile; however, its unfavorable potential for adverse effects compared with other NMBAs often precludes its use in neurocritically ill patients.[94]

TABLE 2.4 Undesirable Neuromuscular Blockers for Neurocritically Ill Patients

Neuromuscular Blocking Agent	Year Available in United States	Undesirable Clinical Effects
Doxacurium (Nuromax)	1991	Long onset of action; prolonged duration of effect. Most potent NMBA
Mivacurium (Mivacron)	1992	Significant histamine release resulting in hypotension
Tubocurarine	1942	Long onset of action
		Prolonged duration of effect
Pancuronium (Pavulon)	1972	Long duration of action
		Duration significantly prolonged with renal dysfunction
		Direct vagolytic properties: causes increases in heart rate, blood pressure, and cardiac output
Pipecuronium (Arduan)	1992	Long duration of action
		Duration significantly prolonged with renal dysfunction
Rapacuronium	1999	High incidence and severity of bronchospasm led to its withdrawal from the US market

Source: Compiled from references 94 and 99.

Adverse Effects. Succinylcholine is often avoided in neurocritically ill patients due to the risk of adverse effects, including a concern for increasing ICPs. Elevations in ICPs with succinylcholine administration have been demonstrated in 2 prospective studies published in the 1980s in patients with mass lesions.[95,96] The findings of a third study failed to demonstrate increases in ICP as a result of succinylcholine administration,[97] so ultimately its use in neurocritically ill patients outside of those with mass lesions remains controversial. Elevations in ICP could be clinically relevant in patients with altered intracranial compliance prior to RSI, and the potential risks of succinylcholine administration should be weighed against the benefits. If used for RSI, providers may consider pretreatment with lidocaine, fentanyl, or defasciculating doses of nondepolarizing NMBAs, although these practices are controversial as well,[98] and elevations in ICPs may not be a result of fasciculations.[99] While succinylcholine may be an unpopular choice for RSI of the neurocritically ill patient, nondepolarizing NMBAs prolong the inability to obtain a meaningful neurologic examination as a result of a longer duration of effect. Although the neurologic examination is lost during neuromuscular blockade, the pupillary response to light is preserved, since the response is primarily mediated by muscarinic receptors that are not routinely affected by NMBAs.[100]

Muscle fasciculations are a common adverse effect of succinylcholine, occurring with high frequency during RSI and seen more often in patients with high muscle mass.[101] To prevent fasciculations, some providers administer a small dose of a nondepolarizing NMBA, also known as a defasciculating dose, prior to the succinylcholine bolus dose. The defasciculating dose is typically one-tenth of the usually RSI dose of the agent and is administered approximately 3 minutes prior to succinylcholine administration. The nondepolarizing NMBA occupies a sufficient amount of receptors to prevent widespread depolarization from succinylcholine channel activation.[99] Fasciculations have been associated with increased intraocular and intragastric pressures as well as hyperkalemia, although other sources suggest that hyperkalemia may not be a result of fasciculations.[99]

Whether a result of fasciculations or some other mechanism, succinylcholine has the potential to cause or exacerbate hyperkalemia. In most patients, modest elevations of 0.5 mmol/L have been documented as a result of muscle depolarization releasing potassium extracellularly; however, in patients with preexisting hyperkalemia, such as those with chronic renal failure, this increase in serum potassium concentration can lead to adverse consequences.[94] Although rare, sudden-onset fatal hyperkalemia has been reported in patients with denervated muscle caused by acute upper and lower motor neuron disease, including spinal cord injury, stroke, demyelinating disease such as Guillain-Barré syndrome, encephalitis, prolonged immobility, chronic progressive neurologic disease, muscular dystrophies, amyotrophic lateral sclerosis, paraplegia, and crush injuries.[101,102] Length of ICU stay (>16 days) and acute cerebral pathology were shown to be associated with the development of hyperkalemia after succinylcholine administration.[103] During such conditions, upregulation of immature nAChR ion channels with altered functionality and placement on the muscle membrane causes patients to be more sensitive to succinylcholine. Caution should be taken in patients with recent histories of these conditions since nAChR sensitivity can persist for 3 to 6 months after the initial insult.[101] In most patients, serum potassium concentration peaks at 5 minutes after succinylcholine administration and resolves by 15 minutes.

Other adverse effects include the potential for malignant hyperthermia, transient increases in intraocular pressure and intragastric pressures, and type I hypersensitivity reactions that can occur in 1 of every 4000 administrations.[94]

TABLE 2.5 Classification, Dosing, and Pharmacokinetic Parameters of Intermediate-Acting, Nondepolarizing Neuromuscular Blocking Agents

Drug	Classification	Suggested Dosing	Onset Time, min	Clinical Duration (min) Bolus Dosing	Clinical Duration (h) Infusion Dosing
Vecuronium (Norcuron)	Aminosteroid	Bolus: 0.08–0.2 mg/kg Infusion: 0.5–1.7 mcg/kg/min	1–1.5	35–45	Mean: 0.75–2 Range: 0.5–48
Rocuronium (Zemuron)	Aminosteroid	Bolus: 0.6–1.2 mg/kg Infusion: 10–16 mcg/kg/min	<2	0.6-mg/kg dose: 20–35 1- to 1.2-mg/kg dose: 30–60	0.25–1
Atracurium (Tracrium)	Benzylisoquinolinium	Bolus: 0.4–0.5 mg/kg Infusion: 0.3–0.6 mg/kg/h	2–2.5	25–35	0.8–1
Cisatracurium (Nimbex)	Benzylisoquinolinium	Bolus: 0.1–0.2 mg/kg Infusion: 0.03–0.6 mg/kg/h	2.5–5	45–60	1.5

Source: Compiled from references 87, 101, 106, 117, and 161.

Masseter rigidity may be a harbinger of malignant hyperthermia, a sometimes fatal syndrome that involves widespread muscle depolarization that can be managed with dantrolene.[99] Elevations in intraocular (usually 5–10 mm Hg)[90,101] and intragastric pressures are not thought to be clinically significant.[94]

Unlike nondepolarizing agents, succinylcholine may also have occasional activity on muscarinic AChRs that yields additional adverse effects. Stimulation of muscarinic receptors of the sinoatrial node can result in bradycardia, particularly in pediatric patients, but can be prevented or treated using atropine.[94]

Plasma cholinesterase activity determines the duration of action of succinylcholine. The duration of action with this agent may be prolonged in the presence of genetically variant enzymes or with conditions that cause reduced synthesis of cholinesterases such as liver disease, cancer, malnutrition, and renal disease. In addition, the development of tachyphylaxis limits its use as a continuous infusion.[99]

Nondepolarizing Neuromuscular Blocking Agents

Pharmacology. Nondepolarizing NMBAs competitively inhibit postsynaptic nAChRs, but upon binding, they do not elicit a conformational change and activation of the receptor prior to inhibition like succinylcholine. Instead, the nondepolarizing NMBAs bind to one or both α subunits and prevent endogenous ACh from binding and activating the receptor. These drugs constantly associate and dissociate from the receptor so that in the presence of increasing amounts of ACh, the competitive inhibition can be overridden. Complete neuromuscular blockade only begins when 92% of the receptors are occupied.[94]

Nondepolarizing NMBAs can further be classified into 2 groups based on their chemical structures. Benzylisoquinolinium compounds (atracurium and cisatracurium) comprise 2 quaternary ammonium compounds connected by methyl groups and are more susceptible to degradation than the aminosteroid compounds. Aminosteroid compounds (pancuronium, rocuronium, and vecuronium) are composed of an androstane skeleton connected to moieties that mimic ACh.[94] Nondepolarizing agents not routinely considered for neurocritically ill patients are represented in Table 2.4. For a detailed comparison of nondepolarizing NMBAs considered for use in neurocritically ill patients, see Table 2.5 and Table 2.6.

Aminosteroid Compounds

Vecuronium. Vecuronium is unstable in solution so it is supplied as a lyophilized powder requiring reconstitution prior to administration, although it goes

TABLE 2.6 Clinical Pharmacokinetic and Pharmacodynamic Characteristics of Intermediate-Acting, Nondepolarizing Neuromuscular Blocking Agent Infusions

Drug	Metabolism	Clinically Active Metabolites	Hemodynamic Effects	Adverse Effects	Therapeutic Hypothermia Concerns	Renal Failure	Hepatic Failure
Vecuronium (Norcuron)	Hepatic (50% biliary excretion) and renal (35%)	Yes, renally excreted	Bradycardia (often not clinically significant)	Prolonged ICU block; tachyphylaxis	Reduced requirements, prolonged duration of action	Increased effect, due primarily to the metabolite accumulation	Variable; mild effects
Rocuronium (Zemuron)	Hepatic primarily (<75% biliary excretion)	No	Bradycardia (often not clinically significant); tachycardia with higher doses due to vagal block	Prolonged ICU block; minimal to none; tachyphylaxis	Reduced requirements, prolonged duration of action	Minimal to no change	± increased effect; moderate
Atracurium (Tracrium)	Hoffman degradation and ester hydrolysis in plasma	No; laudanosine metabolite accumulation possible but rare	Hypotension—as a result of histamine release. Minimal and dose dependent	Seizures—rare. Prolonged ICU block—rare	Reduced requirements, prolonged duration of action	No change	Minimal to no change
Cisatracurium (Nimbex)	Hoffman degradation	No; laudanosine metabolite accumulation not likely	None	Prolonged ICU block—rare	Reduced requirements, prolonged duration of action	No change	Minimal to no change

Source: Compiled from references 87, 101, 106, 117, and 161.

Note: ICU, intensive care unit.

into solution rapidly and completely with 0.9% sodium chloride. As a bolus dose, the onset of action is 3 times that of succinylcholine (3 minutes) and the duration is approximately 30 minutes[94] to 45 minutes.[87] Because of its lipophilicity, vecuronium is significantly taken up by the liver and processed through biliary excretion. Up to 40% of the drug is deacetylated in the liver, resulting in a metabolite with 80% potency of the parent compound. In patients with renal failure, this metabolite can accumulate, resulting in prolonged duration of effect, particularly with long durations of infusion. Vecuronium has no hemodynamic effects and does not release histamine.[94]

Rocuronium. Rocuronium is approximately 7 times less potent than vecuronium. With bolus dosing, the onset of action is approximately 60 to 90 seconds, and it is often used as an alternative to succinylcholine for RSI. Rocuronium is excreted through biliary means even more so than vecuronium since it is more lipophilic, and the only metabolite that results is 20 times less potent than rocuronium. This metabolite is not thought to contribute to clinically significant neuromuscular blocking. In high doses, rocuronium has mild vagolytic effects, and it is more likely than vecuronium to cause anaphylactoid reactions, although rare.[94]

Benzylisoquinolinium Compounds

Atracurium. This agent was designed as a mixture of 10 stereoisomers and geometric isomers. It has no direct cardiovascular effects but can cause the release of histamine, resulting in hypotension. This medication can be used in patients with liver and renal impairment since elimination is driven by Hoffman degradation (45%) and nonspecific ester hydrolysis in the plasma. Ten percent is excreted unchanged in the urine. Metabolism of atracurium by Hoffman degradation results in a tertiary amine metabolite called laudanosine. In high concentrations, this metabolite is thought to lower the seizure threshold[94] and could be of particular concern in hepatically insufficient patients since laudanosine undergoes hepatic metabolism and could accumulate.[87]

Cisatracurium. Cisatracurium is an isolated isomer of atracurium, constituting only 15% of the contents of the atracurium racemic mixture. Cisatracurium is more potent than atracurium and has a slightly longer onset and duration of action. This agent also undergoes Hoffman degradation primarily, with only 15% excreted unchanged in the urine. It lacks vagolytic properties similar to atracurium; however, it is not associated with histamine release. Also, there is minimal to no threat of laudanosine metabolite accumulation with cisatracurium, since less drug is required to achieve desired paralytic effects compared with atracurium. These characteristics make it an ideal agent to consider for use in neurocritically ill patients with renal or hepatic dysfunction, since the agent undergoes an alternative route of elimination and the accumulation of clinically relevant laudanosine concentrations has not been reported.

Nondepolarizing NMBA Adverse Effects

In acidotic conditions, the tertiary amine group of monoquaternary paralytics (vecuronium and rocuronium) can become protonated, resulting in a greater affinity for the nACh receptor. This increase in affinity can potentially increase the potency of these agents, unlike bisquaternary amines such as atracurium, cisatracurium, and succinylcholine, which are already relatively more potent than the monoquaternary agents due to the structural presence of 2 quaternary cations with affinity for the α subunits of the nAChR.[94]

No vagolytic effect has been identified with benzylisoquinolinium compounds, but they may cause histamine release,[94] cisatracurium to a lesser degree than atracurium.

Laudanosine, a neurotoxic metabolite, is produced as a result of Hoffman elimination. If accumulation occurs, the patient may be at increased risk of developing seizures. The maximum concentration (C_{max}) of laudanosine after cisatracurium and atracurium with continuous infusions has been studied in critically ill patients. The C_{max} of laudanosine with atracurium administration was found to be significantly higher than the C_{max} after cisatracurium administration, 4.4 and 1.3 mg/L, respectively, although the clinical significance of this remains in question.[90] NMBAs are hydrophilic compounds that generally do not cross the blood-brain barrier. In the setting of a disrupted or inflamed blood-brain barrier, the potential for neurotoxicity may exist in the setting of laudanosine accumulation.[104] The neurotoxicity of atracurium has been demonstrated in animal studies, but there is only 1 human case report published to date.[88,104]

Tachyphylaxis, defined as a rapid, diminished, or failed pharmacologic response to a drug, may occur when NMBA infusions are administered for at least 72 hours.[105] Tachyphylaxis requiring increasing doses over time is likely a result of increased protein binding and/or ACh receptor upregulation in response to pharmacologic denervation and has been described with all the NMBs, including rocuronium, vecuronium, atracurium, and cisatracurium.[105] Compared with pancuronium, patients receiving cisatracurium required a greater rate of dose increases, resulting in higher drug-related costs.[105] Interestingly, this effect is not generally seen in the diaphragm compared with other voluntary muscles. In addition, upregulation of these immature receptors is a plausible explanation for the resistance and tachyphylaxis seen with nondepolarizing agents in patients with underlying neuromuscular disorders.

ICU-acquired weakness (ICU-AW) includes critical illness polyneuropathy and myopathies and occurs in 5% to 10% of patients on NMBA infusions. Many terms for this condition exist in the literature, including acute quadriplegic myopathy syndrome and prolonged neurogenic weakness. ICU-AW is characterized by electromyographical changes, myonecrosis with elevated creatinine phosphokinase concentrations, and acute paresis. Although many case reports have demonstrated ICU-AW in the presence of NMBA, no prospective, randomized trials have confirmed this relationship, and some providers question a distinct causal relationship.[106,107] In patients with ARDS on a 48-hour infusion of cisatracurium, an increased prevalence of ICU-AW was not identified.[108,109] When ICU-AW occurs, it is associated with significant health care–related costs.[105] The pharmacologic alteration in neuromuscular transmission results in muscle denervation. This denervation causes an upregulation of immature, ACh receptors and redistribution of these receptors on the motor endplate (see Figure 2.1 and Figure 2.2). New receptors are spread throughout the endplate, and the increase in receptors is thought to cause a resistance to NMBAs.[102] The changes in neuromuscular transmission also cause an upregulation of steroid receptors in the cytosol, resulting in an increased sensitivity to steroids.[102] Although NMBAs have been identified as a risk factor for the development of ICU-AW, their role is still uncertain. If this condition occurs, it can significantly prolong the ventilator-weaning period in general ICU patients.[110,111] In neurocritically ill patients, time to rehabilitation may be delayed, which could lead to prolonged neurologic recovery, although this has not been demonstrated in prospective studies.[104]

Another adverse effect that should be distinguished from ICU-AW is prolonged neuromuscular recovery from NMBAs, defined as an increase in recovery time of 50% to 100% anticipated by pharmacokinetic parameters after discontinuation of the paralytic.[87] Prolonged recovery is often a result of NMBA or metabolite accumulation such as that seen after vecuronium administration in obese patients and those with liver dysfunction or end-stage renal disease. The increase in recovery time is likely a result of accumulation of the 3-hydroxy active vecuronium metabolite. Conditions such as prolonged immobility and spinal cord injury can also cause prolonged neuromuscular blockade after discontinuation of NMBAs due to the upregulation of fetal-variant nAChRs that alter neurotransmission at the motor endplate.[87]

Monitoring

Routine monitoring of the NMBAs guides dosing to prevent under- or over-dosing the paralytic and assists with determining onset of action and duration of action. Clinical parameters such as respirations over the ventilator set rate or independent diaphragmatic movements indicate that the patient is underpara-lyzed. Likewise, the Bedside Shivering Assessment Scale can be a useful clinical tool to evaluate for the presence of shivering after initiation of a paralytic. Vital sign monitoring is useful to determine the presence of adverse effects. A more specific and qualitative measure, compared with clinical parameters, of para-lytic efficacy is train-of-four (TOF) monitoring using a peripheral nerve stimulator. This method remains the easiest and most reliable method for measuring the efficacy of NMBAs.[87] With this method, electrodes are placed on the ulnar, facial, or posterior tibial nerve. With TOF monitoring, 4 supra-maximal stimuli are applied every 0.5 seconds. In this manner, tactile and visual measurement of the response is possible.[106] At least 10 to 15 seconds should be allowed between stimulations to allow the nerve to repolarize. While stimu-lating the ulnar nerve at the adductor pollicis is a more sensitive monitoring parameter, the stimulation of the facial nerve at the orbicularis oculi muscle more closely mimics the paralytic effects occurring in the diaphragm. A TOF measurement of 1 or 2 out of 4 twitches is generally acceptable. Values greater than 2 of 4 twitches indicate that the patient is underparalyzed, while a value of 0 of 4 twitches indicates overparalysis.[87] With a TOF of 0 of 4, careful assess-ment of clinical parameters and placement of electrodes should be consid-ered.[101] Results of the TOF should be interpreted carefully in the presence of misplaced electrodes, loss of electrode adhesion, peripheral edema, and hypothermia.[106]

A top concern when initiating NMBAs should be to ensure that the patient is deeply sedated with proper sedatives and analgesics prior to initiating a para-lytic agent. Every attempt should be made to minimize the risk of patient aware-ness during induced paralysis. As such, many institutions have turned to the use of processed encephalogram models such as BIS monitors to continuously evaluate the depth of the patients' sedation while paralyzed. While some stud-ies suggest an appropriate correlation between the BIS values and validated seda-tion scales,[112,113] others do not, and the practice of using BIS values to monitor and titrate sedation during neuromuscular blockade remains controversial.[106] Although patients should be heavily sedated prior to initiating a paralytic agent, it is important to note that NMBAs mask clinical seizure activity, and in high-risk patients, continuous EEG monitoring can be considered if available.

Adjunctive Care

Adjunctive care of the paralyzed patient is necessary for preventing negative sequelae. Adjunctive pharmacologic care typically includes eye lubrication with ophthalmic ointments and eye drops to prevent corneal drying and ulceration since paralysis inhibits the blink reflex and prevents the eyelids from closing. The prevalence of corneal abrasions in critically ill patients can be up to 60%, and prophylactic measures could reduce this risk.[106,114] When ointments are applied, light taping of the eyelids will help maintain ocular moisture. In addition, the patient should be on a bowel regimen to maintain normal stooling. A common misconception among health care providers is that NMBAs inhibit not only skeletal muscle but also gastrointestinal (GI) peristalsis, leading to constipation. The smooth muscle of the GI tract is a site for muscarinic receptors, which are not typically affected by the nondepolarizing NMBs. Paralyzed patients are, however, at risk of constipation since they are immobilized and likely receiving high doses of opioid analgesics.[88] For these reasons, most patients on continuous NMBAs should also receive a laxative regimen. In addition, prolonged immobilization necessitates the use of pharmacologic and non-pharmacologic venous thromboembolism prophylaxis in the absence of contraindications.[101]

Reversal

Ideally, a neurocritically ill patient who has recently received an NMBA should be allowed to spontaneously recover from the paralysis. There are rare instances in which the NMBA must be reversed such as in a scenario when a neurologic examination is essential in dictating further, time-sensitive therapy. Most often, reversal occurs in the setting of postoperative anesthesia recovery.

When reversal is necessary, AChE inhibitors have been used but are only effective against nondepolarizing NMBAs. AChE inhibitors increase ACh concentrations at the NMJ by inhibiting the metabolism of ACh. They are less than optimal reversal agents due to an inability to fully reverse the neuromuscular blocking effects during profound blockade and the potential for cardiac and autonomic side effects since these agents increase ACh concentrations at muscarinic receptors in addition to the nicotinic receptors. When these agents are used, concomitant use of an anticholinergic medication, such as atropine or glycopyrrolate, may be warranted. Side effects that may be seen with anticholinesterase agents include bradyarrhythmias, increased secretions, and bronchoconstriction.[115] Atropine 0.6 to 1.2 mg may be administered 30 seconds prior to or simultaneously with pyridostigmine or neostigmine. Alternatively,

TABLE 2.7 Acetylcholinesterase Inhibitor Neuromuscular Blocking Reversal Agents

Agent	Onset, min	Duration, min	Usual Dose	Maximum Dose	Notes
Edrophonium	0.5–1	10–73	10 mg over 30 to 45 seconds; may be repeated if no response	40 mg	70% renally cleared 30% hepatically cleared
Pyridostigmine	4; peak effects 12–16	30–60	10 mg	20 mg	75% renally cleared 25% hepatically cleared
Neostigmine	1; peak effects 7–11	20–30	0.03–0.07 mg/kg	0.07 mg/kg or 5 mg (whichever is less)	No dose adjustments for renal or hepatic failure

Source: Compiled from references 115, 117, 118, 119, and 120.

IV glycopyrrolate is administered in a dose of 0.2 mg for every 1 mg of neostigmine or every 5 mg of pyridostigmine.[116,117] Neostigmine and pyridostigmine durations of reversal of the neuromuscular blockade are longer than with edrophonium due to a tighter covalent bond with AChE.[106] A "ceiling" effect exists with these types of reversal agents when all AChE enzymes have been inhibited; therefore, additional doses are not effective beyond this point.[118–121] When comparing edrophonium, neostigmine, and pyridostigmine, although they are equally effective at NMBA reversal,[122] there is much variability in the literature as to the time of onset and durations of action of these agents. These parameters likely depend on the dose used, the amount of neuromuscular blockade, and patient-specific factors. It is agreed, however, that edrophonium has the fastest onset and shortest duration of the agents. For a comparison of AChE inhibitor reversal agents, see Table 2.7.

While the pursuit of a nondepolarizing NMBA with a pharmacokinetic profile such as that of succinylcholine has fallen short, investigators have shifted their attention to the development of safe and rapid paralytic reversal agents. Sugammadex (Bridion) is a first-in-class, selective relaxant-binding agent that has recently been FDA approved. Sugammadex, a modified γ-cyclodextrin, only reverses aminosteroid agents (rocuronium more than vecuronium) by tightly encapsulating them at the motor endplate, thereby preventing their ability to bind and inhibit ACh receptors. The sugammadex-aminosteroid complex is then renally excreted. Sugammadex is not associated with the cholinergic effects that limit the AChE inhibitors since it is pharmacologically unrelated to the AChE inhibitors,[123] but it is associated with hypersensitivity reactions.[122,124]

Special Adult Populations

Hypothermia

With therapeutic hypothermia becoming a more commonly employed strategy after cardiac arrest and also being used at times for refractory intracranial hypertension[104] or status epilepticus (limited data),[125] careful consideration of paralytic dosing is imperative. Hypothermia has been shown to impair renal and hepatic elimination of drugs, including NMBAs.[126-128] In general, a reduce muscle twitch response should be expected with reductions in core temperature regardless of the presence of an NMBA.[129,130] When combined with an NMBA, the effects on the twitch response can be even more profound. While most studies of NMBA pharmacokinetics during hypothermia have been conducted in hypothermic, cardiopulmonary bypass patients, important concepts can be extrapolated from this research. Vecuronium concentrations have been shown to gradually increase as central body temperature was reduced from 36° to 34°C, and twitch response was reduced by 20% per degree Celsius in a study of a vecuronium continuous infusion.[131] In addition, the duration of action of a vecuronium bolus dose of 0.1 mg/kg was shown to have almost doubled (28 to 62 minutes) when body temperature was reduced from 36.5° to 34.4°C.[131,132] Atracurium duration of action has also been shown to be prolonged during hypothermia,[133,134] and lower infusion rates were required to maintain a constant level of neuromuscular blockade, likely as a result of reduced enzymatic activity of the plasma esterase during Hoffman elimination.[105,135,136] In a study of 19 neurosurgical patients paralyzed with rocuronium, the presence of hypothermia prolonged the duration of action and delayed recovery, likely as a result of reduced clearance.[126,137] Overall, careful monitoring of NMBA effects should be employed during all phases of induced hypothermia as infusion requirements will likely be reduced during the cooling and maintenance phases and increased during the rewarming phase and at normal body temperatures.

Elderly

Age-related changes in onset of vecuronium and rocuronium may be slower in the elderly, presumably from reductions in cardiovascular output,[99,101] and clearance may be affected by reduced glomerular filtration rates and liver function.[106] No significant changes have been demonstrated in the clearance of atracurium and cisatracurium in this population,[101] although the onsets of action of the benzylisoquinolinium compounds can be prolonged.[138] There is little evidence to suggest any alterations in the action of succinylcholine in elderly patients.[138] More recent data suggest that elderly patients aged 70 to 90 years are at greater risk of prolonged, postoperative neuromuscular block compared with a younger cohort, and this prolonged block is associated with a greater complications.[139] The same may be true after maintenance NMBA use in the ICU.[139] Use in the elderly patients should be closely monitored by clinical parameters and peripheral nerve stimulation, and it should be discontinued as soon as possible.

Pregnancy

Pregnancy has been shown to alter the pharmacokinetics of the NMBAs due to a larger plasma volume leading to decreased concentrations of plasma pseudocholinesterases; however, the clinical duration of succinylcholine has been shown to remain unchanged.[140] There is concern with the NMBAs in general for placental transfer that is highly variable and dependent on the dose, functional state of the placenta, and the molecular weight of the agent. Although data are scarce, rocuronium appears to have the highest maternal-fetal NMBA transfer due to its low molecular weight followed by vecuronium and then atracurium, which has the highest molecular weight.[90] Maternal-fetal transfer parameters have not been extensively studied with cisatracurium. Interestingly, with cisatracurium, mean onset time, and duration of effects are significantly shorter in the immediate postpartum period compared with nonpregnant females.[140,141]

Traumatic Brain Injury

The use of NMBs for ICP management in traumatic brain injury (TBI) dates back to the 1980s and remains controversial due to limited, low-quality, and conflicting data in both animal and human subjects.[104] NMBs are believed to prevent fatal increases in ICP as a result of coughing, suctioning, moving, or ventilator dyssynchrony when deep sedation is ineffective. Six small, prospective studies revealed no increases in ICP when a bolus of an NMBA was administered prior to endotracheal suctioning[104]; however, in a prospective trial of 23 patients who received a bolus of vecuronium prior to fiberoptic bronchoscopy, increases in ICP during the procedure were not prevented.[142] Typically, nondepolarizing NMBAs are used for this indication due to the concern for increased ICPs with bolus administration of succinylcholine. In addition, NMBAs may reduce energy expenditure[104,143]; however, only 1 prospective study (involving atracurium bolus administration) has actually demonstrated significant reductions in ICP.[144] In contrast, a post hoc analysis of a randomized controlled trial conducted in 2000 evaluated prospectively collected data from patients with TBI. This study demonstrated that patients who were prescribed NMBAs experienced greater time with ICPs above 20 mm Hg compared with those who were not taking NMBAs (13.5 hours vs 6.5 hours, respectively; $P < .5$).[145] This result challenges the benefit of NMBAs but should be interpreted cautiously due to trial design. In patients with TBI, NMBAs have been shown to increase ICU length of stay, incidence of pneumonia, and number of severely disabled survivors, although long-term effects have been insufficiently studied.[88,146] The 2007 Brain Trauma Foundation Guidelines for TBI do not offer any recommendations on the use of paralytics for this indication.[1,147] Although firm conclusions cannot be drawn, NMBs for TBI should likely be reserved for refractory, malignant intracranial hypertension, and bolus dosing of nondepolarizing NMBAs may be considered prior to noxious stimuli that may elevate ICPs such as endotracheal suctioning.

Shivering

NMBAs are often included in institutional, antishivering protocols in neurointensive care units. Induced hypothermia or normothermia may be used in neurocritically ill patients to control fevers or refractory ICPs or in the management of refractory status epilepticus. In 2011, Choi and colleagues[2] published a study evaluating the use of an antishivering protocol in a neurointensive care unit. This stepwise protocol emphasized the use of the least sedating drugs first to minimize influence of the medications on the patient's neurologic examination. Dexmedetomidine, opioids, and propofol were the most commonly used first-line agents. Vecuronium boluses were considered the last-line agent in the protocol, and less than 1% of the 213 patients included in the study required paralysis to terminate shivering during induced hypothermia or normothermia. In general, NMBAs should be considered last-line agents to manage refractory shivering in the neurointensive care unit, and this study demonstrated that shivering could often be prevented and managed effectively with alternative agents such as sedatives and analgesics.[2]

Drug Interactions

Several clinically relevant pharmacokinetic and pharmacodynamic drug interactions have been identified with NMBAs. Pharmacokinetic interactions primarily affect onset time or recovery time of the neuromuscular block while pharmacodynamic interactions tend to affect the amount of paralysis produced.[148]

A significant interaction occurs between classes of NMBAs themselves and depends on the class and sequence of administration. The most common indication for combining NMBAs is the use of defasciculating doses of nondepolarizing NMBAs prior to succinylcholine administration to reduce the risk of muscle fasciculations. In reverse sequence, it has been shown that when a nondepolarizing NMBA is administered *after* recovery from a depolarizing neuromuscular block as demonstrated when vecuronium was administered after decamethonium bromide, the paralytic effects of vecuronium were potentiated 7-fold compared to when vecuronium was administered alone.[149] A possible explanation is that the depolarizing NMBA blocks presynaptic nicotinic receptors, resulting in a reduction in the positive feedback that would normally cause increased amounts of ACh to be released into the synapse. In contrast, the administration of a depolarizing NMBA after a nondepolarizing NMBA results in resistance to the blockade, and higher doses of the depolarizing agent may be necessary.[148]

Theophylline, ranitidine, and some older-generation anticonvulsants are also known to antagonize the effects of nondepolarizing NMBAs. In neurosurgical patients, chronic therapy with phenytoin or carbamazepine resulted in higher infusion rate requirements of cisatracurium to maintain the desired paralytic response. These same patients experienced higher clearance rates, leading to more rapid rates of paralytic recovery.[150,151] In the setting of chronic antiepileptic therapy with phenytoin and carbamazepine, higher bolus doses of rocuronium were needed to achieve faster onsets of paralytic action and slower times to recovery during anesthesia to avoid premature recoveries.[152]

Magnesium decreases synaptic concentrations of ACh, presumably from competitive actions with calcium that results in reduced release of ACh from the presynaptic nerve terminal. To a lesser degree, magnesium also reduces muscle fiber excitation and the depolarizing actions of acetylcholine.[99] The interaction of magnesium with vecuronium has been shown to increase the degree of blockade and prolong the duration of action of vecuronium.[148]

Corticosteroids have long been thought to have additive effects with NMBAs in potentiating and prolonging the effects of neuromuscular blockade.[153] This interaction has been demonstrated in experimental models in which the combination of agents yielded pharmacologic denervation[154]; however, this evidence is inconsistent with results from a trial published in 1997 that failed to demonstrate any differences in the incidence of prolonged blockade with the combination of vecuronium and corticosteroids.[155] When possible, clinicians may avoid the combination of corticosteroids and NMBAs, although there are some

TABLE 2.8 Selected Drug Interactions With Neuromuscular Blocking Agents

Drugs Causing Cholinesterase Inhibition	
Metoclopramide	Dose-dependent inhibition of plasma cholinesterases; shown to prolong the action of depolarizing NMBAs
Cyclophosphamide	Inhibits NMBA metabolism
Cyclosporine	Inhibit NMBA metabolism
Oral contraceptives	Significance of clinical effects unknown; case reports only
Competitive Cholinesterase Substrates	
Beta-blockers	Exact mechanism unknown; likely low clinical significance; case reports only
Drugs That Interfere With Muscle Contractility	
Clindamycin	Pre- and postjunctional effects; cannot be reversed with anticholinesterases
Drugs that Interfere With the Postsynaptic AChR	
Polymixins	Prolong neostigmine-resistant block; effects of this interaction are more pronounced with Polymixin B than colistin
Local anesthetics	Multiple mechanisms including a reduction in channel "open time"
Inhaled anesthetics	Reduced nAChR sensitivity; less paralytic effect; higher doses and closer monitoring may be required
Corticosteroids	Multiple mechanisms; may decrease sensitivity of nAChR; likely not clinically significant unless high doses or long duration of use
Drugs That Decrease Production and/or Release of ACh	
Ketamine	Controversial; only shown to increase partial vecuronium block and prolong NMBA effect. Mechanism unclear; could directly affect calcium transport
Tetracycline antibiotics	At high doses can potentiate the extent and duration of block
Aminoglycosides	Depress ACh release and act as a postsynaptic AChR channel blocker. Potentiates the effects of both depolarizing and nondepolarizing NMBAs. Cholinesterase inhibitors (neostigmine/pyridostigmine) only partially reverse paralysis in the setting of an aminoglycoside and NMBA concurrently.
Phenothiazines	High doses can increase sensitivity of nondepolarizing NMBAs
Calcium channel blockers	Effects may not be clinically significant except in high doses
Magnesium sulfate	Dose-related decrease in ACh by competing with calcium at the presynaptic membrane; causes an increase in the degree and duration of block

Source: Compiled from references 87, 94, 106, 118, 148, and 162.

Note: ACh, acetylcholine; AChR, acetylcholine receptor; nAChR, nicotinic acetylcholine receptor; NMBA, neuromuscular blocking agent.

scenarios where the combination cannot be avoided. Careful monitoring and prudent use may mitigate the risk of prolonged recovery.

Other drug-drug interactions that should be considered with the use of NMBAs include metoclopramide, phenothiazines, and antibiotics. These agents and others that are implicated in the potentiation of NMBA effects are listed in Table 2.8

Cost Considerations

Institutional neuromuscular blocking practice and protocols should consider safety first and then cost-effective utilization of these agents. While costs of individual NMBAs vary with time and availability, drug shortages should be considered in addition to changes in local pricing on a routine basis.

Conclusions

Because of its unique structure, each paralytic agent offers a unique pharmacokinetic and pharmacodynamic profile that clinicians should consider when neurocritically ill patients require pharmacologic neuromuscular blockade. These profiles along with patient-specific characteristics should be used to guide the selection of the safest and most cost-effective NMBA for a neurocritically ill patient. Judicious use and careful monitoring is essential for optimizing efficacy and minimizing adverse drug effects.

References

1. Bratton SL, Chestnut RM, Ghajar J, et al. Guidelines for the management of severe traumatic brain injury. XI. Anesthetics, analgesics, and sedatives. *J Neurotrauma*. 2007; 24(suppl 1):S71–S76.
2. Choi HA, Ko SB, Presciutti M, et al. Prevention of shivering during therapeutic temperature modulation: the Columbia anti-shivering protocol. *Neurocrit Care*. 2011;14:389–394.
3. Barr J, Fraser GL, Puntillo K, et al. Clinical practice guidelines for the management of pain, agitation, and delirium in adult patients in the intensive care unit. *Crit Care Med*. 2013;41:263–306.
4. Jacobi J, Fraser GL, Coursin DB, et al. Clinical practice guidelines for the sustained use of sedatives and analgesics in the critically ill adult. *Crit Care Med*. 2002;30:119–141.
5. Chanques G, Sebbane M, Barbotte E, et al. A prospective study of pain at rest: incidence and characteristics of an unrecognized symptom in surgical and trauma versus medical intensive care unit patients. *Anesthesiology*. 2007;107:858–860.
6. Payen JF, Chanques G, Mantz J, et al. Current practices in sedation and analgesia for mechanically ventilated critically ill patients: a prospective multi center patient-based study. *Anesthesiology*. 2007;106(4):687–695.
7. Gélinas C. Management of pain in cardiac surgery ICU patients: have we improved over time? *Intensive Crit Care Nurs*. 2007;23:298–303.

8. Strøm T, Martinussen T, Toft P. A protocol of no sedation for critically ill patients receiving mechanical ventilation: a randomised trial. *Lancet*. 2010;375:475–480.

9. Park G, Lane M, Rogers S, Bassett P. A comparison of hypnotic and analgesic based sedation in a general intensive care unit. *Br J Anaesth*. 2007;98(1):76–82.

10. Albanèse J, Viviand X, Potie F, et al. Sufentanil, fentanyl, and alfentanil in head trauma patients: a study on cerebral hemodynamics. *Crit Care Med*. 1999;27:407–411.

11. Bourgoin A, Albanèse J, Leone M, Sampol-Manos E. Effects of sufentanil or ketamine administered in target-controlled infusion on the cerebral hemodynamics of severely brain-injured patients. *Crit Care Med*. 2005;33(5):1109–1113.

12. Lauer KK, Connolly LA, Schmeling WT. Opioid sedation does not alter intracranial pressure in head injured patients. *Can J Anaesth*. 1997;44:929–933.

13. Smith NT, Benthuysen JL, Bickford RG, et al. Seizures during opioid anesthetic induction—are they opioid-induced rigidity? *Anesthesiology*. 1989;71:852–862.

14. Muellejans B, López A, Cross MH, et al. Remifentanil versus fentanyl for analgesia based sedation to provide patient comfort in the intensive care unit: a randomized, double-blind controlled trial. *Crit Care*. 2004;8:R1–R11.

15. Devlin JW, Roberts RJ. Pharmacology of commonly used analgesics and sedatives in the ICU: benzodiazepines, propofol, and opioids. *Crit Care Clin*. 2009;25:431–449, vii.

16. Wagner BK, O'Hara DA. Pharmacokinetics and pharmacodynamics of sedatives and analgesics in the treatment of agitated critically ill patients. *Clin Pharmacokinet*. 1997; 33:426–453.

17. Puntillo KA, White C, Morris AB, et al. Patients' perceptions and responses to procedural pain: results from Thunder Project II. *Am J Crit Care*. 2001;10:238–251.

18. Preda A, MacLean RW, Mazure CM, Bowers MB. Antidepressant-associated mania and psychosis resulting in psychiatric admissions. *J Clin Psychiatry*. 2001;62:30–33.

19. Matsuura M. Epileptic psychoses and anticonvulsant drug treatment. *J Neurol Neurosurg Psychiatry*. 1999;67:231–233.

20. Patten SB, Neutel CI. Corticosteroid-induced adverse psychiatric effects: incidence, diagnosis and management. *Drug Saf*. 2000;22:111–122.

21. Besag FM. Behavioural effects of the new anticonvulsants. *Drug Saf*. 2001;24:513–536.

22. Sternbach H, State R. Antibiotics: neuropsychiatric effects and psychotropic interactions. *Harv Rev Psychiatry*. 1997;5:214–226.

23. Katz MH. Effect of HIV treatment on cognition, behavior, and emotion. *Psychiatr Clin North Am*. 1994;17:227–230.

24. Dasta DF, Jacobi J, Sesti AM, McLaughlin TP. Addition of dexmedetomidine to standard sedation regimens after cardiac surgery: an outcomes analysis. *Pharmacotherapy*. 2006;26:798–805.

25. Kress JP, Hall JB. Sedation in the mechanically ventilated patient. *Crit Care Med*. 2006;34:2541–2546.

26. Iyer VN, Hoel R, Rabinstein AA. Propofol infusion syndrome in patients with refractory status epilepticus: an 11-year clinical experience. *Crit Care Med*. 2009;37:3024–3030.

27. Riker RR, Shehabi Y, Bokesch PM, et al. Dexmedetomidine vs midazolam for sedation of critically ill patients: a randomized trial. *JAMA*. 2009;301:489–499.

28. Nelson S, Muzyk AJ, Bucklin MH, et al. Defining the role of dexmedetomidine in the prevention of delirium in the intensive care unit. *Biomed Res Int*. 2015;2015:635737.

29. Pandharipande P, Cotton BA, Shintani A, et al. Prevalence and risk factors for development of delirium in surgical and trauma intensive care unit patients. *J Trauma*. 2008; 65:34–41.

30. Griffin CE, Kaye AM, Bueno FR, Kaye AD. Benzodiazepine pharmacology and central nervous system-mediated effects. *Ochsner J*. 2013;13:214–223.
31. Buffett-Jerrott SE, Stewart SH. Cognitive and sedative effects of benzodiazepine use. *Curr Pharm Des*. 2002;8(1):45–58.
32. Sanchez-Izquierdo-Riera JA, Caballero-Cubedo RE, Perez-Vela JL, et al. Propofol versus midazolam: safety and efficacy for sedating the severe trauma patient. *Anesth Analg*. 1998;86:1219–1224.
33. Papazian L, Albanèse J, Thirion X, et al. Effect of bolus doses of midazolam on intracranial pressure and cerebral perfusion pressure in patients with severe head injury. *Br J Anaesth*. 1993;71:267–271.
34. Forster A, Juge O, Morel D. Effects of midazolam on cerebral hemodynamics and cerebral vasomotor responsiveness to carbon dioxide. *J Cereb Blood Flow Metab*. 1983; 3:246–249.
35. Flower O, Hellings S. Sedation in traumatic brain injury. *Emerg Med Int*. 2012;2012:637171.
36. Stewart, SA. The effects of benzodiazepines on cognition. *J Clin Psychiatry*. 2005;66(suppl 2):9–13.
37. Busto U, Sellers EM, Naranjo CA, et al. Withdrawal reaction after long-term therapeutic use of benzodiazepines. *N Engl J Med*. 1986;315:854–859.
38. Forster A, Juge O, Morel D. Effects of midazolam on cerebral blood flow in human volunteers. *Anesthesiology*. 1982;56:453–455.
39. Allonen H, Ziegler G, Klotz U. Midazolam kinetics. *Clin Pharmacol Ther*. 1981; 30:653–661.
40. Yahwak JA, Riker RR, Fraser GL, Subak-Sharpe S. Determination of a lorazepam dose threshold for using the osmol gap to monitor for propylene glycol toxicity. *Pharmacotherapy*. 2008;28:984–991.
41. Laine GA, Hossain SM, Solis RT, Adams SC. Polyethylene glycol nephrotoxicity secondary to prolonged high-dose intravenous lorazepam. *Ann Pharmacother*. 1995; 29:1110–1114.
42. Seay RE, Graves RJ, Wilkin MK. Comment: possible toxicity from propylene glycol in lorazepam infusion. *Ann Pharmacother*. 1997;31:647–648.
43. Arbour RB. Propylene glycol toxicity related to high-dose lorazepam infusion: case report and discussion. *Am J Crit Care*. 1999;8:499–506.
44. Bailie GR, Cockshott ID, Douglas EJ, Bowles BJ. Pharmacokinetics of propofol during and after long-term continuous infusion for maintenance of sedation in ICU patients. *Br J Anaesth*. 1992;68:486–491.
45. Kowalski SD, Rayfield CA. A post hoc descriptive study of patients receiving propofol. *Am J Crit Care*. 1999;8(1):507–513.
46. Chukwuemeka A, Ko R, Ralph-Edwards A. Short-term low-dose propofol anaesthesia associated with severe metabolic acidosis. *Anaesth Intensive Care*. 2006;34:651–655.
47. Merz TM, Regli B, Rothen HU, Felleiter P. Propofol infusion syndrome—a fatal case at a low infusion rate. *Anesth Analg*. 2006;103:1050.
48. Roberts RJ, Barletta JF, Fong JJ, et al. Incidence of propofol-related infusion syndrome in critically ill adults: a prospective, multicenter study. *Crit Care*. 2009;13:R169.
49. Paul BS, Paul G. Sedation in neurological intensive care unit. *Ann Indian Acad Neurol*. 2013;16:194–202.
50. Lee JS, Jang HS, Park BJ. Green discoloration of urine after propofol infusion. *Korean J Anesthesiol*. 2013;65:177–179.
51. Blakey SA, Hixson-Wallace JA. Clinical significance of rare and benign side effects: propofol and green urine. *Pharmacotherapy*. 2000;20:1120–1122.

52. Rawal G, Yadav S. Green urine due to propofol: A case report with review of literature. *J Clin Diagn Res.* 2015;9:OD03–OD04.
53. Mirski MA, Lewin JJ, Ledroux S, et al. Cognitive improvement during continuous sedation in critically ill, awake and responsive patients: the Acute Neurological ICU Sedation Trial (ANIST). *Intensive Care Med.* 2010;36:1505–1513.
54. Venn RM, Hell J, Grounds RM. Respiratory effects of dexmedetomidine in the surgical patient requiring intensive care. *Crit Care.* 2000;4:302–308.
55. Venn M, Newman J, Grounds M. A phase II study to evaluate the efficacy of dexmedetomidine for sedation in the medical intensive care unit. *Intensive Care Med.* 2003;29:201–207.
56. Shehabi Y, Ruettimann U, Adamson H, et al. Dexmedetomidine infusion for more than 24 hours in critically ill patients: sedative and cardiovascular effects. *Intensive Care Med.* 2004;30:2188–2196.
57. Rayner SG, Weinert CR, Peng H, et al. Dexmedetomidine as adjunct treatment for severe alcohol withdrawal in the ICU. *Ann Intensive Care.* 2012;2:12.
58. Dailey RW, Leatherman JW, Sprenkle MD. Dexemedetomidine in the management of alcohol withdrawal and alcohol withdrawal delirium. *Am J Respir Crit Care Med.* 2011;183:A3164.
59. DeMuro JP, Botros DG, Wirkowski E, Hanna AF. Use of dexmedetomidine for the treatment of alcohol withdrawal syndrome in critically ill patients: a retrospective case series. *J Anesth.* 2012;26:601–605.
60. Muzyk AJ, Revollo JY, Rivelli SK. The use of dexmedetomidine in alcohol withdrawal. *J Neuropsychiatry Clin Neurosci.* 2012;24:E45–E46.
61. Morita T, Hitomi S, Saito S, et al. Repeated ketamine administration produces up-regulation of muscarinic acetylcholine receptors in the forebrain, and reduces behavioral sensitivity to scopolamine in mice. *Psychopharmacology (Berl).* 1995;117:396–402.
62. Sarton E, Teppema LJ, Olievier C, et al. The involvement of the mu-opioid receptor in ketamine-induced respiratory depression and antinociception. *Anesth Analg.* 2001;93:1495–1500.
63. Green SM, Andolfatto G, Krauss B. Ketofol for procedural sedation? Pro and con. *Ann Emerg Med.* 2011;57:444–448.
64. Miller AC, Jamin CT, Elamin EM. Continuous intravenous infusion of ketamine for maintenance sedation. *Minerva Anestesiol.* 2011;77:812–820.
65. Mössner LD, Schmitz A, Theurillat R, et al. Inhibition of cytochrome P450 enzymes involved in ketamine metabolism by use of liver microsomes and specific cytochrome P450 enzymes from horses, dogs, and humans. *Am J Vet Res.* 2011;72:1505–1513.
66. Elia N, Tramèr MR. Ketamine and postoperative pain—a quantitative systematic review of randomised trials. *Pain.* 2005;113:61–70.
67. Bourgoin A, Albanèse J, Wereszczynski N, et al. Safety of sedation with ketamine in severe head injury patients: comparison with sufentanil. *Crit Care Med.* 2003;31:711–717.
68. Himmelseher S, Durieux ME. Revising a dogma: ketamine for patients with neurological injury? *Anesth Analg.* 2005;101:524–534.
69. Gaspard N, Foreman B, Judd LM, et al. Intravenous ketamine for the treatment of refractory status epilepticus: a retrospective multicenter study. *Epilepsia.* 2013;54:1498–1503.
70. Roberts I, Sydenham E. Barbiturates for acute traumatic brain injury. *Cochrane Database Syst Rev.* 2012;(12):CD000033.

71. Buchtel HA, Passaro EA, Selwa LM, et al. Sodium methohexital (brevital) as an anesthetic in the Wada test. *Epilepsia*. 2002;43:1056–1061.

72. Patel A, Wordell C, Szarlej D. Alternatives to sodium amobarbital in the Wada test. *Ann Pharmacother*. 2011;45:395–401.

73. Lischke V, Behne M, Doelken P, et al. Droperidol causes a dose-dependent prolongation of the QT interval. *Anesth Analg*. 1994;79:983–986.

74. Misfeldt BB, Jörgensen PB, Spotoft H, Ronde F. The effects of droperidol and fentanyl on intracranial pressure and cerebral perfusion pressure in neurosurgical patients. *Br J Anaesth*. 1976;48:963–968.

75. Riker RR, Picard JT, Fraser GL. Prospective evaluation of the Sedation-Agitation Scale for adult critically ill patients. *Crit Care Med*. 1999;27:1325–1329.

76. Sessler CN, Gosnell MS, Grap MJ, et al. The Richmond Agitation-Sedation Scale: validity and reliability in adult intensive care unit patients. *Am J Respir Crit Care Med*. 2002;166:1338–1344.

77. De Jonghe B, Cook D, Griffith L, et al. Adaptation to the Intensive Care Environment (ATICE): development and validation of a new sedation assessment instrument. *Crit Care Med*. 2003;31:2344–2354.

78. Avripas MB, Smythe MA, Carr A, et al. Development of an intensive care unit bedside sedation scale. *Ann Pharmacother*. 2001;35:262–263.

79. Payen JF, Bru O, Bosson JL, et al. Assessing pain in critically ill sedated patients by using a behavioral pain scale. *Crit Care Med*. 2001;29:2258–2263.

80. Brandl KM, Langley KA, Riker RR, et al. Confirming the reliability of the sedation-agitation scale administered by ICU nurses without experience in its use. *Pharmacotherapy*. 2001;21:431–436.

81. Ryder-Lewis MC, Nelson KM. Reliability of the Sedation-Agitation Scale between nurses and doctors. *Intensive Crit Care Nurs*. 2008;24:211–217.

82. Ely EW, Truman B, Shintani A, et al. Monitoring sedation status over time in ICU patients: reliability and validity of the Richmond Agitation-Sedation Scale (RASS). *JAMA*. 2003;289:2983–2991.

83. Riker RR, Fraser GL, Wilkins ML. Comparing the bispectral index and suppression ratio with burst suppression of the electroencephalogram during pentobarbital infusions in adult intensive care patients. *Pharmacotherapy*. 2003;23:1087–1093.

84. Frenzel D, Greim CA, Sommer C, et al. Is the bispectral index appropriate for monitoring the sedation level of mechanically ventilated surgical ICU patients? *Intensive Care Med*. 2002;28:178–183.

85. Arbour R, Waterhouse J, Seckel MA, Bucher L. Correlation between the Sedation-Agitation Scale and the Bispectral Index in ventilated patients in the intensive care unit. *Heart Lung*. 2009;38:336–345.

86. de Wit M, Epstein SK. Administration of sedatives and level of sedation: comparative evaluation via the Sedation-Agitation Scale and the Bispectral Index. *Am J Crit Care*. 2003;12:343–348.

87. Murray MJ, Cowen J, DeBlock H, et al. Clinical practice guidelines for sustained neuromuscular blockade in the adult critically ill patient. *Crit Care Med*. 2002;30:142–156.

88. Warr J, Thiboutot Z, Rose L, et al. Current therapeutic uses, pharmacology, and clinical considerations of neuromuscular blocking agents for critically ill adults. *Ann Pharmacother*. 2011;45:1116–1126.

89. Prielipp RC. Pharmacology, selection and complications associated with neuromuscular blocking drugs in ICU patients. *Yale J Biol Med*. 1998;71:469–484.

90. Atherton DP, Hunter JM. Clinical pharmacokinetics of the newer neuromuscular blocking drugs. *Clin Pharmacokinet.* 1999;36:169–189.

91. Gonzalez-Freire M, de Cabo R, Studenski SA, Ferrucci L. The neuromuscular junction: aging at the crossroad between nerves and muscle. *Front Aging Neurosci.* 2014;6:208.

92. Jang YC, Van Remmen H. Age-associated alterations of the neuromuscular junction. *Exp Gerontol.* 2011;46:193–198.

93. Engel AG, Fumagalli G. Mechanisms of acetylcholine receptor loss from the neuromuscular junction. In: Evered D, Whelan J, eds. *Ciba Foundation Symposium 90: Receptors, Antibodies and Disease.* Chichester UK: John Wiley; 1982:197–224.

94. Appiah-Ankam J, Hunter JM. Pharmacology of neuromuscular blocking drugs. *Contin Educ Anaesth Crit Care Pain.* 2004;4(1):2–7.

95. Minton MD, Grosslight K, Stirt JA, Bedford RF. Increases in intracranial pressure from succinylcholine: prevention by prior nondepolarizing blockade. *Anesthesiology.* 1986;65:165–169.

96. Stirt JA, Grosslight KR, Bedford RF, Vollmer D. "Defasciculation" with metocurine prevents succinylcholine-induced increases in intracranial pressure. *Anesthesiology.* 1987;67:50–53.

97. Kovarik WD, Mayberg TS, Lam AM, et al. Succinylcholine does not change intracranial pressure, cerebral blood flow velocity, or the electroencephalogram in patients with neurologic injury. *Anesth Analg.* 1994;78:469–473.

98. Stollings JL, Diedrich DA, Oyen LJ, Brown DR. Rapid-sequence intubation: a review of the process and considerations when choosing medications. *Ann Pharmacother.* 2014; 48:62–76.

99. Fisher DM. Clinical pharmacology of neuromuscular blocking agents. *Am J Health Syst Pharm.* 1999;56(11)(suppl 1):S4–S9.

100. Caro DA, Andescavage S, Akhlaghi M, et al. Pupillary response to light is preserved in the majority of patients undergoing rapid sequence intubation. *Ann Emerg Med.* 2011;57:234–237.

101. McManus MC. Neuromuscular blockers in surgery and intensive care, Part 2. *Am J Health Syst Pharm.* 2001;58(24):2381–2395.

102. Latronico N, Shehu I, Seghelini E. Neuromuscular sequelae of critical illness. *Curr Opin Crit Care.* 2005;11:381–390.

103. Blanié A, Ract C, Leblanc PE, et al. The limits of succinylcholine for critically ill patients. *Anesth Analg.* 2012;115:873–879.

104. Sanfilippo F, Santonocito C, Veenith T, et al. The role of neuromuscular blockade in patients with traumatic brain injury: a systematic review. *Neurocrit Care.* 2015;22:325–334.

105. Kanji S, Barletta JF, Janisse JJ, et al. Tachyphylaxis associated with continuous cisatracurium versus pancuronium therapy. *Pharmacotherapy.* 2002;22:823–830.

106. Greenberg SB, Vender J. The use of neuromuscular blocking agents in the ICU: where are we now? *Crit Care Med.* 2013;41:1332–1344.

107. Puthucheary Z, Rawal J, Ratnayake G, et al. Neuromuscular blockade and skeletal muscle weakness in critically ill patients: time to rethink the evidence? *Am J Respir Crit Care Med.* 2012;185:911–917.

108. Forel JM, Roch A, Marin V, et al. Neuromuscular blocking agents decrease inflammatory response in patients presenting with acute respiratory distress syndrome. *Crit Care Med.* 2006;34:2749–2757.

109. Papazian L, Forel JM, Gacouin A, et al. Neuromuscular blockers in early acute respiratory distress syndrome. *N Engl J Med.* 2010;363:1107–1116.

110. de Jonghe B, Bastuji-Garin S, Sharshar T, et al. Does ICU-acquired paresis lengthen weaning from mechanical ventilation? *Intensive Care Med.* 2004;30:1117–1121.

111. Garnacho-Montero J, Amaya-Villar R, García-Garmendía JL, et al. Effect of critical illness polyneuropathy on the withdrawal from mechanical ventilation and the length of stay in septic patients. *Crit Care Med.* 2005;33:349–354.

112. Yaman F, Ozcan N, Ozcan A, et al. Assesment of correlation between bispectral index and four common sedation scales used in mechanically ventilated patients in ICU. *Eur Rev Med Pharmacol Sci.* 2012;16:660–666.

113. Karamchandani K, Rewari V, Trikha A, Batra RK. Bispectral index correlates well with Richmond agitation sedation scale in mechanically ventilated critically ill patients. *J Anesth.* 2010;24:394–398.

114. Honiden S, Siegel MD. Analytic reviews: managing the agitated patient in the ICU: sedation, analgesia, and neuromuscular blockade. *J Intensive Care Med.* 2010; 25:187–204.

115. Dickens MD. Pharmacology of neuromuscular blockade: interactions and implications for concurrent drug therapies. *Crit Care Nurs Q.* 1995;18:1–12.

116. Bevan DR, Donati F, Kopman AF. Reversal of neuromuscular blockade. *Anesthesiology.* 1992;77:785–805.

117. Pyridostigmine: adult dosing. Greenwood Village, CO: Truven Health Analytics; 2016. www.micromedexsolutions.com. Accessed December 22, 2016.

118. Sterling E, Winstead P, Fahy B. Guide to neuromuscular blocking agents. *Anesthesiology News.* 2007;25–30. https://pdfs.semanticscholar.org/63f7/739011654c7ba5763291b39c2 c18c50daf3c.pdf. Accessed March 24, 2017.

119. Srivastava A, Hunter JM. Reversal of neuromuscular block. *Br J Anaesth.* 2009; 103:115–129.

120. Fink H, Hollmann MW. Myths and facts in neuromuscular pharmacology: new developments in reversing neuromuscular blockade. *Minerva Anestesiol.* 2012;78:473–482.

121. Caldwell JE. Clinical limitations of acetylcholinesterase antagonists. *J Crit Care.* 2009;24:21–28.

122. Nicholson WT, Sprung J, Jankowski CJ. Sugammadex: a novel agent for the reversal of neuromuscular blockade. *Pharmacotherapy.* 2007;27:1181–1188.

123. Abad-Gurumeta A, Ripollés-Melchor J, Casans-Francés R, et al. A systematic review of sugammadex vs neostigmine for reversal of neuromuscular blockade. *Anaesthesia.* 2015;70:1441–1452.

124. Tsur A, Kalansky A. Hypersensitivity associated with sugammadex administration: a systematic review. *Anaesthesia.* 2014;69:1251–1257.

125. Brophy G, Bell R, Claassen J, et al. Guidelines for the evaluation and management of status epilepticus. *Neurocrit Care.* 2012;17:3–23.

126. Smeulers NJ, Wierda JM, van den Broek L, et al. Effects of hypothermic cardiopulmonary bypass on the pharmacodynamics and pharmacokinetics of rocuronium. *J Cardiothorac Vasc Anesth.* 1995;9:700–705.

127. Ham J, Miller RD, Benet LZ, et al. Pharmacokinetics and pharmacodynamics of d-tubocurarine during hypothermia in the cat. *Anesthesiology.* 1978;49:324–329.

128. Miller RD, Agoston S, van der Pol F, et al. Hypothermia and the pharmacokinetics and pharmacodynamics of pancuronium in the cat. *J Pharmacol Exp Ther.* 1978; 207:532–538.

129. Ricker K, Hertel G, Stodieck G. Increased voltage of the muscle action potential of normal subjects after local cooling. *J Neurol.* 1977;216:33–38.

130. Bigland-Ritchie B, Thomas CK, Rice CL, et al. Muscle temperature, contractile speed, and motoneuron firing rates during human voluntary contractions. *J Appl Physiol.* 1992;73:2457–2461.

131. Heier T, Caldwell JE. Impact of hypothermia on the response to neuromuscular blocking drugs. *Anesthesiology.* 2006;104:1070–1080.

132. Heier T, Caldwell JE, Sessler DI, Miller RD. Mild intraoperative hypothermia increases duration of action and spontaneous recovery of vecuronium blockade during nitrous oxide-isoflurane anesthesia in humans. *Anesthesiology.* 1991;74:815–819.

133. Leslie K, Sessler DI, Bjorksten AR, Moayeri A. Mild hypothermia alters propofol pharmacokinetics and increases the duration of action of atracurium. *Anesth Analg.* 1995;80:1007–1014.

134. Diefenbach C, Abel M, Buzello W. Greater neuromuscular blocking potency of atracurium during hypothermic than during normothermic cardiopulmonary bypass. *Anesth Analg.* 1992;75:675–678.

135. Flynn PJ, Hughes R, Walton B. Use of atracurium in cardiac surgery involving cardiopulmonary bypass with induced hypothermia. *Br J Anaesth.* 1984;56:967–972.

136. Denny NM, Kneeshaw JD. Vecuronium and atracurium infusions during hypothermic cardiopulmonary bypass. *Anaesthesia.* 1986;41:919–922.

137. Beaufort AM, Wierda JM, Belopavlovic M, et al. The influence of hypothermia (surface cooling) on the time-course of action and on the pharmacokinetics of rocuronium in humans. *Eur J Anaesthesiol Suppl.* 1995;11:95–106.

138. Cope TM, Hunter JM. Selecting neuromuscular-blocking drugs for elderly patients. *Drugs Aging.* 2003;20:125–140.

139. Murphy GS, Szokol JW, Avram MJ, et al. Residual neuromuscular block in the elderly: incidence and clinical implications. *Anesthesiology.* 2015;123:1322–1336.

140. Guay J, Grenier Y, Varin F. Clinical pharmacokinetics of neuromuscular relaxants in pregnancy. *Clin Pharmacokinet.* 1998;34:483.

141. Pan PH, Moore C. Comparison of cisatracurium-induced neuromuscular blockade between immediate postpartum and nonpregnant patients. *J Clin Anesth.* 2001;13:112–117.

142. Kerwin AJ, Croce MA, Timmons SD, et al. Effects of fiberoptic bronchoscopy on intracranial pressure in patients with brain injury: a prospective clinical study. *J Trauma.* 2000;48:878–893.

143. McCall M, Jeejeebhoy K, Pencharz P, Moulton R. Effect of neuromuscular blockade on energy expenditure in patients with severe head injury. *JPEN J Parenter Enteral Nutr.* 2003;27:27–35.

144. Schramm WM, Papousek A, Michalek-Sauberer A, et al. The cerebral and cardiovascular effects of cisatracurium and atracurium in neurosurgical patients. *Anesth Analg.* 1998;86:123–127.

145. Juul N, Morris GF, Marshall SB, Marshall LF. Neuromuscular blocking agents in neurointensive care. *Acta Neurochir Suppl.* 2000;76:467–470.

146. Hsiang JK, Chesnut RM, Crisp CB, et al. Early, routine paralysis for intracranial pressure control in severe head injury: is it necessary? *Crit Care Med.* 1994;22:1471–1476.

147. Carney N, Totten AM, O'Reilly C, Ullman JS, Hawryluk GWJ, Bell MJ, et al. *Guidelines for the Management of Severe Traumatic Brain Injury,* 4th edition. Campbell, CA: Brain trauma foundation; 2016. 1–244.

148. Feldman S, Karalliedde L. Drug interactions with neuromuscular blockers. *Drug Saf.* 1996;15:261–273.

149. Feldman S, Fauvel N. Potentiation and antagonism of vecuronium by decamethonium. *Anesth Analg.* 1993;76:631–634.
150. Richard A, Girard F, Girard DC, et al. Cisatracurium-induced neuromuscular blockade is affected by chronic phenytoin or carbamazepine treatment in neurosurgical patients. *Anesth Analg.* 2005;100:538–544.
151. Koenig MH, Edwards LT. Cisatracurium-induced neuromuscular blockade in anticonvulsant treated neurosurgical patients. *J Neurosurg Anesthesiol.* 2000;12:314–318.
152. Koenig MH, Hoffman WE. The effect of anticonvulsant therapy on two doses of rocuronium-induced neuromuscular blockade. *J Neurosurg Anesthesiol.* 1999;11:86–89.
153. Fischer JR, Baer RK. Acute myopathy associated with combined use of corticosteroids and neuromuscular blocking agents. *Ann Pharmacother.* 1996;30:1437–1445.
154. Kindler CH, Verotta D, Gray AT, et al. Additive inhibition of nicotinic acetylcholine receptors by corticosteroids and the neuromuscular blocking drug vecuronium. *Anesthesiology.* 2000;92:821–832.
155. Rudis MI, Sikora CA, Angus E, et al. A prospective, randomized, controlled evaluation of peripheral nerve stimulation versus standard clinical dosing of neuromuscular blocking agents in critically ill patients. *Crit Care Med.* 1997;25:575–583.
156. Keegan MT. Sedation in the neurologic intensive care unit. *Curr Treat Options Neurol.* 2008;10(2):111–125.
157. Mirski MA, Hemstreet MK. Critical care sedation for neuroscience patients. *J Neurol Sci.* 2007;261(1–2):16–34.
158. Mirski MA, Muffelman B, Ulatowski JA, Hanley DF. Sedation for the critically ill neurologic patient. *Crit Care Med.* 1995;2312:2038–2053.
159. Bilotta F, Guerra C, Rosa G. Update on anesthesia for craniotomy. *Curr Opin Anaesthesiol.* 2013;26(5):517–522.
160. Makii JM, Mirski MA, Lewin JJ. Sedation and analgesia in critically ill neurologic patients. 2013. *J Pharm Pract.* 2010;23(5):455–469.
161. Hemmerling TM, Russo G, Bracco D. Neuromuscular blockade in cardiac surgery: an update for clinicians. *Ann Card Anaesth.* 2008;11(2):80–90.
162. Cammu G. Interactions of neuromuscular blocking drugs. *Acta Anaesthesiol Belg.* 2001;52(4):357–363.

Antithrombotic Therapy for Ischemic Stroke

Eljim P. Tesoro
and Emily Durr

INTRODUCTION

Stroke is a prominent cause of death and remains the primary cause of significant long-term disability among adult Americans. Annually, more than 795,000 individuals in the United States are diagnosed with a stroke (ischemic or hemorrhagic), resulting in over 133,000 deaths in 2014.[1,2] Consequently, the current financial burden of stroke is substantial, carrying an annual cost to the United States of approximately $34 billion. Continued advances in the management of stroke and enhanced public education have contributed to stroke falling from the third leading cause of death prior to 2008 to now the fifth.[2] However, as the aging population increases, the prevalence of stroke will likely also rise.

Acute ischemic stroke (AIS) occurs when a cerebral artery is occluded, resulting in reduced cerebral perfusion distal to the thrombus. AIS comprises approximately 87% of all strokes, making this medical emergency a focus area for prevention and enhanced management strategies.[3] The heterogeneous nature of AIS makes these efforts challenging. Atherosclerosis, leading to local thrombus formation within the cerebral arterial system, is the causative factor in the majority of ischemic strokes. Strokes may also be due to cardiogenic embolism in patients with atrial fibrillation or other cardiac conditions that may lead to clot formation (eg, valvular disease or chronic heart failure). Goals of therapy of AIS include decreasing the morbidity and mortality associated with the event by minimizing the degree of ischemic injury through rapid recanalization, salvaging the area of the penumbra, and preventing stroke recurrence. Guidelines and review articles exist that describe risk factors, prehospital management, and nonpharmacologic therapies.[4,5] This chapter will review the pharmacology of various antithrombotic agents used in the acute management of ischemic stroke in the hospital and agents for secondary stroke prevention. Important advancements in endovascular management were published in 2015, drastically changing the approach to treatment for some patients. Novel agents on the horizon and future directions in the care of patients with AIS will also be addressed.

REPERFUSION/RECANALIZATION STRATEGIES FOR ACUTE ISCHEMIC STROKE

Timely emergency triage of patients is essential given the limited window in which reperfusion therapies can be offered. Within 60 minutes of arrival to the hospital emergency department, patients should be evaluated and fibrinolytic therapy initiated.[4] Despite significant efforts by the American Heart Association/American Stroke Association (AHA/ASA) to enhance public education, improve prehospital management, and establish primary and comprehensive stroke centers, the percentage of patients with AIS treated with a systemic fibrinolytic agent is estimated to remain less than 5%.[6]

Fibrinolytics form an active lytic complex by binding to fibrin within a thrombus, converting plasminogen to plasmin. The first-generation fibrinolytics (streptokinase and urokinase) lack fibrin specificity and are not used in the treatment of AIS. Notably, urokinase has not been available in the United States since October 2010, and streptokinase carries an increased risk of intracranial hemorrhage (ICH) and allergic reactions.

Alteplase

Alteplase (Activase) is a second-generation fibrinolytic, also known as recombinant tissue-type plasminogen activator (rt-PA), which is more fibrin specific and has a shorter half-life than the aforementioned first-generation fibrinolytics. Initially, the US Food and Drug Administration (FDA) approved it in 1987 for the treatment of acute myocardial infarction (AMI), and it has since been approved for use in pulmonary embolism and AIS. Intravenous (IV) alteplase has been the standard of care for AIS over a decade. Published in 1995, the National Institute of Neurological Disorders and Stroke (NINDS) trial proved that IV alteplase could effectively lead to both revascularization and clinical improvement in all subtypes of ischemic strokes when administered within the first 3 hours of symptom onset.[7] The dosing established by the NINDS trial for alteplase in AIS is a total dose of 0.9 mg/kg (maximum 90 mg) with 10% given as an IV bolus over 1 minute followed by the remaining 90% given over 60 minutes as a continuous IV infusion. The alteplase dose was based on actual body weight in this study.

All efforts should be taken to initiate IV fibrinolytic therapy as soon as possible following stroke symptom onset and the exclusion of ICH on head computed tomography (CT), as the greatest benefit is conferred with earlier time to treatment.[8] To aid in a more rapid time to initiation, treatment guidelines advise that the only laboratory result necessary prior to giving alteplase is a blood glucose value greater than 50 mg/dL.[4] Although administration as early as possible is preferred, the most appropriate end of the time window in which to administer alteplase remains an area of investigation. While not part of the FDA-approved indication, the treatment window for IV alteplase may be extended to 4.5 hours following symptom onset for some patients based on the results of the European Cooperative Acute Stroke Study (ECASS) III study.[9] Excluded from this trial were patients older than 80 years, severe stroke as defined by a baseline National Institutes of Health Stroke Score (NIHSS) greater than 25, those with a history of diabetes and stroke, or any anticoagulant use. Since the publication of ECASS III in 2008, data have demonstrated the safety of alteplase administration in the 3- to 4.5-hour window in patients with both diabetes and stroke as well as patients taking warfarin if the INR is less than 1.7.[10] Data also support the safety of alteplase administration in the extended window to patients older than 80 years.[10,11] It is hoped that this expansion of eligibility will increase the number of patients receiving alteplase for AIS. However, alteplase is associated with significant risks of intracerebral hemorrhage, and strict adherence to patient selection criteria is crucial for optimal outcomes.

The list of established contraindications to the administration of IV alteplase outlined in Table 3.1 is extensive yet should be followed closely to minimize the risk of bleeding complications. Seizure occurrence at the time of stroke onset was historically a contraindication to systemic alteplase administration. Current guidelines support initiating fibrinolysis in such patients, provided that any neurologic deficits are secondary to ongoing ischemia rather than a post-ictal state.[12] Patients with AIS who are currently anticoagulated, whether with a vitamin K antagonist (VKA), one of the target-specific oral anticoagulants (TSOACs), unfractionated heparin, or a low molecular weight heparin, pose a therapeutic dilemma if they present within the window of eligibility for fibrinolysis. The potential risk of hemorrhage, particularly ICH, is considerable. However, anticoagulant use does not automatically result in the patient being

TABLE 3.1 Contraindications to Treatment of Acute Ischemic Stroke With Intravenous Alteplase

---

Within 3 hours from symptom onset

Intracranial hemorrhage (current or history of)

Subarachnoid hemorrhage

Active internal bleeding

Recent (within 3 months) intracranial or intraspinal surgery

Serious head trauma

Presence of intracranial conditions that may increase the risk of bleeding

Bleeding diathesis

Current severe uncontrolled hypertension (>185/110 mm Hg)

Blood glucose <50 mg/dL

Platelet count <100,000/mm^3

Current use of anticoagulant with international normalized ratio (INR) >1.7 or prothrombin time >15 seconds

Current use of direct thrombin inhibitors or direct factor Xa inhibitors

Within 3 to 4.5 hours from symptom onset

Age >80 years[a]

History of both stroke and diabetes mellitus[a]

Use of oral anticoagulants regardless of INR[a]

Baseline NIHSS score >25

Greater than one-third MCA territory involvement of ischemic injury

---

[a]No longer absolute contraindications; NIHSS, National Institutes of Health Stroke Scale; MCA, Middle cerebral artery.

ineligible for treatment with alteplase. For those patients taking warfarin and presenting within 3 hours of stroke symptom onset in whom the INR is determined to be less than 1.7, it is reasonable to proceed with IV fibrinolytic therapy.[4,13] Based on the ECASS III trial, current guidelines state that anticoagulant use (even if the INR is <1.7) is a contraindication for alteplase administration in the 3- to 4.5-hour window.[3] However, safety in this patient population has been demonstrated in a subsequent evaluation.[4,10]

The TSOACs include direct thrombin inhibitors (dabigatran) and direct factor Xa inhibitors (rivaroxaban, apixaban, edoxaban). The lack of readily available sensitive laboratory tests to indicate the degree of anticoagulation with the TSOACs results in difficulty assessing patient eligibility for alteplase. The 2013 AHA/ASA guidelines recommend that IV alteplase should not be administered unless it can be confirmed that the patient has normal renal function and has not received a dose of a TSOAC within at least 2 days.[4] The increased utilization of TSOACs has made the attainment of an accurate medication history even more important when considering alteplase for a patient. Unfortunately, the ability to obtain a detailed history is frequently limited by a number of factors, including altered mental status, confusion, or aphasia. Current recommendations suggest that in most circumstances, the use of IV fibrinolytics should be avoided in the setting of recent TSOAC use until further data are available.[4,14]

Once alteplase is infused, strict adherence to the recommended frequency of vital sign monitoring and neurologic examinations over the next 24 hours is important to quickly identify signs or symptoms of ICH. Blood pressure control (<180/105 mm Hg) for the 24 hours following alteplase administration is imperative as deviations are linked to a higher rate of hemorrhagic conversion.[15–18] Antiplatelet therapy for secondary prophylaxis should be initiated with 48 hours but held for 24 hours after rt-PA. It is appropriate to begin pharmacologic prophylaxis for thromboembolism after 24 hours (and negative head computed tomography for hemorrhagic conversion). Anticoagulation should not be initiated (or reinitiated) within 24 hours of IV alteplase administration (Table 3.2).[4]

The greatest risk associated with the use of fibrinolytics in AIS is symptomatic intracranial hemorrhage (sICH). This occurred at a rate of 6.4% in the treatment arm of the NINDS alteplase trial compared with 0.6% in controls but did not lead to an increase in mortality.[7] Subsequent observational studies and pooled analysis demonstrated that the occurrence of substantial neurological decline resulting from intracerebral bleeding was relatively low (<2.5%). In the event that a patient experiences an ICH within the first 24 hours following alteplase administration, antifibrinolytic agents such as aminocaproic acid (4–5 g IV) and tranexamic acid (10–15 mg/kg IV over 20 minutes) are treatment options that can be considered.

Additional adverse events that may occur include major or minor systemic bleeding and myocardial rupture in the setting of subacute AMI. Although extremely rare, potential risk also exists for the development of angioedema or anaphylaxis. If angioedema occurs, it is generally mild, is transient, and can be treated with histamine blockade (diphenhydramine plus an H2 receptor antagonist such as famotidine) and systemic corticosteroids such as methylprednisolone.[19] Alteplase should be discontinued if symptoms occur while the dose is infusing.

Although the current evidence for IV fibrinolytics in the treatment of AIS is strongest for alteplase, there are additional agents in existence. Tenecteplase

TABLE 3.2 Recommendations for the Specific Treatment of Acute Ischemic Stroke

Intravenous alteplase (0.9 mg/kg body weight, maximum 90 mg) is recommended within the first 3 hours (in selected cases also between the first 3 and 4.5 hours) of the ischemic stroke. Ten percent of the calculated dose is given as an intravenous (IV) bolus injection, and 90% is given over 60 minutes as an IV infusion.
Lower blood pressure under 185/110 mm Hg before initiating thrombolysis.
Intravenous alteplase may be used in patients with seizures at stroke onset, if the neurological deficit is related to acute cerebral ischemia.
Intravenous alteplase may also be administered in selected patients younger than 18 years and older than 80 years.
Intra-arterial treatment of acute MCA occlusion within a 6-hour time window with alteplase is an option.
Acute basilar occlusion: intra-arterial thrombolysis is recommended for selected patients and IV thrombolysis is acceptable even after 3 hours.
If thrombolytic therapy is given, prophylactic antithrombotic therapy should be initiated 24 hours or more from thrombolytic administration.
Aspirin (160- to 325-mg loading dose) should be given within the first 48 hours of ischemic stroke. The use of other antiplatelet drugs is not accepted in acute stroke.
Early administration of unfractionated heparin or low molecular weight heparin is not recommended.

Note: MCA, middle cerebral artery.

(TNKase), reteplase (Retavase), and desmoteplase are the result of research efforts to create more highly fibrin-specific agents that have a longer half-life than alteplase, thereby removing the necessity for a prolonged infusion. All 3 agents have been at least preliminarily evaluated for the indication of AIS.[20–28]

Tenecteplase

Tenecteplase, a third-generation thrombolytic agent, is a recombinant product created by making 3 DNA substitutions to the human tissue plasminogen activator molecule. In vitro, tenecteplase exhibits increased fibrin selectivity compared with alteplase. The mean plasma clearance in most patients treated with tenecteplase is up to 6 times that of alteplase.[29] Currently, it is only FDA approved for the management of acute ST elevation myocardial infarction. Its use should be restricted to those patients who are unable to be transferred to a percutaneous coronary intervention (PCI)-capable hospital and receive intervention within 2 hours.[30] When used in the treatment of AMI, tenecteplase dosing is based on patient weight, ranging from 30 mg to a maximum of 50 mg. A recent small phase II trial (n = 104) that randomized patients with AIS to tenecteplase 0.25 mg/kg (maximum 25 mg) or alteplase 0.9 mg/kg (maximum

90 mg) had similar efficacy and safety findings.[22] Larger scale future trials will determine if tenecteplase has a comparable role to alteplase in the treatment of AIS.

Reteplase

Reteplase is a recombinant product derived from tissue-type plasminogen activator produced in *Escherichia coli*.[31] Similar to tenecteplase, it possesses a longer half-life than that of alteplase and is currently only indicated for the treatment of AMI. Reteplase has been evaluated in the setting of AIS but only when administered intra-arterially and typically in conjunction with systemic fibrinolytic therapy and/or mechanical thrombectomy.[23,24,32–34] Reteplase has not been available in the United States since 2015.

Desmoteplase

Desmoteplase is the most recently developed recombinant fibrinolytic agent, originally isolated from vampire bat saliva. Proposed advantages of this agent include a high fibrin specificity (approximately 180-fold more selective than alteplase), lack of neurotoxicity, and a long half-life relative to alteplase. All trials thus far have evaluated desmoteplase in the management of patients with AIS presenting beyond 3 hours from stroke onset.[25–28] The initial phase II trial (Desmoteplase in Acute Ischemic Stroke Trial [DIAS]) evaluated fixed doses of 25 mg, 37.5 mg, and 50 mg of IV desmoteplase.[27] Unacceptably high rates of symptomatic ICH within 72 hours (23.5%–30.8%) led to a protocol amendment, and the trial continued with a revised dosing strategy. Part 2 of the study used a weight-based dose escalation of 62.5 mcg/kg, 90 mcg/kg, or 125 mcg/kg IV desmoteplase. Initial studies (DIAS, DIAS-2, and the Dose Escalation Study of Desmoteplase in Acute Ischemic Stroke [DEDAS]) indicated a potentially promising role for IV desmoteplase in patients 3 to 9 hours following AIS onset.[25,27,28] The phase III trial (DIAS-3) failed to demonstrate a significant clinical benefit.[26] Based on the results of DIAS-3, the additional phase III trial DIAS-4 has been terminated given the unlikely ability to reach the primary end point.

INTRA-ARTERIAL FIBRINOLYTIC ADMINISTRATION

Important advancements in the endovascular management of AIS were published in early 2015, drastically changing the approach to treatment for some patients.[35–39] Most of the recent data center on mechanical clot retrieval devices; however, a component of this growing body of positive literature also includes intra-arterial (IA) administration of fibrinolytics. Theoretical advantages of IA application include local fibrinolysis without the need for systemic therapy, reducing the risk of bleeding complications as well as an extended time window for intervention. This is countered with potential drawbacks, including a longer time to initiation and the chance of arterial injury or procedural complication. Case series providing anecdotal evidence that IA application can achieve cerebral vessel recanalization date back to the 1980s. Minimal data, however, exist from both an efficacy and safety standpoint to guide dosing of IA fibrinolytics since there has been considerable variability in the agents and doses used. Pro-urokinase, urokinase, reteplase, and alteplase have all been studied for IA administration in the setting of AIS. The high rates of sICH coupled with variable recanalization success from initial investigations were disappointing. The Prolyse in Acute Cerebral Thromboembolism (PROACT) I and II trials, published in 1998 and 1999, respectively, used pro-urokinase 6 mg and 9 mg administered intra-arterially within 6 hours of AIS onset. Symptomatic ICH occurred in 10% and 15.4% of patients, which is substantially higher than the 6.4% rate of sICH observed in the NINDS trial that led to FDA approval of systemic alteplase for AIS.[7,40,41] A meta-analysis published in 2002 assessed 27 studies from 1988 to 2002 of IA fibrinolytic use in AIS. Compared with control subjects, IA therapy had a more favorable outcome (41.5% vs 23%, $P = .002$) as well as higher rate of sICH (9.5% vs 3%, $P = .046$).[42] Doses used for IA reteplase administration have ranged from 0.5 to 8 mg.[23,24,32–34] Sugg et al completed a retrospective analysis of IA reteplase and urokinase in patients with large vessel occlusion. The reteplase group received a mean dose of 2.5 mg and had a recanalization rate of 82% with a rate of sICH of 12%.[33] Another retrospective evaluation by Misra et al[24] assessed safety outcomes of high IA doses of reteplase and urokinase (median doses were 2 mg and 200,000 U, respectively). Most (>90%) patients enrolled received IV thrombolytic prior to IA therapy. The reteplase group experienced sICH at a rate of 8%. IA alteplase has also been evaluated in AIS, with doses typically ranging from 20 to 60 mg.[42] A study comparing IA alteplase doses of less than 50 mg to doses of 50 to 100 mg found that higher doses were associated with greater ICH frequency but also a higher rate of reperfusion and improved patient outcomes.[43] The Interventional Management of Stroke (IMS) III study randomized patients with moderate to severe stroke (NIHSS≥10) to endovascular therapy following IV alteplase or standard treatment with IV alteplase only in a 2:1 ratio within 3 hours of stroke symptom onset. The endovascular treatment modalities were not uniform, with IA alteplase administration occurring in 37.8% of patients (median dose, 40 mg). The trial was stopped for futility.[44] A recent retrospective study found that IA thrombolytic doses ranging between 1.5 and 69 mg of alteplase equivalents (using dose conversion of 10 mg alteplase = 2 units reteplase = 6.3 units tenecteplase) within 6 hours of symptom onset yielded similar rates of both recanalization and ICH.[33] Optimal IA fibrinolytic dosing is yet to be determined.

The most notable recent information regarding IA thrombolysis is from the Multicenter Randomized Clinical Trial of Endovascular Treatment for Acute Ischemic Stroke in the Netherlands (MR CLEAN) trial comparing IA treatment (IA thrombolysis, mechanical treatment, or both) plus usual care to usual care alone for an anterior circulation occlusion within 6 hours of stroke onset. In the treatment arm, 10.3% of patients received an IA thrombolytic (alteplase or urokinase) in addition to mechanical intervention. Significant improvement in the rate of favorable outcome occurred in the IA plus usual care group (modified Rankin score [mRs] at 90 days: 3 vs 4; 95% confidence interval [CI], 1.21–2.28).[39] The positive findings of this and subsequent similar trials have led to widespread adoption of endovascular intervention in patients with AIS due to a proximal arterial occlusion.[35–38]

Intra-arterial strategies widen the window of opportunity to treat stroke victims up to 6 hours from the onset of symptoms. Given the profoundly low rates of patients experiencing AIS who receive IV fibrinolytic therapy, the option for intra-arterial intervention(s) is attractive. Consideration should be given to select cases when systemic alteplase is contraindicated or the patient is outside of the 3- to 4.5-hour window for IV therapy. Careful assessment of potential contraindications and risks to intra-arterial use should be assessed similarly to that of IV alteplase. Post-administration monitoring for 24 hours should also be implemented as it would be for systemic fibrinolysis.

Glycoprotein IIB/IIIA Inhibitors

The glycoprotein (GP) IIb/IIIa inhibitors were developed to block the final pathway of platelet aggregation. This medication class includes abciximab (a human/murine monoclonal antibody), eptifibatide (a synthetic peptide), and tirofiban, lamifiban, xemilofiban, orbofiban, and sibrafiban (synthetic nonpeptides). The positive findings of additional antiplatelet therapy with GP IIb/IIIa inhibitors in the setting of AMI led to evaluation of these agents in a number of AIS trials since 2000. The phase III Abciximab in Emergency Stroke Treatment Trial-II (AbESTT-II) trial evaluated IV abciximab vs placebo within 5 hours of AIS onset (NIHSS 4-22) in adult patients who had not received IV thrombolytic therapy. The study was terminated early due to a lack of outcomes benefit and a significantly higher rate of sICH in the abciximab arm (5.5% vs

0.5%, $P=.002$).[45] Tirofiban (0.6 mcg/kg/min for 30 minutes, then 0.15 mcg/kg/min for 72 hours) was compared with IV aspirin (300 mg/d for 3 days) in patients presenting within 6 hours of AIS onset. The trial was halted following an interim analysis that concluded that finding a treatment effect would be unfeasible.[46] The phase II Safety of Tirofiban in acute Ischemic Stroke (trial assessed initiation of tirofiban (0.4 mcg/kg/min for 30 minutes, then 0.1 mcg/kg/min for 48 hours) vs placebo within 3 to 22 hours after symptom onset in moderate-severity AIS. No difference in the rate of ICH or functional outcome was found between groups; however, mortality at 5 months was significantly lower in the tirofiban group (2% vs 8%, $P=.03$).[47] The phase II Combined Approach to Lysis Utilizing Eptifibatide and rt-PA in Acute Ischemic Stroke -Enhanced Regimen (CLEAR-ER) trial of eptifibatide (135-mcg/kg bolus and 0.75-mcg/kg/min infusion for 2 hours) given in combination with reduced-dose alteplase (0.6 mg/kg) compared with standard-dose alteplase (0.9 mg/kg) within 3 hours of stroke onset had a higher rate of sICH in the alteplase-alone group (12% vs 2%, $P=.053$). There was no difference in functional outcomes at 90 days.[48] Based on these findings, a phase III trial will likely be undertaken to further evaluate the role of eptifibatide in AIS. This class of antiplatelet agents may eventually have a role as an adjunctive therapy in AIS; however, none of the available GP IIb/IIIa inhibitors are currently indicated, although their use in thrombotic complications during endovascular treatment of cerebral aneurysms is under investigation.

SECONDARY PREVENTION OF ISCHEMIC STROKE

Antiplatelets

Antiplatelet agents are the cornerstone pharmacologic agents used for secondary stroke prevention while anticoagulant drugs are used specifically to prevent embolic stroke, typically from nonvalvular atrial fibrillation (Table 3.3). After acute ischemic stroke, antiplatelet agents are recommended to be initiated within 48 hours (holding for 24 hours if thrombolytics are given or longer if decompressive craniectomy is anticipated); for stroke due to nonvalvular atrial fibrillation, anticoagulant therapy may be started within 14 days. While these agents are not commonly used in the acute treatment of critically ill patients, it is crucial for clinicians to be familiar with their pharmacokinetic and pharmacodynamic aspects to effectively deal with hemorrhagic complications that may result in admission to intensive care. Guidelines for the treatment of antithrombotic-induced hemorrhage have been published and include information on specific reversal agents.[49]

Aspirin

Aspirin or acetylsalicylic acid (ASA) remains the drug of choice to prevent secondary stroke due to its low cost and extensive history of use. It can decrease the risk of non-cardioembolic stroke by about 20%.[50] Two large trials reported a decrease in recurrent stroke and the combination of death and nonfatal stroke with aspirin when given within 48 hours of acute stroke—the Chinese Acute Stroke Trial and International Stroke Trial.[51,52] It is a nonselective cyclooxygenase (COX) inhibitor that produces platelet inhibition in a non-dose-dependent manner. However, many of its adverse effects such as bleeding are seen more at higher doses. As a result, the most recommended dose of aspirin for prevention of non-cardioembolic stroke is 81 mg.

Aspirin is absorbed rapidly in the gastrointestinal tract and produces an irreversible inhibition of thromboxane A2 formation, which is directly involved in platelet activation, aggregation, and subsequent thrombosis. This thromboxane inhibition is sustained until the platelet is removed from the circulation (approximately 10 days). The serum half-life is relatively short at 15 to 20 minutes, and onset of action occurs within 60 minutes. Enteric-coated formulations have decreased bioavailability of aspirin and should probably be avoided unless patients have gastrointestinal issues that would limit adherence to therapy. If enteric-coated aspirin is used, larger doses (>300 mg) should be used to optimize antiplatelet effects.[53] For patients who are unable to take aspirin orally, rectal formulations are available. One clinically relevant interaction occurs with ibuprofen, which may compete with aspirin for binding sites on platelets. If given concomitantly, ibuprofen should be separated from aspirin administration (8 hours before or 2 hours after) to fully optimize antiplatelet effects.

The concept of aspirin resistance has been introduced but not yet fully elucidated in the setting of ischemic stroke. Resistance can be described in terms of clinical recurrence while on aspirin therapy as well as platelet non-responsiveness as assessed by laboratory testing with a variety of agonists.[54] Clinical resistance has been reported to range between 6% and 60% depending on the definition and method of evaluation used. Aspirin nonresponse is reported to be 6% to 26% depending on the specific laboratory assay, with no single method considered a universal standard. There is no consensus on improving non-responsiveness to aspirin therapy or recommendations for routine screening. Various explanations of resistance include drug interactions, non-adherence, and genetic polymorphisms of the COX-1 enzyme. Approaches to this apparent resistance include increasing doses or adding or switching antiplatelet agents. So far, platelet function-guided antiplatelet therapy for stroke

TABLE 3.3 Antithrombotic Agents Used in Stroke Prevention

Name	Dose	Dosing Adjustments	Major Side Effects	Monitoring	Reversal Strategies	Comments
Aspirin (ASA)	75 to 325 mg PO daily	None	Gastritis, bleeding, bronchospasm	Platelet aggregometry	DDAVP 0.4 mcg/kg IV × 1	May give PR if no enteral access
Clopidogrel (Plavix)	75 mg PO daily	None	Bleeding	Platelet aggregometry	DDAVP 0.4 mcg/kg IV × 1	Pharmacogenetic dosing may be useful in some circumstances
ASA/extended-release dipyridamole (Aggrenox)	25 mg/200 mg PO twice daily	Avoid if CLcr < 10 mL/min	Headache, bleeding		DDAVP 0.4 mcg/kg IV × 1	Do not substitute with individual components; do not crush/open capsules
Warfarin (Coumadin)	Adjusted to INR 2 to 3 (high-risk patients may aim for 2.5–3.5)	Consider lower doses in hepatic impairment	Bleeding, bruising, skin necrosis	INR (goal 2–3)	Phytonadione (vitamin K) 1 to 10 mg PO/IV; 4PCC 25 to 50 U/kg IV based on INR	Consider CYP2C9 or VKORC1 genotyping to guide dosing; hold >5 days before invasive procedures
Dabigatran (Pradaxa)	150 mg PO twice daily	75 mg PO twice daily if CLcr 15 to 30 mL/min	Bleeding, dyspepsia	PTT, TT (screening)	Idarucizumab (Praxbind) 5 g IV × 1	Do not open/crush capsule; hold 1 to 2 days before surgery (3–5 days if CLcr < 50 mL/min); avoid use with rifampin; adjust/avoid with P-glycoprotein inhibitors
Rivaroxaban (Xarelto)	20 mg PO daily	15 mg PO daily if CLcr 15 to 50 mL/min; avoid if CLcr < 15 mL/min; avoid use if Child-Pugh class B or C	Bleeding	PT, anti-Xa (agent specific)	FEIBA or 4PCC 50 U/kg IV (andexanet alfa is not approved currently)	Hold at least 24 hours before invasive procedures; avoid giving with strong inducers/inhibitors of CYP3A4 and P-glycoprotein

TABLE 3.3 *Continued*

Name	Dose	Dosing Adjustments	Major Side Effects	Monitoring	Reversal Strategies	Comments
Apixaban (Eliquis)	5 mg PO twice daily	2.5 mg PO twice daily if any 2 of the following: age ≥ 80 years, SCr ≥ 1.5 mg/dL, weight ≤ 60 kg	Bleeding	Anti-Xa (agent specific)	FEIBA or 4fPCC 50 U/kg IV (andexanet alfa is not approved currently)	Hold at least 24 hours before low-risk invasive procedures or 48 hours before high-risk invasive procedures; adjust dosing if given with strong inducers/inhibitors of CYP3A4 and P-glycoprotein
Edoxaban (Savaysa)	60 mg PO daily	Avoid use if Clcr >95 mLLmin or < 15 mL/min; 30 mg PO daily if Clcr is 15 to 30 mL/min; avoid use if Child-Pugh B or C	Bleeding, anemia, elevated ALT/AST	Anti-Xa (agent specific)	FEIBA or 4fPCC 50 U/kg IV (andexanet alfa is not approved currently)	Hold at least 24 hours before invasive procedures; avoid use with rifampin

Note: ALT, alanine aminotransferase; ASA, acetylsalicylic acid; AST, aspartate aminotransferase; Clcr, creatinine clearance; CYP3A4, cytochrome P450 3A4 enzyme; DDAVP, desmopressin; FEIBA, factor VIII inhibitor bypassing agent; 4fPCC, 4-factor prothrombin complex concentrate; INR, international normalized ratio; IV, intravenous; PO, per os; PR, per rectum; SCr, serum creatinine; VKORC1, vitamin K epoxide reductase complex 1.

prevention has not resulted in any improved outcomes.[55] Its utilization in the setting of neuroendovascular stenting is under continued investigation.[56–58]

Clopidogrel

Clopidogrel is an oral thienopyridine inhibitor of the P2Y12 receptor on platelets. Platelet inhibition occurs within 48 hours of starting maintenance dosing of 75 mg/d. Oral loading doses of 300 to 600 mg result in a more immediate antiplatelet effect within 2 hours. After being absorbed in the duodenum, the majority (85%) of clopidogrel is deactivated in the liver by carboxylesterase 1 (CES1). The remaining parent drug is metabolized to an active metabolite via cytochrome P450 enzymes, most notably by CYP2C19 and CYP3A4. The most notable alteration in clopidogrel metabolism occurs with the CYP2C19 enzyme, the major pathway of biotransformation. The wild-type normal function allele is *1, with the most common loss-of-function allele being *2 and the most common gain-of-function allele being *17. Thus, patients may be categorized based on their allele pair genotype as poor metabolizers (e.g., *2/*2), intermediate metabolizers (e.g., *1/*2), extensive metabolizers (*1/*1), or ultra-rapid metabolizers (*17/*17). Patients who are poor metabolizers may have high on-treatment platelet reactivity resulting in more thrombotic events due to a decrease in the active metabolite while ultra-rapid metabolizers may be at risk of hemorrhagic events due to higher than expected antiplatelet activity. Patients displaying a heterogeneous genotype (e.g., *1/*2) may have platelet reactivity between the 2 extremes. Guidelines have been published to help clinicians navigate pharmacogenomic testing for clopidogrel therapy.[59] Individual testing may be of greatest utility in high-risk populations (i.e., patients experiencing thrombotic events despite therapy or poor metabolizers) and not for routine use.[60] Alternative antiplatelet agents may be recommended for poor or intermediate metabolizers of clopidogrel. Resources are available to assist clinicians in evaluating genotype effects for specific drugs, including online websites (www.pharmgkb.org, accessed December 19, 2016). It should be noted that there is limited evidence for using genotype-based antiplatelet therapy in stroke prevention, with most studies focused on patients with acute coronary syndromes undergoing percutaneous coronary interventions. Genetic alterations in other metabolic pathways (e.g., CES1) also occur, but the significance of testing for these variants is presently unclear.

Clopidogrel is just as effective as aspirin for the secondary prevention of stroke based on the results of Clopidogrel versus Aspirin in Patients at Risk of Ischaemic Events (CAPRIE).[61] Clopidogrel has also been compared with ASA/extended-release (ER) dipyridamole as well and found to be similar with regard to stroke recurrence (8.8% vs 9.0%) but better in terms of ICH (1.0% vs 1.4%, $P<.006$).[62] For patients allergic to aspirin, clopidogrel is a viable alternative.

Prasugrel/Ticagrelor

The newer generation oral P2Y12 inhibitors, prasugrel and ticagrelor, provide more potent antiplatelet effects compared with clopidogrel. However, prasugrel is not recommended for use in patients with prior stroke due to higher risk of ICH.

Like clopidogrel, prasugrel requires biotransformation to an active metabolite. After rapid absorption, prasugrel is quickly hydrolyzed by intestinal esterases before activation by P450 enzymes, mainly via CYP3A4 and CYP2B6. Despite this, prasugrel is not affected by genomic variants or drug interactions usually associated with this enzyme system. Prasugrel therapy results in irreversible inhibition of the P2Y12 receptor within 30 minutes of a loading dose of 60 mg. The offset of action is prolonged and similar to clopidogrel (7–10 days).

Ticagrelor is the first orally available cyclopentyl triazolopyrimidine P2Y12 receptor inhibitor that does not bind to an adenosine diphosphate binding site like the thienopyridines.[63] It has a rapid onset of action with 40% platelet inhibition seen within 30 minutes and peak effects seen at 2 hours. Ticagrelor's binding is reversible, producing a quicker offset of action compared with other antiplatelet agents. The plasma half-life is 8 to 12 hours with both parent drug and metabolites having antiplatelet activity. Drug interactions occur with CYP3A4 inducers and inhibitors and should be assessed. Decreased doses of CYP3A4 substrates (e.g., simvastatin) should be used if given with ticagrelor, which inhibits CYP3A4.

In the Acute Stroke Or Transient IsChaemic Attack TReated with Aspirin or Ticagrelor and Patient OutcomES (SOCRATES) trial, ticagrelor (180 mg followed by 90 mg/d) was not found to be superior to aspirin (300 mg followed by 100 mg/d) in reducing the composite end point of stroke, myocardial infarction, and death after 90 days (hazard ratio [HR], 0.89; 95% CI, 0.79–1.01, $P=.07$). Rates of major bleeding, ICH, and fatal bleeding were no different between the groups.[64]

Aspirin/Extended-Release Dipyridamole (ASA/ERD)

Dipyridamole is an oral pyrimidopyrimidine that reversibly inhibits cyclic nucleotide phosphodiesterase, adenosine uptake, and subsequent activation of platelets. It is thought that the combination of this agent with aspirin would increase antiplatelet activity due to the inclusion of multiple mechanisms of action, resulting in improved stroke prevention. The combination of aspirin 25 mg and extended-release dipyridamole 200 mg given twice daily has been evaluated for both agents alone and placebo for secondary stroke prevention. After 2 years of treatment, combination therapy produced a 37% relative risk reduction (RRR) in stroke ($P<.001$) compared with placebo; aspirin provided an 18% RRR ($P<.013$), while dipyridamole provided a 16% RRR ($P<.039$) compared with placebo. Risk of bleeding was similar among all groups and mortality was not affected. Headache was reported in approximately 40% of patients and resulted in early discontinuation of therapy in 10% of patients taking dipyridamole. Women and Hispanic patients have been reported to have a higher incidence of headache from ASA/ERD.[65] A slow titration has been recommended to help patients tolerate this transient side effect when starting on ASA/ERD.[66,67]

Due to the extended-release formulation, ASA/ERD should not be crushed and therefore should not be given in patients who are unable to swallow. It is not recommended to replace ASA/ERD with the individual components due to the additive benefit seen with the parent compound. Patients who require a higher daily dose of aspirin for cardiovascular protection or other indications may need to take additional tablets since this compound provides only 50 mg of aspirin per day.

Dual Antiplatelet Therapy

Traditionally, dual antiplatelet therapy (DAPT) has been used only clinically in the setting of acute coronary syndromes or intravascular stenting. For stroke prevention, it has been recognized in large clinical trials to increase bleeding events without improvement in overall recurrent stroke risk, especially in patients with lacunar stroke.[68–70] Recent data have suggested there may be a benefit of early (<24 hours) or short-term (90 days) DAPT for patients presenting with minor ischemic stroke or high-risk transient ischemic attack (TIA). Investigators reported that the combination of clopidogrel (loading dose of 300 mg, followed by 75 mg/d for 90 days) with aspirin 75 mg/d for the first 21 days resulted in less ischemic stroke compared with aspirin 81 mg/d for 90 days (7.9% vs 11.4%, $P<.001$).[71] The rates of hemorrhagic stroke and moderate or severe bleeding were not different between the groups. A 1-year follow-up did not uncover any evidence of rebound risk of stroke after DAPT was stopped and suggests that patients are at higher risk of subsequent stroke in the weeks following the initial stroke or TIA.[72] The risk of hemorrhagic events may only be realized after the first few months of continued DAPT, past the time of perceived benefit.[73] A short duration of DAPT followed by chronic monotherapy, as seen in patients after coronary stenting, may be appropriate in this subset of stroke patients. Clinical trials to confirm these findings are under way.[74]

For patients with stroke symptoms due to severe intracranial artery stenosis (70%-99%), the use of early DAPT for 90 days may also be beneficial. Treatment with intracranial stents has included DAPT, supported by evidence garnered from coronary stent literature.[56] Further studies exploring the use of newer agents and platelet function testing will further highlight this practice.

Vorapaxar, a selective, oral platelet thrombin protease-activated receptor 1 blocker, is indicated for the prevention of atherothrombotic complications after myocardial infarction and in peripheral artery disease in combination with other antiplatelet agents. Although the incidence of ICH was higher when used as DAPT, there may be some benefit as monotherapy in stroke prevention.[75]

Anticoagulants

Prevention of cardioembolic stroke from nonvalvular atrial fibrillation requires full anticoagulation with either VKAs or TSOACs (see Table 3.3). Warfarin is the standard VKA in clinical practice today. The TSOACs provide several benefits over VKAs, including predictable and timely antithrombotic activity with rapid offset, minimal to no routine laboratory monitoring, and less drug and food interactions. Recent advances in reversal agents for the TSOACs have begun to address the concerns for managing patients with life-threatening hemorrhage.

The choice of antithrombotic to use in patients with atrial fibrillation can be evaluated using the $CHADS_2$-VASC score, which evaluates patient risk factors for stroke: 1 point for Congestive heart failure, 1 point for Hypertension, 2 points if Age is greater than 75 years, 1 point for Diabetes, 2 points for Stroke, 1 point for Vascular disease, 1 point for Age 65–74 years, and 1 point for female Sex Category. A $CHADS_2$-VASC score of 0 requires no antithrombotic treatment while a score of 1 would require either aspirin or anticoagulation. A score of 2 or higher mandates anticoagulation. The risk of hemorrhage may be determined by using various schemes such as HAS-BLED (Hypertension, Abnormal Renal/Liver Function, Stroke, Bleeding History or Predisposition, Labile INR, Elderly, Drugs/Alcohol Concomitantly), HEMORR$_2$HAGES (Hepatic or Renal Disease, Ethanol Abuse, Malignancy, Older Age, Reduced Platelet Count or Function, Re-Bleeding, Hypertension, Anemia, Genetic Factors, Excessive Fall Risk and Stroke), or ATRIA (Anticoagulation and Risk Factor in Atrial Fibrillation), but HAS-BLED has been reported to be more predictive of the three.[76–79] HAS-BLED assigns 1 point to hypertension (systolic blood pressure >160 mm Hg), abnormal liver function (cirrhosis, bilirubin >2 times normal, or aspartate aminotransferase/alanine aminotransferase/alkaline phosphatase >3 times normal), abnormal renal function (dialysis, transplant, or serum creatinine >2.6 mg/dL), stroke history, bleeding disposition, labile INR (time in therapeutic range <60%), elderly (age >65 years), and drug or alcohol (>8 drinks/wk) use.

Warfarin

Since 1954, warfarin has been the traditional anticoagulant of choice to prevent embolic stroke, especially in the setting of atrial fibrillation, where it can decrease the risk of stroke by 70%. Warfarin therapy causes a decrease in vitamin K–dependent clotting factors—II, VII, IX, and X—through inhibition of vitamin K epoxide reductase complex 1 (VKORC1). As active vitamin K is depleted, these factors along with the endogenous anticoagulants protein C and protein S are no longer made and are slowly metabolized out of the system. Full anticoagulation therefore takes several days to be complete and is dependent on the half-lives of the factors. Maintenance doses are determined using laboratory or point-of-care blood testing of the INR, with the goal range being 2 to 3 for most cases. The INR may start to increase in as little as 1 day due to the depletion of factor VII but typically takes 5 to 7 days for full effect. For this reason, it is reasonable to bridge therapy with titrated, IV heparin until the INR is above 2.

Warfarin is a mixture of 2 racemic forms, with S-warfarin being up to 5 times more potent than R-warfarin. Warfarin is administered orally and is readily absorbed from the gastrointestinal tract, with peak serum concentrations seen at 4 hours. Metabolism is primarily hepatic, with CYP2C9 as the main pathway for the S-enantiomer, but other enzymes include CYP1A2 and CYP3A4. Serum half-life is reported to be around 40 hours. Many drugs interact with warfarin in a variety of mechanisms, including decreased absorption (e.g., cholestyramine), increased metabolism (e.g., rifampin, phenobarbital), or inhibited clearance (e.g., metronidazole, trimethoprim-sulfamethoxazole). Foods rich in vitamin K will also attenuate the effect of warfarin by replenishing the vitamin K–dependent clotting factors. Overuse of broad-spectrum antibiotics may augment the effect of warfarin by decreasing the normal gut flora that produces vitamin K.

The individual dosing of warfarin can be affected by multiple factors, including diet, smoking, drug interactions, and genetic variations in enzymes or target proteins. Two genomic variants have been associated with 50% of the variability seen in patient dosing: CYP2C9 and VKORC1.[80] Variants of CYP2C9 can be categorized as poor, intermediate, or extensive metabolizers of warfarin while variants of VKORC1 can be categorized as low, intermediate, or high sensitivity to warfarin. Taken together, results of genomic testing may assist clinicians in individualizing regimens by identifying those who may require higher or lower than normal doses of warfarin (~5 mg/d). Although promising in concept, results of recent genotype-based dosing trials for warfarin have not fully supported this practice compared with traditional dosing.[81–83] However, applications to specific patient populations (e.g., African Americans) may bear some utility. Using both clinical factors such as age and drug interactions along with genetic dosing algorithms may provide the best approach in timely achievement of goal INR while minimizing hemorrhagic events. Online dosing algorithms are also available (www.warfarindosing.org) that integrate previous dosing/INR results to estimate future doses. The use of genetic information if available seems reasonable to consider when dosing warfarin, especially in high-risk populations, but whether it is beneficial to obtain genotype data in all patients has yet to be determined.

The treatment of severe warfarin-induced hemorrhagic complications (e.g., ICH) has historically been the administration of parenteral phytonadione (vitamin K) and fresh-frozen plasma. However, these do not provide immediate correction of the INR and therefore may not provide timely reversal required for emergent invasive interventions. With the introduction of factor products (i.e., activated factor VII) and prothrombin complex concentrates (PCCs), the time to correct the coagulopathy has decreased substantially (see Table 3.3). A new product, Kcentra, a 4-factor PCC (4fPCC) is approved for episodes of acute major bleeding due to vitamin K antagonists. Kcentra contains the inactivated vitamin K–dependent clotting factors II, VII, IX, and X, as well as the endogenous anticoagulants protein C and protein S. Other 3-factor PCCs contain small amounts or no factor VII and may be considered a reversal option when 4fPCCs are not available. Intravenous dosing is based on pretreatment INR and patient weight (individual dosing should be rounded to the nearest vial size); correction of the INR can be seen within 30 minutes after a single dose. There is limited information on repeat dosing, but there is concern over inducing thrombotic events. Kcentra is contraindicated in patients with disseminated intravascular coagulopathy or heparin-induced thrombocytopenia as it is formulated with small amounts of heparin. Vitamin K therapy should still be implemented with Kcentra to prevent potential rebound increases in the INR.

Dabigatran

Dabigatran etexilate was the first nonwarfarin anticoagulant available to patients with nonvalvular atrial fibrillation for stroke prevention. At a dose of 150 mg per os (PO) twice daily, dabigatran was shown to be superior to warfarin in the prospective, randomized, multicenter, Randomized Evaluation of Long-Term Anticoagulation Therapy (RE-LY) trial (relative risk [RR], 0.66; 95% CI, 0.53–0.82; $P<.001$ for superiority).[84] Dosing of 110 mg PO twice daily was reported to be noninferior to warfarin (RR, 0.91; 95% CI, 0.74–1.11, $P<.001$ for noninferiority).[84]

Dabigatran etexilate is an oral direct thrombin inhibitor that is formulated with tartaric acid to facilitate a low pH for optimal absorption. It is a substrate of P-glycoprotein, and there can be significant interactions with other drugs that are inhibitors (i.e., dronadarone, ketoconazole, verapamil) or inducers (i.e., rifampin) of this transport protein. Its half-life is 12 to 17 hours, resulting in twice-daily dosing. The majority of dabigatran is renally excreted while the remaining portion is hepatically metabolized to active agents, although none via significant P450 enzymes. As a result, dosing depends on renal function, and patients with creatinine clearance less than 15 mL/min or receiving dialysis should not receive this drug.

No widely used laboratory monitoring test coincides directly with the anticoagulant effect of dabigatran. Thrombin time (TT), prothrombin time (PT), and activated partial thromboplastin time (aPTT) are elevated in a dose-responsive fashion but may not be consistent across all laboratories. If elevated, they provide evidence of the presence of dabigatran in the blood but do not reflect a quantitative level of anticoagulation. The TT is more sensitive than aPTT, and a normal aPTT does not necessarily reflect the absence of dabigatran.[85] Thrombin time is becoming more used to detect the presence of dabigatran for clinical decision making. Dilute thrombin time (dTT) and ecarin clotting time (ECT) have the potential for use in quantitative measurement of the anticoagulant activity of dabigatran (i.e., drug concentration), but further investigation is warranted. For institutions that may have dabigatran assays, it has been suggested that a trough level of more than 200 ng/mL may indicate increased bleeding risk.[86]

Common side effects of dabigatran etexilate include bleeding and gastritis. Results of the RE-LY trial reported no difference in major bleeding with the 150-mg dose compared with warfarin (RR, 0.93; 95% CI, 0.81–1.07; $P=.31$) and less bleeding with the 110-mg dose (RR, 0.80; 95% CI, 0.69–0.93; $P=.003$). Dyspepsia was reported more with dabigatran than with warfarin (11% vs 5.8%). Risk factors for increased bleeding risk include advanced age (>75 years), renal dysfunction, and antiplatelet use, including chronic nonsteroidal anti-inflammatory drug therapy. Gastrointestinal bleed rates were higher with the

150-mg dose of dabigatran (RR, 1.5; 95% CI, 1.19–1.89; $P < .001$) while ICH rates were lower compared with warfarin for both doses (for 110 mg: RR, 0.31; 95% CI, 0.2–0.41, $P < .001$; for 150 mg: RR, 0.40; 95% CI, 0.27–0.60; $P < .001$).[84]

The special formulation of dabigatran etexilate may degrade when exposed to humidity, so it must be stored in the original packaging with the integrated desiccant. Patients may not prefer a twice-daily dosing or the high incidence of gastritis that is associated with this drug. Due to the special formulation for stability issues, this drug should not be crushed or opened for administration via a feeding tube, and an alternative anticoagulant should be used. Crushing the capsule shell can increase oral bioavailability by 75%, potentially increasing bleeding risk.

Patients who develop life-threatening bleeding while taking dabigatran may benefit from reversal using idarucizumab, a parenteral monoclonal antibody fragment that binds to both the parent drug and its metabolites to neutralize the anticoagulant effects. Idarucizumab irreversibly binds to both free and thrombin-bound dabigatran with an affinity that is 350 times more potent that dabigatran has for thrombin.[87] By itself, idarucizumab does not have any anticoagulant or prothrombotic effects. In a study of 90 patients experiencing uncontrollable or emergent bleeding or requiring invasive surgery within 8 hours, a fixed dose of idarucizumab 5 g IV (given as two 2.5-g doses no more than 15 minutes apart) was effective in normalizing ECT and dTT in up to 98% of patients within 30 minutes of dosing. Thirty-five percent of the emergent bleeds were ICH in this series, with the remainder constituting trauma-related, gastrointestinal, or nonspecified bleeding. Rebound increases in unbound dabigatran concentrations and clotting times were reported after 12 and 24 hours in some patients, highlighting the potential need for continued monitoring and possible redosing. Idarucizumab offers a rapid and safe reversal treatment for patients with emergent bleeding who are taking dabigatran. Data that should be obtained in these patients to help guide therapy include time of most recent dose, renal function, location and severity of bleed, and aPTT or TT. Idarucizumab may not be necessary if 3 to 5 effective half-lives have passed since the last dose. Other strategies for episodes of dabigatran toxicity include activated charcoal for recent ingestions of less than 2 hours or emergent hemodialysis. There are concerns with potential aspiration of charcoal, especially in nonintubated patients with altered mental status from intracranial bleeding. The challenges with dialysis include obtaining timely intravascular access and lack of immediate response in the setting of emergent surgery.

Rivaroxaban

Rivaroxaban is an oral selective Xa inhibitor that inhibits the conversion of prothrombin to thrombin. It is administered once daily for prevention of stroke in nonvalvular atrial fibrillation. In the Rivaroxaban Once Daily Oral Direct Factor Xa Inhibition Compared with Vitamin K Antagonism for Prevention of Stroke and Embolism Trial in Atrial Fibrillation (ROCKET-AF) trial, rivaroxaban 20 mg was noninferior to dose-adjusted warfarin (goal INR 2-3) in the prevention of stroke or systemic embolism (HR, 0.79; 95% CI, 0.66–0.96; $P < .001$ for noninferiority). A decreased dose of 15 mg once daily was given to patients with creatinine clearance 30 to 50 mL/min. Bleeding rates were better with rivaroxaban compared with warfarin, especially with ICH (0.5% per year vs 0.7% per year, $P = .02$). Rivaroxaban was associated with less fatal bleeding than warfarin (0.2% per year vs 0.5% per year; HR, 0.5; 95% CI, 0.31–0.79).[88]

Rivaroxaban has good oral bioavailability (66%) that is increased when taken with food, and maximum concentrations are seen within 2 to 4 hours after ingestion. It is highly protein bound (95%), mainly to serum albumin. The parent drug is metabolized via CYP450 oxidation and hydrolysis in the liver (51%) to inactive moieties that are then predominately excreted renally. Serum half-life is reported to be 5 to 9 hours and is prolonged in the elderly to 11 to 13 hours. Obesity does not appear to have an effect on dosing (there were no weight exclusions in ROCKET-AF).

Rivaroxaban should not be given concomitantly with inhibitors of P-glycoprotein or CYP3A4 (e.g., diltiazem, verapamil, dronedarone, erythromycin) due to increased risk of bleeding due to elevated serum levels. Patients with moderate to severe liver disease (Child-Pugh class B–C) should not take rivaroxaban due to potential existing coagulopathy and additional bleeding risk.

Laboratory monitoring for rivaroxaban therapy can be performed with PT, which is sensitive enough to detect the presence of drug in the serum and therefore is useful for screening purposes. Anti-Xa assays that are calibrated to rivaroxaban may be useful in quantifying amount of drug, but their use is not yet widely available for clinical use.

For patients who cannot swallow, rivaroxaban tablets may be crushed and suspended in 50 mL of water (stable up to 4 hours) for administration via a feeding tube into the stomach (sites distal to the stomach may have decreased absorption), followed by enteral nutrition. No IV preparation of rivaroxaban (or any of the other new Xa inhibitors) is commercially available.

Apixaban

Apixaban is an oral, direct, reversible inhibitor of factor Xa. Like the others in this class, it has good bioavailability (50%), a fast onset with a half-life range of 9 to 14 hours, and high protein binding (87%). Apixaban was proven to be superior to warfarin in patients with atrial fibrillation in the prevention of stroke or systemic embolism (1.27% per year vs 1.60% per year; HR, 0.79; 95% CI, 0.66–0.95; $P=.01$). The rates of intracranial bleeding were lower with apixaban (0.33% per year vs 0.80% per year; HR, 0.42; 95% CI, 0.30–0.58; $P<.001$) and included hemorrhagic stroke and fatal ICH. Mortality was also reported to be improved with apixaban compared with warfarin (3.52% per year vs 3.94% per year; HR, 0.89; 95% CI, 0.80–0.99; $P=.047$). Gastrointestinal bleeding was not found to be different between the agents (HR, 0.89; 95% CI, 0.7–1.14).[89]

Monitoring apixaban therapy using an agent-specific anti-Xa assay seems to be the most promising and effective method since both PT and aPTT are only mildly sensitive to its presence and therefore not useful for screening. For patients with renal impairment (serum creatinine > 1.5g/dL), decreased dosage is only recommended if in combination with an age greater than or equal to 80 years or a weight less than or equal to 60kg. However, recent data supports the safe and efficacious use of full-dose apixaban as an alternative agent to warfarin for use in patients with renal failure or who are receiving hemodialysis.[90]

Patients who are unable to take apixaban orally may have their doses crushed and suspended in 60 mL of water, 5% dextrose in water, or apple juice and administered via a nasogastric tube. These crushed formulations are stable for 4 hours.

Edoxaban

Edoxaban is the latest oral, reversible, direct Xa inhibitor to come on the market for stroke prevention in patients with nonvalvular atrial fibrillation. It has predictable, linear kinetics with a half-life of 10 to 14 hours, and peak concentrations as well as pharmacodynamic effects are seen at 2 hours after ingestion. It has moderate protein binding (55%) and is predominantly renally excreted as unchanged drug (50%) with the remaining elimination via bile. Edoxaban dosing should be decreased at creatinine clearances of 15 to 30 mL/min; it should be avoided in patients with creatinine clearance less than 15 mL/min or with moderate to severe hepatic injury.

Two doses of edoxaban (30 mg and 60 mg) were compared with warfarin (goal INR 2-3) for the prevention of stroke and systemic emboli and found to be noninferior, but the smaller dose was found to be less effective in preventing ischemic stroke. Increased stroke rates were also seen in patients with creatinine clearances more than 95 mL/min, a reflection of decreased serum concentrations seen with higher renal function. Edoxaban was associated with less intracranial bleeding (30 mg: HR, 0.47; 95% CI, 0.34–0.63; $P<.001$; 60 mg: HR, 0.30; 95% CI, 0.21–0.43; $P<.001$).[91]

As with all of the TSOACs, there is a risk of thrombotic events after abrupt discontinuation (not due to acute bleeding), and consideration of bridging with an alternative anticoagulant should be made if the appropriate treatment duration has not been completed. None of these agents are approved for use in patients with mechanical or bioprosthetic heart valves or in patients with acute coronary syndromes.[92] Concerns for treatment of emergent bleeding from Xa inhibitors may be addressed by emerging antidotes, most notably andexanet alfa, a recombinant factor Xa decoy protein that binds and inactivates factor Xa inhibitors. A study in older healthy volunteers taking rivaroxaban or apixaban reported a 94% reduction in anti-Xa activity following a single IV bolus of andexanet alfa.[93] Reversal effects were seen within 5 minutes of the dose and lasted up to 3 hours after the end of infusion. No clinical evidence of thromboses was reported; however, its use in critically ill patients with acute hemorrhage remains to be formally evaluated. Its use may be beneficial in patients taking factor Xa with acute intracerebral hemorrhage or who require emergent surgery. Anticoagulant activity may be restored once the andexanet infusion is stopped because of its short half-life. Because of the high level of protein binding, none of the Xa inhibitors are effectively removed by dialysis. Until andexanet is formally approved for clinical use, 3 to 4fPCCs remain the main options for treatment of life-threatening bleeding from Xa inhibitors (see Table 3.3). However, clinicians should consider product half-life, patient's renal function, drug interactions, and time of last dose when deciding the need for PCC administration. Factor Xa assays are currently not recommended to evaluate the reversal activity of PCCs.[94]

CONCLUSION

Antithrombotic therapy is used for the prevention of ischemic and cardioembolic stroke. The TSOACs have been shown to be at least as equivalent in stroke prevention and have a lower risk of intracranial bleeding compared with warfarin and may be a useful alternative in patients with nonvalvular atrial fibrillation at high risk of bleeding. Although these agents are not used extensively in acute illness, patients currently on these therapies may experience hemorrhagic events, and knowledge of their individual properties can guide subsequent treatment. The ARAMIS (Addressing Real-World Anticoagulation Management Issues in Stroke) Registry is collecting ongoing data on TSOAC management in patients suffering from acute ischemic stroke and acute intracranial hemorrhage to help improve clinical decision making in the future.[95] Newer agents are being studied for both stroke prevention (e.g., vorapaxar) and anticoagulant reversal (e.g., aripazine) and may provide improved outcomes for these patients.

References

1. Centers for Disease Control and Prevention, National Center for Health Statistics. Underlying cause of death 1999–2014 on CDC WONDER Online Database, released 2015. http://wonder.cdc.gov/ucd-icd10.htm. Accessed December 23, 2016.

2. Mozaffarian D, Benjamin EJ, Go AS, et al. Heart disease and stroke statistics—2016 update: a report from the American Heart Association. *Circulation*. 2016;133(4): e38–e360.

3. Jauch EC, Saver JL, Adams HP Jr, et al. Guidelines for the early management of patients with acute ischemic stroke: a guideline for healthcare professionals from the American Heart Association/American Stroke Association. *Stroke*. 2013;44:870–947.

4. Baldwin K, Orr S, Briand M, et al. Acute ischemic stroke update. *Pharmacotherapy*. 2010;30:493–514.

5. Miller DJ, Simpson JR, Silver B. Safety of thrombolysis in acute ischemic stroke: a review of complications, risk factors, and newer technologies. *Neurohospitalist*. 2011;1: 138–147.

6. The National Institute of Neurological Disorders and Stroke rt-PA Stroke Study Group. Tissue plasminogen activator for acute ischemic stroke. *N Engl J Med*. 1995;333: 1581–1587.

7. Marler JR, Tilley BC, Lu M, et al. Early stroke treatment associated with better outcome: the NINDS rt-PA stroke study. *Neurology*. 2000;55:1649–1655.

8. Hacke W, Kaste M, Bluhmki E, et al. Thrombolysis with alteplase 3 to 4.5 hours after acute ischemic stroke. *N Engl J Med*. 2008;359:1317–1329.

9. Cronin CA, Sheth KN, Zhao X, et al. Adherence to Third European Cooperative Acute Stroke Study 3- to 4.5-hour exclusions and association with outcome: data from Get with the Guidelines-Stroke. *Stroke*. 2014;45:2745–2749.

10. The IST-3 Collaborative Group. The benefits and harms of intravenous thrombolysis with recombinant tissue plasminogen activator within 6 h of acute ischaemic stroke: a randomised controlled trial. *Lancet*. 2012;379:2352–2363.

11. Selim M, Kumar S, Fink J, et al. Seizure at stroke onset: should it be an absolute contraindication to thrombolysis? *Cerebrovasc Dis*. 2002;14:54–57.

12. Adams HP Jr, del Zoppo G, Alberts MJ, et al. Guidelines for the early management of adults with ischemic stroke: a guideline from the American Heart Association/American Stroke Association Stroke Council, et al. *Stroke*. 2007;38:1655–1711.

13. Hankey GJ, Norrving B, Hacke W, Steiner T. Management of acute stroke in patients taking novel oral anticoagulants. *Int J Stroke*. 2014;9:627–632.

14. The NINDS t-PA Stroke Study Group. Intracerebral hemorrhage after intravenous t-PA therapy for ischemic stroke. *Stroke*. 1997;28:2109–2118.

15. Tanne D, Kasner SE, Demchuk AM, et al. Markers of increased risk of intracerebral hemorrhage after intravenous recombinant tissue plasminogen activator therapy for acute ischemic stroke in clinical practice: the Multicenter rt-PA Stroke Survey. *Circulation*. 2002;105:1679–1685.

16. Lansberg MG, Albers GW, Wijman CA. Symptomatic intracerebral hemorrhage following thrombolytic therapy for acute ischemic stroke: a review of the risk factors. *Cerebrovasc Dis*. 2007;24:1–10.

17. Wahlgren N, Ahmed N, Eriksson N, et al. Multivariable analysis of outcome predictors and adjustment of main outcome results to baseline data profile in randomized controlled trials: Safe Implementation of Thrombolysis in Stroke-MOnitoring STudy (SITS-MOST). *Stroke*. 2008;39:3316–3322.

18. Hill MD, Barber PA, Takahashi J, et al. Anaphylactoid reactions and angioedema during alteplase treatment of acute ischemic stroke. *CMAJ*. 2000;162:1281–1284.

19. Parsons MW, Miteff F, Bateman GA, et al. Acute ischemic stroke: imaging-guided tenecteplase treatment in an extended time window. *Neurology*. 2009;72:915–921.

20. Haley EC Jr., Lyden PD, Johnston KC, Hemmen TM. A pilot dose-escalation safety study of tenecteplase in acute ischemic stroke. *Stroke*. 2005;36:607–612.

21. Huang X, Cheripelli BK, Lloyd SM, et al. Alteplase versus tenecteplase for thrombolysis after ischaemic stroke (ATTEST): a phase 2, randomised, open-label, blinded endpoint study. *Lancet Neurol*. 2015;14:368–376.

22. Qureshi AI, Harris-Lane P, Kirmani JF, et al. Intra-arterial reteplase and intravenous abciximab in patients with acute ischemic stroke: an open-label, dose-ranging, phase I study. *Neurosurgery*. 2006;59:789–797.

23. Misra V, El Khoury R, Arora R, et al. Safety of high doses of urokinase and reteplase for acute ischemic stroke. *Am J Neuroradiol*. 2011;32:998–1001.

24. Hacke W, Furlan AJ, Al-Rawi Y, et al. Intravenous desmoteplase in patients with acute ischaemic stroke selected by MRI perfusion-diffusion weighted imaging or perfusion CT (DIAS-2): a prospective, randomised, double-blind, placebo-controlled study. *Lancet Neurol*. 2009;8:141–150.

25. Albers GW, von Kummer R, Truelsen T, et al. Safety and efficacy of desmoteplase given 3–9 h after ischaemic stroke in patients with occlusion or high-grade stenosis in major cerebral arteries (DIAS-3): a double-blind, randomised, placebo-controlled phase 3 trial. *Lancet Neurol*. 2015;14:575–584.

26. Hacke W, Albers G, Al-Rawi Y, et al. The Desmoteplase in Acute Ischemic Stroke Trial (DIAS): a phase II MRI-based 9-hour window acute stroke thrombolysis trial with intravenous desmoteplase. *Stroke*. 2005;36:66–73.

27. Furlan AJ, Eyding D, Albers GW, et al. Dose Escalation of Desmoteplase for Acute Ischemic Stroke (DEDAS): evidence of safety and efficacy 3 to 9 hours after stroke onset. *Stroke*. 2006;37:1227–1231.

28. TNKase [package insert]. San Franscico, CA: Genentech, Inc; 2011.

29. O'Gara PT, Kushner FG, Ascheim DD, et al. 2013 ACCF/AHA guideline for the management of ST-elevation myocardial infarction: a report of the American College of Cardiology Foundation/American Heart Association Task Force on Practice Guidelines. *J Am Coll Cardiol*. 2013;61:e78–e140.

30. Martin U, Kaufmann B, Neugebauer G. Current clinical use of reteplase for thrombolysis: a pharmacokinetic-pharmacodynamic perspective. *Clin Pharmacokinet*. 1999;36:265–276.

31. Qureshi AI, Hussein HM, Janjua N, et al. Postprocedure intravenous eptifibatide following intra-arterial reteplase in patients with acute ischemic stroke. *J Neuroimaging.* 2008;18:50–55.

32. Hassan AE, Abd-Allah F, Chaudhry SA, et al. A critical analysis of intra-arterial thrombolytic doses in acute ischemic stroke treatment. *Neurocrit Care.* 2014;21:119–123.

33. Sugg RM, Noser EA, Shaltoni HM, et al. Intra-arterial reteplase compared to urokinase for thrombolytic recanalization in acute ischemic stroke. *Am J Neuroradiol.* 2006;27:769–773.

34. Goyal M, Demchuk AM, Menon BK, et al. Randomized assessment of rapid endovascular treatment of ischemic stroke. *N Engl J Med.* 2015;372:1019–1030.

35. Campbell BC, Mitchell PJ, Kleinig TJ, et al. Endovascular therapy for ischemic stroke with perfusion-imaging selection. *N Engl J Med.* 2015;372:1009–1018.

36. Saver JL, Goyal M, Bonafe A, et al. Stent-retriever thrombectomy after intravenous t-PA vs. t-PA alone in stroke. *N Engl J Med.* 2015;372:2285–2295.

37. Jovin TG, Chamorro A, Cobo E, et al. Thrombectomy within 8 hours after symptom onset in ischemic stroke. *N Engl J Med.* 2015;372:2296–2306.

38. Berkhemer OA, Fransen PS, Beumer D, et al. A randomized trial of intraarterial treatment for acute ischemic stroke. *N Engl J Med.* 2015;372:11–20.

39. del Zoppo GJ, Higashida RT, Furlan AJ, et al. PROACT: a phase II randomized trial of recombinant pro-urokinase by direct arterial delivery in acute middle cerebral artery stroke. PROACT Investigators. Prolyse in Acute Cerebral Thromboembolism. *Stroke.* 1998;29:4–11.

40. Furlan A, Higashida R, Wechsler L, et al. Intra-arterial prourokinase for acute ischemic stroke. The PROACT II study: a randomized controlled trial. Prolyse in Acute Cerebral Thromboembolism. *JAMA.* 1999;282:2003–2011.

41. Lisboa RC, Jovanovic BD, Alberts MJ. Analysis of the safety and efficacy of intra-arterial thrombolytic therapy in ischemic stroke. *Stroke.* 2002;33:2866–2871.

42. Christoforidis GA, Slivka AP, Karakasis C, et al. Hemorrhage rates and outcomes when using up to 100 mg intra-arterial t-PA for thrombolysis in acute ischemic stroke. *Interv Neuroradiol.* 2010;16:297–305.

43. Broderick JP, Palesch YY, Demchuk AM, et al. Endovascular therapy after intravenous t-PA versus t-PA alone for stroke. *N Engl J Med.* 2013;368:893–903.

44. Adams HP Jr, Effron MB, Torner J, et al. Emergency administration of abciximab for treatment of patients with acute ischemic stroke: results of an international phase III trial: Abciximab in Emergency Treatment of Stroke Trial (AbESTT-II). *Stroke.* 2008; 39:87–99.

45. Torgano G, Zecca B, Monzani V, et al. Effect of intravenous tirofiban and aspirin in reducing short-term and long-term neurologic deficit in patients with ischemic stroke: a double-blind randomized trial. *Cerebrovasc Dis.* 2010;29:275–281.

46. Siebler M, Hennerici MG, Schneider D, et al. Safety of Tirofiban in acute Ischemic Stroke: the SaTIS trial. *Stroke.* 2011;42:2388–2392.

47. Pancioli AM, Adeoye O, Schmit PA, et al. Combined approach to lysis utilizing eptifibatide and recombinant tissue plasminogen activator in acute ischemic stroke-enhanced regimen stroke trial. *Stroke.* 2013;44:2381–2387.

48. Frontera JA, Lewin Iii JJ, Rabinstein AA, et al. Guideline for reversal of antithrombotics in intracranial hemorrhage: a statement for healthcare professionals from the Neurocritical Care Society and Society of Critical Care Medicine. *Neurocrit Care.* 2016; 24:6–46.

49. Antiplatelet Trialists' Collaboration. Collaborative overview of randomised trials of anti-platelet therapy, I: prevention of death, myocardial infarction, and stroke by prolonged antiplatelet therapy in various categories of patients. *BMJ*. 1994;308:81–106.

50. CAST Collaborative Group. CAST: randomised placebo-controlled trial of early aspirin use in 20,000 patients with acute ischaemic stroke. *Lancet*. 1997;349:1641–1649.

51. International Stroke Trial Collaborative Group. The International Stroke Trial (IST): a randomised trial of aspirin, subcutaneous heparin, both, or neither among 19435 patients with acute ischaemic stroke. *Lancet*. 1997;349:1569–1581.

52. Awtry EH, Loscalzo J. Aspirin. *Circulation*. 2000;101:1206–1218.

53. Mijajlovic MD, Shulga O, Bloch S, et al. Clinical consequences of aspirin and clopido-grel resistance: an overview. *Acta Neurol Scand*. 2013;128:213–219.

54. Depta JP, Fowler J, Novak E, et al. Clinical outcomes using a platelet function-guided approach for secondary prevention in patients with ischemic stroke or transient ischemic attack. *Stroke*. 2012;43:2376–2381.

55. Fiorella D, Thiabolt L, Albuquerque FC, et al. Antiplatelet therapy in neuroendovascu-lar therapeutics. *Neurosurg Clin North Am*. 2005;16:517–540, vi.

56. Oran I, Cinar C, Bozkaya H, and Korkmaz M. Tailoring platelet inhibition according to multiple electrode aggregometry decreases the rate of thrombotic complications after intracranial flow-diverting stent implantation. *J Neurointerv Surg*. 2015;7:357–362.

57. Flechtenmacher N, Kammerer F, Dittmer R, et al. Clopidogrel resistance in neurovas-cular stenting: correlations between light transmission aggregometry, VerifyNow, and the multiplate. *Am J Neuroradiol*. 2015;36:1953–1958.

58. Scott SA, Sangkuhl K, Stein CM, et al. Clinical Pharmacogenetics Implementation Consortium guidelines for CYP2C19 genotype and clopidogrel therapy: 2013 update. *Clin Pharmacol Ther*. 2013;94:317–323.

59. Beitelshees AL, Voora D, Lewis JP. Personalized antiplatelet and anticoagulation ther-apy: applications and significance of pharmacogenomics. *Pharmgenomics Pers Med*. 2015;8:43–61.

60. Committee CS. A randomised, blinded, trial of clopidogrel versus aspirin in patients at risk of ischaemic events (CAPRIE). CAPRIE Steering Committee. *Lancet*. 1996; 348:1329–1339.

61. Sacco RL, Diener HC, Yusuf S, et al. Aspirin and extended-release dipyridamole versus clopidogrel for recurrent stroke. *N Engl J Med*. 2008;359:1238–1251.

62. Husted S, van Giezen JJ. Ticagrelor: the first reversibly binding oral P2Y12 receptor antagonist. *Cardiovasc Ther*. 2009 ;27:259–274.

63. Johnston SC, Amarenco P, Albers GW, et al. Ticagrelor versus aspirin in acute stroke or transient ischemic attack. *N Engl J Med*. 2016;375:35–43.

64. Lipton RB, Bigal ME, Kolodner KB, et al. Acetaminophen in the treatment of headaches associated with dipyridamole-aspirin combination. *Neurology*. 2004;63:1099–1101.

65. Theis JG, Deichsel G, Marshall S. Rapid development of tolerance to dipyridamole-associated headaches. *Br J Clin Pharmacol*. 1999;48:750–755.

66. Douen AG, Medic S, Sabih M, et al. Titrated initiation of acetylsalicylic acid-dipyridamole therapy reduces adverse effects and improves tolerance in patients with stroke. *J Stroke Cerebrovasc Dis*. 2008;17:356–359.

67. Diener HC, Bogousslavsky J, Brass LM, et al. Aspirin and clopidogrel compared with clopidogrel alone after recent ischaemic stroke or transient ischaemic attack in high-risk patients (MATCH): randomised, double-blind, placebo-controlled trial. *Lancet*. 2004; 364:331–337.

68. Bhatt DL, Topol EJ; Clopidogrel for High Atherothrombotic Risk and Ischemic Stabilization, Management, and Avoidance Executive Committee. Clopidogrel added to aspirin versus aspirin alone in secondary prevention and high-risk primary prevention: rationale and design of the Clopidogrel for High Atherothrombotic Risk and Ischemic Stabilization, Management, and Avoidance (CHARISMA) trial. *Am Heart J.* 2004; 148:263–268.

69. Investigators SPS, Benavente OR, Hart RG, et al. Effects of clopidogrel added to aspirin in patients with recent lacunar stroke. *N Engl J Med.* 2012;367:817–825.

70. Wang Y, Wang Y, Zhao X, et al. Clopidogrel with aspirin in acute minor stroke or transient ischemic attack. *N Engl J Med.* 2013;369:11–19.

71. Wang Y, Pan Y, Zhao X, et al. Clopidogrel With Aspirin in Acute Minor Stroke or Transient Ischemic Attack (CHANCE) trial: one-year outcomes. *Circulation.* 2015; 132:40–46.

72. Liu F, Tantry US, Gurbel PA. P2Y12 receptor inhibitors for secondary prevention of ischemic stroke. *Expert Opin Pharmacother.* 2015;16:1149–1165.

73. Johnston SC, Easton JD, Farrant M, et al. Platelet-oriented inhibition in new TIA and minor ischemic stroke (POINT) trial: rationale and design. *Int J Stroke.* 2013;8: 479–483.

74. Serebruany VL, Kim MH, Hanley DF. Vorapaxar monotherapy for secondary stroke prevention: a call for randomized trial. *Int J Stroke.* 2016;11(6):614–617.

75. Pisters R, Lane DA, Nieuwlaat R, de Vos CB, Crijns HJ, Lip GY. A novel user-friendly score (HAS-BLED) to assess 1-year risk of major bleeding in patients with atrial fibrillation: the Euro Heart Survey. *Chest.* 2010;138:1093–1100.

76. Gage BF, Yan Y, Milligan PE, et al. Clinical classification schemes for predicting hemorrhage: results from the National Registry of Atrial Fibrillation (NRAF). *Am Heart J.* 2006;151:713–719.

77. Fang MC, Go AS, Chang Y, et al. A new risk scheme to predict warfarin-associated hemorrhage: The ATRIA (Anticoagulation and Risk Factors in Atrial Fibrillation) Study. *J Am Coll Cardiol.* 2011;58:395–401.

78. Caldeira D, Costa J, Fernandes RM, Pinto FJ, Ferreira JJ. Performance of the HAS-BLED high bleeding-risk category, compared to ATRIA and HEMORR2HAGES in patients with atrial fibrillation: a systematic review and meta-analysis. *J Interv Card Electrophysiol.* 2014;40:277–284.

79. International Warfarin Pharmacogenetics Committee, Klein TE, Altman RB, et al. Estimation of the warfarin dose with clinical and pharmacogenetic data. *N Engl J Med.* 2009;360:753–764.

80. Pirmohamed M, Burnside G, Eriksson N, et al. A randomized trial of genotype-guided dosing of warfarin. *N Engl J Med.* 2013;369:2294–2303.

81. Kimmel SE, French B, Kasner SE, et al. A pharmacogenetic versus a clinical algorithm for warfarin dosing. *N Engl J Med.* 2013;369:2283–2293.

82. Verhoef TI, Redekop WK, Veenstra DL, et al. Cost-effectiveness of pharmacogenetic-guided dosing of phenprocoumon in atrial fibrillation. *Pharmacogenomics.* 2013;14: 869–883.

83. Connolly SJ, Ezekowitz MD, Yusuf S, et al. Dabigatran versus warfarin in patients with atrial fibrillation. *N Engl J Med.* 2009;361:1139–1151.

84. Favaloro EJ, Lippi G. Laboratory testing in the era of direct or non-vitamin K antagonist oral anticoagulants: a practical guide to measuring their activity and avoiding diagnostic errors. *Semin Thromb Hemost.* 2015;41:208–227.

85. van Ryn J, Stangier J, Haertter S, et al. Dabigatran etexilate—a novel, reversible, oral direct thrombin inhibitor: interpretation of coagulation assays and reversal of anticoagulant activity. *Thromb Haemost.* 2010;103:1116–1127.

86. Eikelboom JW, Quinlan DJ, van Ryn J, Weitz JI. Idarucizumab: the antidote for reversal of dabigatran. *Circulation.* 2015;132:2412–2422.

87. Patel MR, Mahaffey KW, Garg J, et al. Rivaroxaban versus warfarin in nonvalvular atrial fibrillation. *N Engl J Med.* 2011;365:883–891.

88. Granger CB, Alexander JH, McMurray JJ, et al. Apixaban versus warfarin in patients with atrial fibrillation. *N Engl J Med.* 2011;365:981–992.

89. Giugliano RP, Ruff CT, Braunwald E, et al. Edoxaban versus warfarin in patients with atrial fibrillation. *N Engl J Med.* 2013;369:2093–2104.

90. Stanton BE, Barasch NS, Tellor KB. Comparison of the safety and effectiveness of apixaban versus warfarin in patients with severe renal impairment. *Pharmacotherapy.* 2017;doi:10.1002/phar.1905

91. Siegal DM, Curnutte JT, Connolly SJ, et al. Andexanet alfa for the reversal of factor Xa inhibitor activity. *N Engl J Med.* 2015;373:2413–2424.

92. Trikha R, Kowey PR. Practical considerations for the nonvitamin K antagonist oral anticoagulants. *Cardiology.* 2017;136:115–124.

93. Demaerschalk BM, Kleindorfer DO, Adeoye OM, et al. Scientific rationale for the inclusion and exclusion criteria for intravenous alteplase in acute ischemic stroke: a statement for healthcare professionals from the American Heart Association/American Stroke Association. *Stroke.* 2016;47:581–641.

94. Brown KS, Zahir H, Grosso MA, et al. Nonvitamin K antagonist oral anticoagulant activity: challenges in measurement and reversal. *Critical Care.* 2016;20:273–282.

95. Xian Y, Hernandez AF, Harding T, et al. Acute management of stroke patients taking nonvitamin K antagonist oral anticoagulants addressign real-world anticoagulant management issues in stroke (ARAMIS) registry: design and rationale. *Am Heart J.* 2016;182:28–35.

Coagulopathy Reversal Agents for Intracranial Hemorrhage

4

Karen Berger, Nicholas G. Panos,
and John J. Lewin III

INTRODUCTION

Anticoagulants, antiplatelet agents, and thrombolytics are frequently used to treat or decrease the risk of thrombotic or embolic events in a wide variety of medical conditions. Use of these agents is expected to increase as the population ages.[1] As new therapeutic options to prevent stroke and treat clotting disorders become available, it is imperative that clinicians remain up to date on how to best manage bleeding complications associated with antithrombotics. As it relates to the management of intracranial hemorrhage (ICH), the presence of a coagulopathy can complicate management and affect outcomes. Compared with patients experiencing spontaneous ICH without anticoagulation, those on antithrombotics have a higher likelihood of secondary hematoma expansion, and an increased risk of death or poor functional outcome.[2,3] Given the high morbidity and mortality associated with ICH, immediate reversal of the effects of the offending antithrombotic is typically advised.[4]

PATHOPHYSIOLOGY OF HEMOSTASIS IN INTRACRANIAL HEMORRHAGE

The concept of the coagulation cascade, wherein a cascade of enzymes is activated, which in turn further activate other enzymes downstream resulting in the formation of a stable fibrin clot, dates back to 1964.[5] This system is divided into the extrinsic and intrinsic pathways, which are interconnected. Blood coming into contact with injured endothelium (and the exposure of tissue factor) activates the extrinsic pathway, initiating the cascade that results in the conversion of prothrombin (factor II) to thrombin (factor IIa). Since the inception of the concept of this cascade, the scientific understanding of clotting has continued to evolve. It is now recognized that platelets play a critical role in the cascade.[6] In addition to providing an initial physical barrier to bleeding (by aggregating at the bleeding site and adhering to endovascular collagen), the platelet surface serves as a catalyst to amplify the activation of factors within the cascade, perpetuating a burst of thrombin. This results in the eventual formation of the fibrin mesh around the aggregated platelets and the formation of a stable clot. A detailed review of the evolving pathophysiologic understanding of thrombus formation is beyond the scope of this chapter, and the reader is referred to other references.[6] It is important that clinicians possess a fundamental understanding of these pathways, as well as the mechanism of action of antithrombotics, as this background knowledge is important to understanding the physiologic basis for many of the reversal strategies employed and discussed in this chapter.

As ICH occurs within the fixed space of the cranial vault, it was initially thought that ICH was in large part a singular event that stopped quickly as a result of tamponade.[7] However, multiple studies suggest that continued hematoma expansion is common, usually occurring in the early phase of ICH, and is a major determinant of early deterioration and death.[3,8,9] Aside from the fact that antithrombotics increase the risk of ICH in and of themselves, when ICH does occur, their presence in a patient further complicates the clinical picture. The increased morbidity and mortality (compared with ICH patients not on antithrombotics) is thought to be a result of the increased ICH volumes,[10] increased rate of hematoma expansion,[3] and increased number of underlying comorbidities in patients on anthithrobotics.[11]

LABORATORY ASSESSMENT OF SELECTED ANTITHROMBOTIC AGENTS

Interpretation of laboratory coagulation assays must take into consideration the individual patient's current clinical status, comorbid disease states, and medication history. Using laboratory values as the sole source of information to determine whether or not coagulopathy should be reversed, as well as how much of a given reversal agent to administer, could lead to underdosing or overdosing of reversal agents. Indeed, administration of some hemostatic agents may slow bleeding without affecting laboratory parameters. For example, one case report demonstrated the impact of factor VIII inhibitor bypassing agent (FEIBA, 26 units/kg) in achieving hemostasis in a patient on dabigatran with a transeptal perforation occurring during an ablation procedure.[12] Hemostasis (as measured by blood output via the pericardial window) noticeably slowed and eventually stopped as a result of a low-dose FEIBA. In this case, the measured laboratory parameters (ecarin chromogenic assay) did not correct immediately or in concert with the observed hemostasis. Conversely, while recombinant factor VIIa (rFVIIa) has been shown to effectively and rapidly correct an elevated INR in the setting of warfarin therapy, it is known that the international normalized ratio (INR) is particularly sensitive to factor VII levels. In the setting of warfarin, an observed INR reduction from rFVIIa administration may occur despite inadequate hemostasis and correction of the other vitamin K–dependent clotting factors.[13]

The laboratory monitoring techniques clinically employed to monitor the effects of warfarin (ie, the INR) and unfractionated heparin (UFH) (ie, activated partial thromboplastin time [aPTT], anti–factor Xa assay, and the activated clotting time [ACT]), are well understood and routinely used. Therefore, this chapter will focus on those laboratory assays used to monitor the more recently available antithrombotics. The reader is thus referred to the American College of Chest Physicians guidelines on *Antithrombotic Therapy and Prevention of Thrombosis*, ninth edition, for further details on monitoring of warfarin, low molecular weight heparins (LMWHs), and UFH.[14,15] For comparison purposes, Table 4.1 provides a list of selected laboratory parameters and their relative utility for warfarin and direct oral anticoagulants (DOACs).

Direct Factor Xa Inhibitors

Oral direct factor Xa inhibitors, such as rivaroxaban, apixaban, and edoxaban, typically do not require routine monitoring of their anticoagulant effect. Indeed, this is one of the potential benefits of these agents. However, in the setting of ICH, a rapidly available laboratory assessment of the presence and intensity of anticoagulation is desired. These agents do prolong the prothrombin time (PT), but the sensitivity of the PT can vary substantially.[16–18] The effects on the aPTT are even more variable.[18,19] Given the variability in sensitivity, it is important to understand that while these measures may be elevated, they might also be normal in the presence of a therapeutic drug concentration.

The most accurate tests to measure the levels of a direct factor Xa inhibitor are the chromogenic anti–factor Xa assays. Studies demonstrate reproducibility and a linear correlation of the laboratory result with the concentration of the factor Xa inhibitor.[20,21] Ideally, the anti–Xa assay employs a drug-specific

TABLE 4.1 Laboratory Tests to Consider When Assessing Warfarin and Direct Oral Anticoagulants (DOACs)

Laboratory Test	Warfarin	Dabigatran	Rivaroxaban, Apixaban, and Edoxaban	Comments
SCr and CBC with platelets	Potentially useful	Potentially useful	Potentially useful	Monitor serum calcium concentration if transfusing blood
INR or PT	Potentially useful; value increased	Potentially useful; value increased; use central laboratory because point-of-care test can give much higher values	Potentially useful; value may be increased	PT may be considered because INR may not be calibrated for the DOACs; PT more responsive to factor Xa inhibitors than to dabigatran; limited ability to quantify amount of drug
aPTT	Potentially useful; value somewhat increased	Potentially useful; value increased, but aPTT response flattens at higher serum drug concentration	Potentially useful; value increased	aPTT more responsive to dabigatran than to factor Xa inhibitors; limited ability to quantify amount of drug
TT	Clinical use limited	Potentially useful; very sensitive at low concentration but not useful at higher concentration	Inadequate measure	Limited ability to quantify amount of dabigatran
ECT	Clinical use limited	Potentially useful if available; potential ability to quantify amount of drug present	Inadequate measure	Limited availability; potential quantitative test
Diluted TT	Clinical use limited	Potentially useful if available; potential ability to quantify amount of drug present	Inadequate measure	Lack of standardization and potential differences in measured results among laboratories; may have limitations at low dabigatran concentration
Chromogenic antifactor Xa assay	Inadequate measure	Inadequate measure	Potentially useful; value increased	Limited availability; nonstandardized; results may vary among laboratories where available

Source: Adapted from Nutescu EA, Dager WE, Kalus JS, et al. Management of bleeding and reversal strategies for oral anticoagulants: clinical practice considerations. *Am J Health Syst Pharm.* 2013;70:1914–1929, with permission.

Note: aPTT, activated partial thromboplastin time; CBC, complete blood count; ECT, ecarin clotting time; INR, international normalized ratio; PT, prothrombin time; SCr, serum creatinine; TT, thrombin time.

calibrator. However, anti-Xa assays calibrated for the newer agents are rarely available in the clinical setting in a timely fashion in order to be of use in the setting of ICH. It has been suggested that the anti-Xa assays more commonly available (ie, for UFH or LMWH) could be used to exclude the existence of significant levels of the direct factor Xa inhibitors, as the presence of the drug would be detected regardless of the calibrator used.[22]

Direct Thrombin Inhibitors

The aPTT is fairly sensitive to the anticoagulant effects of intravenous direct thrombin inhibitors (eg, argatroban and bivalirudin). This assay is used routinely in their monitoring, dose titration, and management. However, while the aPTT is more responsive to dabigatran than is the PT, the aPTT is a less sensitive marker for the anticoagulant effect of dabigatran compared with other direct thrombin inhibitors (DTIs).[23] It has been suggested that a normal aPTT may reasonably exclude a highly significant drug effect for dabigatran.[23,24] However, others have demonstrated that a normal aPTT can be observed in the setting of measurable dabigatran levels.[25] The thrombin time in particular can be of clinical relevance, in that it is exquisitely sensitive to dabigatran. A normal thrombin time suggests no or minimal presence of dabigatran.[25–27]

Other assays may provide a more quantitative assessment of dabigatran serum concentrations. The dilute thrombin time (dTT) in general demonstrates a linear, concentration–dependent relationship with dabigatran and other DTIs.[26,28] A potential downside of this assay in the context of ICH is the lack of immediate availability and rapid turnaround time in many centers. The ecarin clotting time (ECT) and ecarin chromogenic assays also demonstrate a reliable concentration-dependent, linear relationship with direct thrombin inhibitors.[29,30] Similar to the dTT, the clinical applicability of these assays is often limited by availability and turnaround time.

Antiplatelet Agents

A plethora of platelet function tests are available. These tests of platelet function can be grouped into the different methods employed in the testing. Light transmission platelet aggregometry (LTA) is the gold standard but requires expert interpretation and may not be available in most centers. More recently, point-of-care measures have been developed such as VerifyNow (Acumetrics) and PFA-100 (Dade-Behring) which correlate with LTA and can be used to evaluate the presence of antiplatelet therapy and antiplatelet resistance. The pros and cons of the various platelet aggregation tests are reviewed in detail elsewhere.[4,31] Recent guidelines recommend the use of platelet function testing in patients with ICH undergoing neurosurgical evacuation,[4] based on a trial demonstrating the benefit of platelet transfusion in those taking aspirin and who were also aspirin sensitive as determined by the PFA-100.[32] A single-center prospective cohort study conducted by Naidech et al[33] demonstrated that reduced platelet activity (as measured by VerifyNow) was associated with early ICH volume growth and worse functional outcome. A separate single-center prospective cohort study also conducted by Naidech et al[34] demonstrated that platelet activity (VerifyNow) is increased in patients receiving platelet transfusions. The most recent guidelines for reversal of antithrombotics in ICH suggest platelet transfusion only in those patients undergoing a neurosurgical procedure and that platelet function testing prior to platelet transfusion is recommended when feasible.[4]

REVERSAL AGENTS

A broad armamentarium of reversal agents can be used to acutely manage a patient with ICH depending on the type of anticoagulant, thrombolytic, or antiplatelet contributing to the expansion of a hematoma. Table 4.2 provides a recommended approach for the major classes of antithrombotic agents.

Plasma

Plasma, or fresh-frozen plasma (FFP), contains all the coagulation factors necessary to reverse the effects of vitamin K antagonists (VKAs) in the setting of a life-threatening hemorrhage from VKAs. Animal studies and case series have described the use of FFP in DOAC-associated hemorrhage, which found no reduction in mortality.[35–37] In addition, the use of FFP in the setting of an LMWH-associated hemorrhage is not recommended due to the lack of effect.[4] The dose of FFP for VKA-associated hemorrhage ranges between 5 and 30 mL/kg, with higher volumes achieving greater correction of factor levels. Currently, a dose of 10 to 15 mL/kg is recommended to provide factor replacement in the setting of an ICH.[4] Despite its low cost and widespread availability compared with prothrombin complex concentrates (PCCs) and rFVIIa, FFP may place patients at risk for delayed reversal and adverse effects.[38] Complications associated with administration of the required volume of FFP are pulmonary edema and transfusion-related lung injury.[39,40] In regards to delayed reversal, studies have shown it can take up to 30 hours to reverse the effects of VKAs when FFP is used.[39,41,42] This may be unfavorable when a patient presents with an ICH as expansion of the hematoma may occur the longer it takes to correct the INR.[9,43] In a few retrospective cohort studies of patients with ICH, failure

TABLE 4.2 Approach to the Emergent Reversal of ICH

Warfarin (if INR ≥ 1.4)	DTI	Factor Xa Inhibitors	UFH	LMWH	Pentasaccharides	Thrombolytics	Antiplatelet Agents
1. Withhold drug	1. Withhold drug	1. Withhold drug	1. Withhold drug	1. Withhold drug	1. Withhold drug	1. Withhold drug	1. Withhold drug
2. IV vitamin K 10 mg	2. Activated charcoal if ingestion within 2 hours of presentation. For dabigatran: consider emergent hemodialysis if idarucizumab not available	2. Activated charcoal if ingestion within 2 hours of presentation and consider emergent hemodialysis	2. Protamine sulfate based on the total dose of heparin infused over the last 2 hours (maximum: 50 mg)	2. Protamine sulfate within 8 hours of enoxaparin or 3 to 5 half-lives of dalteparin, nadroparin, and tinzaparin administration	2. aPCC 20 unit/kg	2. Cryoprecipitate 10 units if received thrombolytic in the last 24 hours. If cryoprecipitate contraindicated or patient has religious restrictions, consider aminocaproic acid or tranexamic acid.	2. If patient to receive emergent surgical intervention, give platelet transfusion immediately prior to surgery. Consider holding platelet transfusion if patient is not a candidate for surgery.
3. Any of the following in order of preference: • PCC4 • aPCC4 • PCC3 + rFVIIa • PCC3 • RFVIIa • Plasma	3. Any of the following in order of preference: • Dabigatran ∘ Idarucizumab • IV DTIs ∘ aPCC4 ∘ PCC4 • PCC3 + rFVIIa	3. Any of the following in order of preference: • PCC4 • aPCC4 • PCC3 + rFVIIa	3. If aPTT prolonged after administration of protamine, another dose of protamine (half dose) may be considered	3. If bleeding persists or patient has renal insufficiency, consider another dose of protamine (half dose).	3. If aPCC contraindicated, use rFVIIa 90 mcg/kg × 1 dose.	3. If fibrinogen level <150 mg/dL after replacement, consider an additional 10 units of cryoprecipitate.	3. If unable to give platelets due to contraindication or religious restrictions, consider DDAVP 0.3 to 0.4 mcg/kg × 1 dose.

Source: Compiled from references 4, 53, 62, and 102.

Note: aPCC4, activated 4-factor prothrombin complex concentrate; aPTT, activated partial thromboplastin time; DDAVP, desmopressin; DTI, direct thrombin inhibitor; ICH, intracranial hemorrhage; INR, international normalized ratio; IU, international unit; IV, intravenous; LMWH, low molecular weight heparin; PCC3, 3-factor prothrombin complex concentrate; PCC4, inactivated 4-factor prothrombin complex concentrate; rFVIIa, recombinant activated factor VII; UFH, unfractionated heparin.

to reverse INR was an independent predictor of mortality and severe disability.[9,44] Recently, the Fresh Frozen Plasma Versus Prothrombin Complex Concentrate in Patients With Intracranial Haemorrhage Related to Vitamin K Antagonists trial determined that 30 international units/kg of PCC was superior to 20 mL/kg of FFP in reducing the INR to less than 1.2 within 3 hours ($P > .0003$).[45] This is the first prospective, randomized trial conducted in ICH patients comparing FFP to PCCs. In this study, the mean time to reversal was 24.7 hours for FFP vs 40 minutes with PCC ($P = .05$). Although hematoma expansion in the FFP group was statistically significant ($P = .023$), mortality and functional outcome did not differ between the 2 groups. When analyzing the incidence of thromboembolism, this study found no difference between the 2 agents, which was also described in other randomized trials.[46,47] Therefore, FFP should be considered a reversal agent for VKAs when PCCs are not readily available or when patients have a confirmed allergy to PCCs or any of the excipients. Furthermore, the use of FFP is not recommended in the setting of DOAC- or LMWH-associated hemorrhage based on a lack of clinical evidence showing benefit.

Cryoprecipitate

Cryoprecipitate is the preferred blood product in the setting of recombinant tissue plasminogen activator (rt-PA)–induced hemorrhage since it contains fibrinogen.[4] Cryoprecipitate contains fibrinogen, factor XIII, and von Willebrand factor. Fibrinogen levels can decrease after rt-PA administration, and severe hypofibrinogenemia may occur in up to 5% of stroke patients receiving rt-PA.[48] This reduction in fibrinogen after rt-PA administration is a strong predictor of the increased risk of intraparenchymal hemorrhage (IPH) and hematoma expansion.[49,50] As such, replacement of fibrinogen in the setting of rt-PA–induced hemorrhage is a reasonable approach. Therefore, when providing care to a patient presenting with a fibrinolytic-associated hemorrhage, it would be reasonable to start with 10 units of cryoprecipitate to raise the fibrinogen level in the plasma with a fibrinogen target greater than 150 mg/dL.[50]

Platelets

Two randomized trials have investigated the utility of platelet transfusions in the setting of antiplatelet-related ICH. In one study, 780 patients with acute hypertensive basal ganglia hemorrhages undergoing craniotomy and hematoma evacuation were evaluated.[32] Patients who had been on aspirin and were deemed to be aspirin sensitive by way of a platelet aggregation test were randomized to receive no transfusion, 6 units of platelets before surgery, or 12 units of platelets

(6 units before surgery and 6 units 24 hours later). In those who received platelets, there was less ICH recurrence (14% vs 35 %, P = .02) and lower postoperative hematoma volume (35 ± 20 cm^3 in treated groups vs 57 ± 20 cm^3 in the untreated group, P = .001). In addition, a significant reduction in mortality was observed in those who received platelets (15.5% vs 34.2%, P = .02). Notably, this study had several limitations, making it challenging to extrapolate to all patients with antiplatelet-related ICH. The cohort was divided into multiple subgroups with multiple statistical analysis performed, and all patients underwent neurosurgery for hematoma evacuation regardless of ICH size or presence of mass effect.

A second more recent trial evaluated 190 patients at 60 hospitals in an open-label, masked-endpoint, randomized trial of patients receiving antiplatelet therapy for at least 7 days before admission for supratentorial ICH.[51] Patients were randomized to standard of care or standard of care plus platelet transfusion within 90 minutes of diagnostic brain imaging. The odds of death or dependence at 3 months were higher in the platelet transfusion arm (odds ratio, 2.05; 95% confidence interval, 1.15–3.56; P = .0114), with a higher percentage of patients in the platelet transfusion arm having a serious adverse event during hospitalization (42% vs 29%).

Based on the results of these trials, combined with the fact that it is unclear as to whether the presence of antiplatelets influences outcomes in ICH,[4] platelet transfusion as a means of reversing antiplatelet agents cannot be routinely recommended. Consideration can be given to using platelet transfusion in the subset of patients undergoing neurosurgical hematoma evacuation.

Prothrombin Complex Concentrates

Prothrombin complex concentrates were originally approved by the US Food and Drug Administration (FDA) for use in patients presenting with acute bleeding due to hemophilia A or B. With the adaptation of concentrated factor products such as PCCs for anticoagulant reversal, the effective dosing volume is decreased and the risk for adverse events from fluid overload is diminished compared with plasma, but there continues to be a risk of thrombotic complications. Over time, their use in VKA and DOAC reversal increased, with Kcentra being the first PCC in the United States to be approved by the FDA for the urgent reversal of VKA in patients with major bleeding or need for an urgent invasive procedure.[46,47,52] Prothrombin complex concentrates can be further classified as activated (aPCC) and inactivated (PCC). The inactivated PCCs are classified as 3-factor (PCC3) or 4-factor (PCC4), which contain vitamin K–associated factors in varying concentrations (factors II, VII, IX, and X and proteins C and S).[53] The PCC3 contain factors II, IX, and X with zero to trace amounts of inactivated factor VII. Four-factor PCC contains factors II, VII, IX, and X. The aPCC is a 4-factor PCC that contains factors II, IX, and X and activated VII. All nonactivated PCCs are dosed based on units of factor IX. FEIBA is dosed based on units of factor VIII bypassing activity, with 500 units of FEIBA containing 500 units of factor VIII bypassing activity. Examples of available PCC formulations in the United States are provided in Table 4.3. Of note, Kcentra, a PCC4 approved for use in the United States in 2013, and Bebulin (PCC3) both contain heparin.[54,55] Use of Kcentra should be avoided in patients with a recent history of heparin-induced thrombocytopenia or hypersensitivity reaction to heparin. If immediate reversal of VKA is required in a patient with a recent history of heparin intolerance, the PCC3, Profilnine, or aPCC, FEIBA, may be considered a replacement to Kcentra since they do not contain heparin. When dosing any of the PCCs for VKA reversal, the pretreatment INR should be assessed to determine an efficacious weight-based dose to prevent overcorrecting.[46] On the other hand, varying doses of aPCC and PCCs have been used in clinical practice to reverse factor Xa inhibitors or direct thrombin inhibitors. The doses are based on studies in healthy human subjects and in vitro analysis of various coagulation laboratory parameters.[56–59] Currently, no clinical trials have established a safe and effective dose. Moreover, it is difficult to predict the true duration of PCC since most clinical trials administer it concomitantly with vitamin K. One retrospective study found a 25% rate in INR rebound (defined as INR $\geq$1.5 within 24 hours after INR correction was previously achieved) after the administration of PCC4 for warfarin reversal. Of those, 57% did not receive concomitant vitamin K.[60] This demonstrates a potential for a rebound effect of PCCs as the duration weans off. Thus, patients should be monitored closely even after hemostasis has been achieved. Randomized clinical trials have reported a thrombosis rate of 6.8% to 7.8% in patients who were reversed for warfarin.[46,47] Based on the available evidence, using a maximum dose of either aPCC or PCC4 (if new reversal agents are not available) of 50 units/kg is suggested.[4]

Recombinant Activated Factor VII

Like some of the first PCCs, rFVIIa was FDA approved for bleeding episodes associated with hemophilia A or B.[61] When used for VKA reversal, rFVIIa immediately decreases INR comparable to PCCs.[39] One of the limitations of rFVIIa is that the other vitamin K–dependent factors II, IX, and X must be replaced using plasma or a PCC3 to fully achieve adequate hemostasis. Consequently, adequate hemostasis may not be achieved when using rFVIIa alone, and rebound INR elevations may occur as the medication effect wears off. Given the short half-life of rFVIIa, a potential rebound may occur within hours. With guideline recommendations promoting the use of PCCs for the immediate reversal of VKAs, rFVIIa may be used as an alternative to PCCs in patients with religious objections to human blood products.[4,62] Doses typically ranging from 20 to 80 mcg/kg have been reported in the literature, but an optimal dosing target has not been defined.[4] In addition, rFVIIa has been used for the reversal of factor Xa inhibitors, direct thrombin inhibitors, LMWHs, and fondaparinux.[4] When considering rFVIIa, one of the major adverse effects associated with its use is thrombosis. Patients with a preexisting history of hypercoagulability are at greater risk for developing thrombotic complications.[63]

Vitamin K (Phytonadione)

Vitamin K (phytonadione) is the antidote for VKAs and works by promoting the hepatic synthesis of vitamin K–associated factors (factors II, VII, IX, and X).[64] The dose and route of administration of vitamin K are an important consideration when patients present with a life-threatening hemorrhage. In the setting of ICH, higher doses (10 mg) are recommended to completely reverse the anticoagulant effect of warfarin.[4] In rare instances, when early re-anticoagulation with warfarin is expected, it may be reasonable to use a lower dose of vitamin K. Retrospective data suggest intravenous (IV) doses as low as 2 mg may be as effective as 10 mg in lowering the INR, which presumably would result in shorter anticoagulation bridge times when reinitiating therapy.[65] Subcutaneous administration of vitamin K results in erratic and incomplete absorption, whereas the enteral administration will delay normalization of INR due to the delayed absorption in the gastrointestinal tract.[66,67] The IV route of administration is preferred in the setting of an acute hemorrhage from VKA due to the quicker onset of effect.[68] However, there is a risk of an anaphylactoid reaction when giving vitamin K via the IV route.[69] Diluting the vitamin K dose in an IV piggyback and infusing the dose no faster than 1 mg/min can potentially mitigate the anaphylactoid reaction risk.

Desmopressin

Desmopressin (DDAVP) is a vasopressin analogue that increases the endothelial release of von Willebrand factor and factor VIII, promoting platelet adhesion to the endothelium. In the setting of hemorrhage where antiplatelets are contributing to expansion of a hematoma, DDAVP may be useful in promoting platelet activation, adhesion, and aggregation to further reduce bleeding at the site of vascular injury. In the setting of ICH in patients exposed to

Table 4.3 Selected Characteristics of Reversal Agents

Reversal Agent	Mechanism of Action	Dose	Onset of Effect	Adverse Effects
Blood products • Plasma • Platelets • Cryoprecipitate	Replaces vitamin K–dependent factors Replaces platelets Replaces fibrinogen, vWF, factor VIII, factor XIII, fibronectin	10 to 15 mL/kg 6 to 12 units or 1 to 2 pooled units 10 units	Delayed and dose dependent; up to 24 hours	TRALI, volume overload, thrombosis
PCC3 • Bebulin • Profilnine SD	Replaces factors II, IX, and X with low or trace amount of factor VII (inactivated)	25 to 50 IU/kg of factor IX	Immediate	Thrombosis, HIT (Bebulin)
PCC4 • Kcentra	Replaces factors II, VII (inactivated), IX, and X and proteins C and S	25 to 50 IU/kg of factor IX	Immediate	Thrombosis, HIT, hypersensitivity reaction to heparin
aPCC4 • FEIBA	Replaces factors II, VII (activated), IX, and X and protein C	20 to 50 IU/kg or 500 IU for INR less than 5, 1000 IU for INR greater than 5	Immediate	Thrombosis
rFVIIa (Novoseven)	Recombinant activated factor VII	10 to 90 mcg/kg	Immediate	Thrombosis, rebound PT/INR
Phytonadione (vitamin K)	Promotes liver synthesis of factors II, VII, IX, and X	2 to 10 mg	Delayed; intial, 2 hours; peak, 24 hours	Anaphylactoid reaction
Desmopressin (DDAVP)	Increases plasma levels of vWF and factor VIII and increases platelet glycoprotein expression	0.3 to 0.4 mcg/kg	Immediate	Facial flushing, hyponatremia
Antifibrinolytics • Aminocaproic acid • Tranexamic acid	Binds to plasminogen, inhibiting conversion to plasmin and inhibiting fibrin degradation	Aminocaproic acid: 4- to 5-g IV bolus, then 1 g/h Tranexamic acid: 1000-mg IV bolus every 8 hours × 2 doses	Rapid, within 1 hour	Hypotension, thrombosis

Table 4.3 *Continued*

Reversal Agent	Mechanism of Action	Dose	Onset of Effect	Adverse Effects
Protamine	Forms stable complex with heparin	1 mg/100 units heparin given in last 2 to 3 hours 1 mg/1 mg if enoxaparin given in last 8 hours 0.5 mg/1 mg if enoxaparin given within 8 to 12 hours 1 mg/100 units anti-Xa of LMWH within 3 to 5 half-lives	Immediate	Hypotension, hypersensitivity reaction
Idarucizumab	Monoclonal antibody that selectively binds to dabigatran	2.5 g × 2 doses for a total of 5 g	Immediate	Hypokalemia
Andexanet alfa[a]	Modified recombinant factor Xa, which selectively binds factor Xa inhibitors	Apixaban: 400-mg IV bolus, then 4 mg/min for 120 minutes Rivaroxaban: 800-mg IV bolus, then 8 mg/min for 120 minutes	Immediate	Flushing, infusion site reactions
Ciraparantag[a]	Small molecule that binds to UFH, LMWH, factor Xa, and direct thrombin inhibitors	Phase I/II trials in process	Immediate	Unknown at this time

Source: Compiled from references 4, 32, 39, 50, 53, 72, 80, 83, 86, 100 to 103.

Note: aPCC4, activated 4-factor prothrombin complex concentrate; DDAVP, desmopressin; FEIBA, factor VIII inhibitor bypassing agent; INR, international normalized ratio; IU, international unit; IV, intravenous; HIT, heparin-induced thrombocytopenia; LMWH, low molecular weight heparin; PCC3, 3-factor prothrombin complex concentrate; PCC4, inactivated 4-factor prothrombin complex concentrate; PT, prothrombin time;; rFVIIa, recombinant activated factor VII; TRALI, transfusion-related acute lung injury; UFH, unfractionated heparin; vFW, von Willebrand factor.

[a]Investigational agent, not Food and Drug Administration approved.

antiplatelet medications, DDAVP 0.3 to 0.4 mcg/kg may be administered to promote platelet activation and decrease the volume of hematoma expansion.[70,71] DDAVP may also be combined with a platelet infusion prior to surgery in patients with history of recent use of an antiplatelet medication.[4] Caution needs to be taken when administering DDAVP as it can cause hypotension upon rapid administration, bradycardia, decreased urine output, and hyponatremia. In addition, tachyphylaxis can be seen after repeat dosing due to depletion of von Willebrand factor and factor VIII from the endothelial compartment.

Antifibrinolytic Agents

Antifibrinolytics, such as aminocaproic acid and tranexamic acid, can be used as an alternative to cryoprecipitate where either a contraindication is present or a patient refuses it due to religious concerns.[72] These agents work by binding to plasminogen and inhibiting the conversion to plasmin and subsequent fibrin degradation. Experience is limited to case reports in the setting of ICH after rt-PA administration for an ischemic stroke.[72,73] The potential adverse effects of using this agent include infusion-related reactions (hypotension) and increased risk for thrombosis.

Protamine

Protamine sulfate is a cationic peptide derived from fish sperm nuclei that binds to heparin sodium to form a stable salt. This, in turn, inactivates heparin and reverses its anticoagulant effect. Dosing of protamine is dependent on the cumulative amount of heparin administered in the preceding 2 to 3 hours.[74] Caution should be used when determining the appropriate dose, as protamine itself in high concentrations can act as an anticoagulant. Protamine can also be used for the reversal of LMWH, but it does not completely bind to the LMWHs to reverse the anti–factor IIa and anti–factor Xa activity.[75,76] In addition, each of the LMWHs binds differently to protamine due to their molecular weight and sulfate charge density. Since tinzaparin has the highest sulfate charge density of the LMWHs, it will bind better to protamine than dalteparin and enoxaparin. Some adverse effects to monitor for include anaphylaxis, pulmonary hypertension, hypotension, and bronchoconstriction.

Idarucizumab

Idarucizumab is the first FDA-approved antidote for a direct-acting oral anticoagulant, specifically targeted against dabigatran, an oral direct thrombin inhibitor. Idarucizumab is a humanized monoclonal antibody fragment that binds to dabigatran with a very high affinity (350 times higher affinity than that of dabigatran to thrombin) and neutralizes dabigatran activity.[77] Idarucizumab rapidly neutralizes the anticoagulation effect of dabigatran in a concentration-dependent manner, with complete neutralization at equimolar concentrations of idarucizumab and dabigatran.[77] Idarucizumab is specific to dabigatran and does not reverse the effects of other direct thrombin inhibitors such as argatroban or bivalirudin. A range of doses has been studied and shown to be effective in phase I studies.[78,79] In a prospective, single arm trial which included 18 patients with ICH, patients received a dose of 5 g administered as 2 consecutive 2.5-g doses given as 50-mL boluses.[80] While idarucizumab is structurally similar to thrombin, it does not functionally mimic thrombin activity. In vitro studies and in vivo animal studies have found no effect of idarucizumab on coagulation times, thrombin generation, conversion of fibrinogen to fibrin, or platelet aggregation, suggesting a lack of prothrombotic activity with idarucizumab.[77] However, in a prospective study of patients with life-threatening bleed or need of urgent procedure, thrombotic events occurred in 5 of 90 patients, although there was no control arm for comparison.[77,80]

Prior to the approval of idarucizumab, many reversal guidelines recommended supportive therapy with 3- or 4-factor PCC or aPCC (FEIBA) for life-threatening bleeds or emergent surgery in patients receiving dabigatran.[12,81] With the availability of a targeted antidote, there no longer seems to be a role for the routine administration of adjunctive concentrated factors. However, although idarucizumab normalized the dTT and ECT in 88% to 98% of patients studied in the prospective REVERSE-AD trial, the median time to cessation of bleed in the 35 evaluable patients was 11.4 hours.[80] This is likely a result of the trial design and timing of follow-up radiographic studies to determine cessation of bleeding, as opposed to the actual onset of hemostasis. The small number of patients evaluated in this analysis, strict definitions of hemostasis employed, and lack of correlation with the more immediate changes seen in the dTT and ECT laboratory parameters make it difficult to predict whether such a delay will be seen when the drug is used in clinical practice. If so, some cases may still require adjunctive concentrated factors if hemostasis cannot be achieved quickly.[80]

Andexanet Alfa

Andexanet alfa is a modified recombinant protein that rapidly binds to direct factor Xa inhibitors and neutralizes their anticoagulant effect by reducing the fraction of free drug available. Andexanet alfa is structurally similar to factor Xa and has a similar binding affinity to direct Xa inhibitors as factor Xa, allowing it to act as a decoy for factor Xa inhibitors. In contrast to idarucizumab, which is a drug-specific antidote, andexanet alfa is a class-specific antidote, targeted against all of the direct oral factor Xa inhibitors (apixaban, rivaroxaban, and edoxaban). Andexanet alfa also reverses indirect factor Xa inhibitors such as enoxaparin and fondaparinux by competing with factor Xa for the antithrombin III (ATIII) binding site, which prevents formation of the active ATIII-heparin complex. Andexanet alfa has several mutations at its active sites, making it enzymatically inactive.[82] In ex vivo clotting assays, there was no difference in thrombin generation in the presence of andexanet alfa, demonstrating its lack of procoagulant activity.[82] In a study of 145 healthy, older volunteers who received apixaban 5 mg twice daily or rivaroxaban 20 mg daily, patients were randomized to placebo or andexanet alfa as a bolus alone or a bolus followed by a 2-hour continuous infusion.[83] Patients in the apixaban group received a bolus of 400 mg IV or a bolus followed by a continuous infusion (400 mg IV, then 4 mg per minute for 120 minutes), and patients in the rivaroxaban group received a bolus of 800 mg IV or a bolus followed by a continuous infusion (800 mg IV, then 8 mg per minute for 120 minutes). A higher dose was administered for rivaroxaban reversal due to the higher initial maximum plasma concentrations and larger volume of distribution of rivaroxaban. Anti–factor Xa activity was significantly reduced with the bolus alone (94% reduction in apixaban group, 92% reduction in rivaroxaban group) and with the bolus plus continuous infusion (92% in apixaban group, 97% in rivaroxaban group) compared with placebo. In addition, thrombin generation was restored to above the lower limit of normal within 2 to 5 minutes after administration of andexanet in almost all patients. In all groups, anti–factor Xa activity returned to that of placebo levels 1 to 2 hours after completion of the infusion. No thrombotic events or serious adverse events were reported in this study. Depending on the half-life of the anticoagulant, longer infusions or repeat boluses may be necessary for patients with continued bleeding to allow for elimination of the anticoagulant.[84] Studies in patients with life-threatening bleeds are needed to confirm that the positive surrogate changes seen in healthy volunteers correlate with clinical outcomes in a real-world setting.[85,86]

Ciraparantag (PER977)

Ciraparantag (previously referred to as aripazine) is a water-soluble, cationic synthetic molecule that combines with anticoagulants through noncovalent hydrogen bonding to neutralize their activity.[86] Ciraparantag binds to UFH, LMWH, the oral factor Xa inhibitors (apixaban, rivaroxaban, and edoxaban), and the oral thrombin inhibitor (dabigatran). Animal studies have shown a decrease in blood loss in animals receiving rivaroxaban, apixaban, and dabigatran, and ex vivo human studies with apixaban and rivaroxaban have shown a decrease in anticoagulant activity as measured by aPTT and anti–factor Xa levels.[86] In a randomized, controlled study of 80 healthy volunteers who received 1 dose of edoxaban 60 mg followed by placebo or a single dose of ciraparantag 100 to 300 mg, whole-blood clotting time decreased to baseline values within 10 minutes and was sustained for 24 hours in the ciraparantag group. There were no changes in D-dimer, prothrombin fragments, or tissue factor pathway inhibitor, indicating a lack of procoagulant activity. Side effects included transient flushing, dysgeusia, and headache.[87] Ciraparantag is not yet FDA approved, but clinical investigations are ongoing.

Extracorporeal Removal

Extracorporeal removal of the offending agent may be a helpful option in some scenarios, particularly for antithrombotics that do not have targeted reversal agents. Hemodialysis may also be helpful for patients with renal insufficiency who are on medications that are renally cleared. In these cases, the expected half-life of the medication is prolonged and a rebound effect may occur, wherein the hemostatic interventions wear off before the antithrombotic has been fully eliminated. Drugs with a low molecular weight, low protein binding, and low volume of distribution are more amenable to removal by hemodialysis. The antiplatelet agents clopidogrel, prasugrel, and ticagrelor (or their active metabolites) are highly protein bound (≥98%) and are not candidates for dialysis. Aspirin is highly protein bound (90%), but protein binding decreases with higher concentrations (to 30% after an overdose). Hemodialysis is currently recommended in aspirin overdose cases to manage the acid/base disturbances, not to reverse bleeding.[88] Aspirin irreversibly inhibits platelets for their life span (~10 days), so extracorporeal removal of aspirin in an overdose setting would not expect to reverse its antiplatelet effects or decrease bleeding. Apixaban and rivaroxaban are highly protein bound (87% and 90%, respectively) and are not candidates for hemodialysis. Edoxaban has lower protein binding of 55%, but a study of 10 patients with end-stage renal disease who received one 15-mg dose of edoxaban showed no difference in mean total edoxaban area under the curve after hemodialysis compared with no hemodialysis.[89] Dabigatran exhibits low protein binding (35%), has a low molecular weight, is hydrophilic, and is primarily renally eliminated (80%), making it a potential candidate for hemodialysis.[90] In a study of 35 healthy volunteers who received a single dose of 150 mg (normal renal function and mild, moderate, or severe renal impairment) or 50 mg (end-stage renal disease on hemodialysis), 1 session of hemodialysis removed 62% of dabigatran after 2 hours and 68% after 4 hours.[91] Another study of patients with end-stage renal failure who received 3 days of dabigatran followed by a 4-hour hemodialysis session found that hemodialysis removed 49% of dabigatran at a rate of 200 mL/min and 59% of dabigatran at a rate of 400 mL/min with a linear reduction in its anticoagulation activity. Mean plasma dabigatran concentrations increased by 7.2% (200-mL/min group) and 15.5% (400-mL/min group) after the end of hemodialysis perhaps due to the moderate volume of distribution (60–70 L) of dabigatran resulting in redistribution.[92] One case report showed a significant decrease in dabigatran concentrations immediately following a 3-hour hemodialysis session (from 49 ng/mL at hour 1 of hemodialysis to 29 ng/mL at hour 3), although a notable rebound 2 hours posthemodialysis (43 ng/mL) was also reported.[93] Hemodialysis may be a useful option when the patient is stable enough to be dialyzed, the patient has acute or existing renal dysfunction resulting in a prolonged half-life of dabigatran, and access to hemodialysis and placement of lines can be provided in a timely manner.[26] Hemodialysis carries additional risks in patients with intracranial hemorrhage and may worsen cerebral edema and intracranial pressure due to dramatic fluid shifts and a decrease in serum urea. For these reasons, hemodialysis should be used judiciously in patients with ICH, even when used to remove antithrombotics that are considered dialyzable. Continuous renal replacement therapy may carry a lower risk of complications in these cases, but the reduced flow rates may produce ineffective elimination of the antithrombotic.[4] One case series that used hemodialysis for dabigatran reversal reported a case where continuous veno-venous hemodialysis (CVVHD) was initiated after a 2-hour session of hemodialysis. A rebound in dabigatran concentrations the day after hemodialysis was reported (632 ng/mL from 420 ng/mL), but no rebound increase was noted after CVVHD (follow-up concentration was 121 ng/mL).[37] Another case series that included 1 patient who received initial treatment with continuous veno-venous hemofiltration (CVVH) showed a rebound increase in dabigatran concentrations during CVVH (60 ng/mL to 22 ng/mL to 63 ng/mL), which subsequently decreased after initiation of hemodialysis.[94] Data are lacking on the efficacy of continuous renal replacement therapy alone for dabigatran-related life-threatening bleeds.

Plasmapheresis has been reported in 2 patients receiving oral direct acting anticoagulants. In 1 case, a patient on dabigatran, aspirin, and ibuprofen presented with a gastrointestinal bleed and remained hemodynamically unstable with a downtrending hemoglobin despite receiving blood, plasma, platelets, PCC, an esomeprazole infusion, and endoscopic treatment with topical epinephrine. After 1 session of plasmapheresis, the hemoglobin and vital signs stabilized and the patient was extubated the following day.[95] Another case report describes a patient on apixaban who developed hemorrhagic tamponade following a pacemaker implantation. The patient declined PCC due to the potential thrombotic risk, was ineligible for activated charcoal as the time from his last ingestion was more than 6 hours, and was not a candidate for hemodialysis since apixaban is poorly dialyzable. The patient received a 2-hour session of plasma exchange with 3 L of plasma (1 plasma volume) with a subsequent reduction in his anti-Xa levels (UFH assay: 0.22 units/mL from 0.76 units/mL; LMWH assay: 0.35 units/mL from 0.84 units/mL) and was able to undergo a pericardiocentesis.[96] Plasmapheresis may be a potential consideration for some patients with limited treatment options, but currently the efficacy of plasma exchange for the reversal of life-threatening bleeds is limited to case reports. Generally, drugs with a low volume of distribution and high protein binding are more likely to be removed by plasmapheresis.[97]

GENERAL PRINCIPLES OF REVERSING THE EFFECTS OF ANTICOAGULANTS

Most guidelines for the reversal of life-threatening bleeds recommend similar basic management principles such as cessation of any antithrombotic agents; supportive treatment with blood products, concentrated factors, pharmacologic hemostatic agents, or vasopressors when indicated; and extracorporeal removal strategies such as hemodialysis when clinically appropriate.[4] Targeted reversal agents such as phytonadione (vitamin K) for patients receiving vitamin K antagonists and idarucizumab for those on dabigatran are a relatively straightforward treatment option. Other treatments such as concentrated blood factors, pharmacologic therapy, and blood products are more controversial with regards to their role in therapy, dose, and clinical effectiveness. In these cases, clinicians must use a combination of available evidence, the pharmacokinetic and pharmacodynamic properties of the antithrombotic, patient-specific factors such as age and renal function, and an overall assessment of the risk of hemorrhagic expansion vs risk of a thrombotic event to guide management of these complex scenarios. Timing since last ingestion is a very important consideration and requires extensive knowledge about not only the drug's pharmacokinetic parameters but also the patient's history, including last known ingestion, renal and hepatic function, age, interacting medications, and laboratory measurements such as PT, aPTT, INR, and thrombin time when available. Timing will also determine if there is a benefit to administering activated charcoal. Drug-specific properties such as the route of elimination (hepatic vs renal), half-life, and protein binding may help individualize therapy, predict the expected duration of anticoagulation, and determine if there is a role for extracorporeal removal or repeat dosing of reversal agents. While the direct-acting oral anticoagulants have a shorter half-life than warfarin, they are all, to some extent, renally eliminated, with dabigatran being the most highly dependent on renal function (80% renally eliminated) and apixaban being the least dependent (25% renally eliminated). In patients with severe renal impairment (creatinine clearance <30 mL/min), the terminal half-life of dabigatran was doubled (28 vs 14 hours) and aPTT and ECT prolonged after a single dose compared with patients with normal renal function.[91] In elderly patients with seemingly normal serum creatinine levels, a certain degree of renal dysfunction should be considered, thus prolonging the half-life.

Balancing the Risk of Continued Hemorrhage and ICH Expansion vs Thrombotic Risk

Careful consideration should be used when developing a plan for anticoagulant reversal in patients with various comorbidities, which increase the risk of thrombotic complications. In addition, understanding the intensity of anticoagulation, time of bleed onset, and risk for hematoma expansion will help determine the priority level for reversal to achieve adequate hemostasis and reduce the risk of a thromboembolic event. For example, smaller intracranial hemorrhages with normal neurological examinations may not warrant the use of aggressive reversal of the anticoagulant in a patient who presents greater than 6 hours after the initial ictus. Therefore, a clinician needs to consider a number of factors, which include but are not limited to the following[53]:

- Medication history
  - Dose and frequency of anticoagulant
  - Time since last dose
  - Use of medications that contribute to thrombosis
  - Allergies or concern for heparin-induced thrombocytopenia
- Medical/surgical history
  - History of hypercoagulable condition
  - Nonvalvular atrial fibrillation
  - Presence of cardiac thrombus on recent echocardiogram
  - Positive history or at high risk for developing venous thromboembolism
  - Type and position of cardiac valve
  - Recent administration of concentrated clotting factors
  - Mechanical device or vascular hardware
  - Arterial thromboembolic disease

- Physical and neurological examination
  - Vital signs
  - External evidence of hemorrhage
  - Clinical status
- Imaging
  - Diagnosis of internal hemorrhage
  - Access to bleeding site
- Laboratory tests
  - Level of anticoagulation
  - Markers for blood loss
  - Organ function

Clinical Pathways, Protocols, and Order Sets

Although life-threatening bleeds commonly occur in the emergency department, operating room, and intensive care unit, they are prevalent throughout the hospital setting. It is necessary to develop guidelines to ensure quick and efficient pathways to appropriate treatment. National guidelines are helpful in providing summarized recommendations based on the best available data, but they may offer multiple different treatment strategies and dosing regimens for a specific scenario and usually provide more general recommendations. Moreover, the agents they recommend may not be available in every hospital setting. Institutional protocols streamline the process by guiding providers to the preferred management strategies within the institution, the available formulary options and doses, and the approval mechanism for specific treatments. Institutional protocols also provide standardization and consistency by drawing consensus from key stakeholders on the desired therapy for specific indications, a standardized algorithm for care, and case-specific options for challenging scenarios. The ideal protocols will outline a process that enables any prescriber to easily submit orders for the recommended treatments; guide the pharmacy or blood bank to review, verify and prepare the order; and provide instructions on how the product will be emergently delivered. There may be different processes for different areas of the hospital such as the emergency department or operating room as well as for different types of bleeds (intracranial vs gastrointestinal) and procedures (cardiac surgery vs neurosurgery).

Despite the availability of guidelines and protocols, some patients do not receive the recommended treatment often due to lack of adherence to the guidelines or unsatisfactory knowledge of the appropriate treatment strategies.[98,99] Due to the wide array of available anticoagulants and antiplatelets and differences in their pharmacokinetic and pharmacodynamic profiles, an electronic pathway or order set can provide both general management strategies and targeted, individualized therapy recommendations for unique scenarios. Electronic order sets with prepopulated doses, automatic dosing calculations, rounding strategies, and inclusion of adjunctive therapy allow for easy, more accurate ordering of treatments. For example, the reversal of warfarin requires both blood products or concentrated factors and vitamin K. The focus is generally placed on the blood products and concentrated factors because of their faster onset of action; however, this may lead to the omission of vitamin K. Moreover, the confusion surrounding concentrated factor preparations (the amount of factors vary from vial to vial) may lead to incorrect initial dosing. For example, a 500-unit vial of Kcentra may actually only contain 485 units. Depending on the institution's protocol, an order for 500 units may be delayed while the pharmacist recommends a change to the correct vial content of 485 units. An order set with prepopulated treatment recommendations that include the dose of concentrated factors and vitamin K as prechecked or auto-calculated items will help prevent the omission of vitamin K and ensure that both medications are ordered correctly. Protocols that allow for dose rounding to the nearest vial may decrease delays resulting from having to call, clarify, and rewrite the orders. These logistical barriers can be removed by allowing a pharmacist to automatically change the dose to the nearest vial size.

Expedited Consultation and Approval

When uncertainty exists, consultation with an expert such as a critical care pharmacist, hematologist, or critical care or transfusion medicine physician is ideal, but these resources are not always available 24/7. In addition, waiting for a consultation may lead to unnecessary delays in straightforward cases, such as those that have a targeted reversal recommendation (eg, idarucizumab for dabigatran). Setting up a 24/7 expedited consultative and approval process can speed up treatment turnaround time and facilitate a management plan. It may also prevent a patient from receiving unnecessary blood products (such as FFP for reversal of warfarin in a patient who will receive PCC4). The inherent risk of a continuing life-threatening bleed, hemorrhagic expansion of an ICH, or need for emergent surgery requires a sense of urgency and the application of interventions rapidly. The risks associated with severity of bleed often make the decision to reverse the patient's antithrombotic while accepting the thrombotic risks more straightforward. The decision becomes more complex for major bleeds that are non–life-threatening and urgent but not emergent procedures where the benefit of hemostasis may no longer outweigh the major thrombotic risks such as pulmonary embolism, myocardial infarction, and stroke. Having an emergency consultant in place can help provide expert guided treatment recommendations in these more challenging cases.

Practice Pearls

Formulary availability is a major consideration whenever access to treatment is needed emergently. In the case of life-threatening bleeds, the acuity of the bleed requires emergent therapy with a readily accessible agent. Formulary options and alternatives should be decided in advance, with consensus from key players such as intensivists, hematologists, surgeons, and pharmacists. Guideline-driven therapy is critical and may prevent major delays that stem from knowledge deficits about available products, the appropriate ordering process, recommended dosing, and source of medication (ie, pharmacy, blood bank, automated dispensing cabinet). Waste control is necessary considering the high cost and short stability of many of these agents. Implementing a stewardship program with an expedited approval system in conjunction with guidelines on product preparation can help decrease inappropriate use and waste of these products. Institutions should determine who prepares the medications (pharmacy vs nursing) in advance. Benefits to pharmacy preparation include a labeled, ready-to-use product with instructions and preparation in a clean room or hood. For example, the PCC4 product, Kcentra, may require reconstitution of up to 10 vials for a single dose, which may take up significant nursing time to both reconstitute and administer. Pharmacy can help by reconstituting the vials and pooling together in an empty bag that can be hung as a rapid infusion with an IV pump. Issues surrounding pharmacy preparation include perceived delay to obtaining the medication and wasted drug in scenarios where the vial is reconstituted and subsequently not used by the time the medication reaches the patient. For these reasons, some institutions advocate for bedside preparation of concentrated factors. Settings such as the operating room where patients have rapidly changing hemodynamics and close monitoring by multiple physicians and nurses may be better suited for medication preparation outside of the pharmacy. Any process should be reviewed to ensure that it provides the medication in a safe way that improves the speed and ease of administration while minimizing waste. Whether the drug will be picked up at the pharmacy or blood bank or delivered should also be clarified in advance as well as the location the drug should be delivered to, particularly for patients en route to the operating room. Many of these seemingly easy processes account for some of the most significant barriers to rapid treatment. Finally, quality assessments on guideline adherence and outcomes should be performed routinely to ensure that best practices are followed.

CONCLUSION

Rapidly reversing anticoagulation in patients with severe, life-threatening bleeds or those in need of emergent surgery is critical, but the optimal treatment strategy remains controversial. Even the term *bleeding reversal* is a misnomer, especially in the case of irreversible antithrombotics where bleeding is managed supportively with hemostatic agents rather than through reversal of the offending agent.

Conflicting data exist regarding many of the pharmacologic interventions and blood product selections for the reversal of life-threatening hemorrhages. With only a few large, well-designed, randomized controlled trials available, much of the treatment has been left up to expert opinion and institutional protocols. As such, successful reversal of antithrombotics in patients with ICH requires knowledge of the offending drug's pharmacokinetic and pharmacodynamic properties, available interventions and agents for reversal, and risk-benefit analyses. Rapid decision making and in many instances aggressive treatment are necessary to prevent hemorrhagic expansion and/or allow for emergent procedures or surgery. In the absence of a substantive evidence base, patient-specific characteristics such as severity of bleed, risk of thrombosis, antithrombotic regimen, last known time of ingestion, age, and renal function should guide therapy. Factoring in the logistical issues related to engagement of the multiprofessional team of experts and establishing expedited pathways and protocols (with frequent updates) that streamline the correct therapies to the patient in a timely manner are pragmatic steps that can help optimize care of these patients. As new agents are approved and the armamentarium of data continues to evolve, guidelines and protocols will have to be updated to reflect best practices.

References

1. Flaherty ML, Kissela B, Woo D, et al. The increasing incidence of anticoagulant-associated intracerebral hemorrhage. *Neurology*. 2007;68:116–121.
2. Rosand J, Eckman MH, Knudsen KA, et al. The effect of warfarin and intensity of anticoagulation on outcome of intracerebral hemorrhage. *Arch Intern Med*. 2004; 164:880–884.
3. Flibotte JJ, Hagan N, O'Donnell J, et al. Warfarin, hematoma expansion, and outcome of intracerebral hemorrhage. *Neurology*. 2004;63:1059–1064.
4. Frontera JA, Lewin JJ III, Rabinstein AA, et al. Guideline for reversal of antithrombotics in intracranial hemorrhage: a statement for healthcare professionals from the Neurocritical Care Society and Society of Critical Care Medicine. *Neurocrit Care*. 2016;24: 6–46.

5. Davie EW, Ratnoff OD. Waterfall sequence for intrinsic blood clotting. *Science.* 1964;145:1310–1312.

6. Furie B, Furie BC. Mechanisms of thrombus formation. *N Engl J Med.* 2008; 359:938–949.

7. Qureshi AI, Tuhrim S, Broderick JP, et al. Spontaneous intracerebral hemorrhage. *N Engl J Med.* 2001;344:1450–1460.

8. Davis SM, Broderick J, Hennerici M, et al. Hematoma growth is a determinant of mortality and poor outcome after intracerebral hemorrhage. *Neurology.* 2006;66:1175–1181.

9. Kuramatsu JB, Gerner ST, Schellinger PD, et al. Anticoagulant reversal, blood pressure levels, and anticoagulant resumption in patients with anticoagulation-related intracerebral hemorrhage. *JAMA.* 2015;313:824–836.

10. Franke CL, de Jonge J, van Swieten JC, et al. Intracerebral hematomas during anticoagulant treatment. *Stroke.* 1990;21:726–730.

11. Fogelholm R, Eskola K, Kiminkinen T, et al. Anticoagulant treatment as a risk factor for primary intracerebral haemorrhage. *J Neurol Neurosurg Psychiatry.* 1992; 55:1121–1124.

12. Dager WE, Gosselin RC, Roberts AJ. Reversing dabigatran in life-threatening bleeding occurring during cardiac ablation with factor eight inhibitor bypassing activity. *Crit Care Med.* 2013;41:e42–e46.

13. Skolnick BE, Mathews DR, Khutoryansky NM, et al. Exploratory study on the reversal of warfarin with rFVIIa in healthy subjects. *Blood.* 2010;116:693–701.

14. Garcia DA, Baglin TP, Weitz JI, Samama MM. Parenteral anticoagulants: Antithrombotic Therapy and Prevention of Thrombosis, 9th ed: American College of Chest Physicians Evidence-Based Clinical Practice Guidelines. *Chest.* 2012;141:e24S-43S.

15. Ageno W, Gallus AS, Wittkowsky A, et al. Oral anticoagulant therapy: Antithrombotic Therapy and Prevention of Thrombosis, 9th ed: American College of Chest Physicians Evidence-Based Clinical Practice Guidelines. *Chest.* 2012;141:e44S-e88S.

16. Barrett YC, Wang Z, Frost C, Shenker A. Clinical laboratory measurement of direct factor Xa inhibitors: anti-Xa assay is preferable to prothrombin time assay. *Thromb Haemost.* 2010;104:1263–1271.

17. Samama MM, Martinoli JL, LeFlem L, et al. Assessment of laboratory assays to measure rivaroxaban—an oral, direct factor Xa inhibitor. *Thromb Haemost.* 2010;103:815–825.

18. Hillarp A, Gustafsson KM, Faxalv L, et al. Effects of the oral, direct factor Xa inhibitor apixaban on routine coagulation assays and anti-FXa assays. *J Thromb Haemost.* 2014;12:1545–1553.

19. Hillarp A, Baghaei F, Fagerberg Blixter I, et al. Effects of the oral, direct factor Xa inhibitor rivaroxaban on commonly used coagulation assays. *J Thromb Haemost.* 2011; 9:133–139.

20. Asmis LM, Alberio L, Angelillo-Scherrer A, et al. Rivaroxaban: quantification by anti-FXa assay and influence on coagulation tests: a study in 9 Swiss laboratories. *Thromb Res.* 2012;129:492–498.

21. Becker RC, Yang H, Barrett Y, et al. Chromogenic laboratory assays to measure the factor Xa-inhibiting properties of apixaban—an oral, direct and selective factor Xa inhibitor. *J Thromb Thrombolysis.* 2011;32:183–187.

22. Adcock DM, Gosselin R. Direct oral anticoagulants (DOACs) in the laboratory: 2015 review. *Thromb Res.* 2015;136:7–12.

23. Lindahl TL, Baghaei F, Blixter IF, et al. Effects of the oral, direct thrombin inhibitor dabigatran on five common coagulation assays. *Thromb Haemost.* 2011;105:371–378.

24. Weitz JI, Quinlan DJ, Eikelboom JW. Periprocedural management and approach to bleeding in patients taking dabigatran. *Circulation*. 2012;126:2428–2432.

25. Hawes EM, Deal AM, Funk-Adcock D, et al. Performance of coagulation tests in patients on therapeutic doses of dabigatran: a cross-sectional pharmacodynamic study based on peak and trough plasma levels. *J Thromb Haemost*. 2013;11:1493–1502.

26. van Ryn J, Stangier J, Haertter S, et al. Dabigatran etexilate—a novel, reversible, oral direct thrombin inhibitor: interpretation of coagulation assays and reversal of anticoagulant activity. *Thromb Haemost*. 2010;103:1116–1127.

27. Dager WE, Gosselin RC, Kitchen S, Dwyre D. Dabigatran effects on the international normalized ratio, activated partial thromboplastin time, thrombin time, and fibrinogen: a multicenter, in vitro study. *Ann Pharmacother*. 2012;46:1627–1636.

28. Stangier J, Feuring M. Using the HEMOCLOT direct thrombin inhibitor assay to determine plasma concentrations of dabigatran. *Blood Coagul Fibrinolysis*. 2012;23:138–143.

29. Lange U, Nowak G, Bucha E. Ecarin chromogenic assay—a new method for quantitative determination of direct thrombin inhibitors like hirudin. *Pathophysiol Haemost Thromb*. 2003;33:184–191.

30. Douxfils J, Mullier F, Robert S, et al. Impact of dabigatran on a large panel of routine or specific coagulation assays: laboratory recommendations for monitoring of dabigatran etexilate. *Thromb Haemost*. 2012;107:985–997.

31. Paniccia R, Priora R, Liotta AA, Abbate R. Platelet function tests: a comparative review. *Vasc Health Risk Manag*. 2015;11:133–148.

32. Li X, Sun Z, Zhao W, et al. Effect of acetylsalicylic acid usage and platelet transfusion on postoperative hemorrhage and activities of daily living in patients with acute intracerebral hemorrhage. *J Neurosurg*. 2013;118:94–103.

33. Naidech AM, Jovanovic B, Liebling S, et al. Reduced platelet activity is associated with early clot growth and worse 3-month outcome after intracerebral hemorrhage. *Stroke*. 2009;40:2398–2401.

34. Naidech AM, Liebling SM, Rosenberg NF, et al. Early platelet transfusion improves platelet activity and may improve outcomes after intracerebral hemorrhage. *Neurocrit Care*. 2012;16:82–87.

35. Zhou W, Schwarting S, Illanes S, et al. Hemostatic therapy in experimental intracerebral hemorrhage associated with the direct thrombin inhibitor dabigatran. *Stroke*. 2011;42:3594–3599.

36. Zhou W, Zorn M, Nawroth P, et al. Hemostatic therapy in experimental intracerebral hemorrhage associated with rivaroxaban. *Stroke*. 2013;44:771–778.

37. Kumar R, Smith RE, Henry BL. A review of and recommendations for the management of patients with life-threatening dabigatran-associated hemorrhage: a single-center university hospital experience. *J Intensive Care Med*. 2015;30:462–472.

38. Steiner T, Rosand J, Diringer M. Intracerebral hemorrhage associated with oral anticoagulant therapy: current practices and unresolved questions. *Stroke*. 2006;37:256–262.

39. Woo CH, Patel N, Conell C, et al. Rapid warfarin reversal in the setting of intracranial hemorrhage: a comparison of plasma, recombinant activated factor VII, and prothrombin complex concentrate. *World Neurosurg*. 2014;81:110–115.

40. Cervera A, Amaro S, Chamorro A. Oral anticoagulant-associated intracerebral hemorrhage. *J Neurol*. 2012;259:212–224.

41. Lee SB, Manno EM, Layton KF, Wijdicks EF. Progression of warfarin-associated intracerebral hemorrhage after INR normalization with FFP. *Neurology*. 2006;67:1272–1274.

42. Chapman SA, Irwin ED, Beal AL, et al. Prothrombin complex concentrate versus standard therapies for INR reversal in trauma patients receiving warfarin. *Ann Pharmacother.* 2011;45:869–875.

43. Goldstein JN, Thomas SH, Frontiero V, et al. Timing of fresh frozen plasma administration and rapid correction of coagulopathy in warfarin-related intracerebral hemorrhage. *Stroke.* 2006;37:151–155.

44. Huttner HB, Schellinger PD, Hartmann M, et al. Hematoma growth and outcome in treated neurocritical care patients with intracerebral hemorrhage related to oral anticoagulant therapy: comparison of acute treatment strategies using vitamin K, fresh frozen plasma, and prothrombin complex concentrates. *Stroke.* 2006;37:1465–1470.

45. Steiner T, Poli S, Griebe M, et al. Fresh frozen plasma versus prothrombin complex concentrate in patients with intracranial haemorrhage related to vitamin K antagonists (INCH): a randomised trial. *Lancet Neurol.* 2016;15:566–573.

46. Sarode R, Milling TJ Jr, Refaai MA, et al. Efficacy and safety of a 4-factor prothrombin complex concentrate in patients on vitamin K antagonists presenting with major bleeding: a randomized, plasma-controlled, phase IIIb study. *Circulation.* 2013;128:1234–1243.

47. Goldstein JN, Refaai MA, Milling TJ Jr, et al. Four-factor prothrombin complex concentrate versus plasma for rapid vitamin K antagonist reversal in patients needing urgent surgical or invasive interventions: a phase 3b, open-label, non-inferiority, randomised trial. *Lancet.* 2015;385:2077–2087.

48. Matrat A, De Mazancourt P, Derex L, et al. Characterization of a severe hypofibrinogenemia induced by alteplase in two patients thrombolysed for stroke. *Thromb Res.* 2013;131:e45–e48.

49. Sun X, Berthiller J, Trouillas P, et al. Early fibrinogen degradation coagulopathy: a predictive factor of parenchymal hematomas in cerebral rt-PA thrombolysis. *J Neurol Sci.* 2015;351:109–114.

50. Yaghi S, Boehme AK, Dibu J, et al. Treatment and outcome of thrombolysis-related hemorrhage: a multicenter retrospective study. *JAMA Neurol.* 2015;72:1451–1457.

51. Baharoglu MI, Cordonnier C, Al-Shahi Salman R, et al. Platelet transfusion versus standard care after acute stroke due to spontaneous cerebral haemorrhage associated with antiplatelet therapy (PATCH): a randomised, open-label, phase 3 trial. *Lancet.* 2016; 387:2605–2613.

52. Pabinger I, Brenner B, Kalina U, et al. Prothrombin complex concentrate (Beriplex P/N) for emergency anticoagulation reversal: a prospective multinational clinical trial. *J Thromb Haemost.* 2008;6:622–631.

53. Nutescu EA, Dager WE, Kalus JS, et al. Management of bleeding and reversal strategies for oral anticoagulants: clinical practice considerations. *Am J Health Syst Pharm.* 2013; 70:1914–1929.

54. Kcentra (prothrombin complex concentrates, human) [prescribing information]. Kankakee, IL: CSL Behring, LLC; 2014.

55. Bebulin (factor IX complex) [prescribing information]. Westlake Village, CA: Baxter Healthcare Corporation; 2012.

56. Eerenberg ES, Kamphuisen PW, Sijpkens MK, et al. Reversal of rivaroxaban and dabigatran by prothrombin complex concentrate: a randomized, placebo-controlled, crossover study in healthy subjects. *Circulation.* 2011;124:1573–1579.

57. Dinkelaar J, Molenaar PJ, Ninivaggi M, et al. In vitro assessment, using thrombin generation, of the applicability of prothrombin complex concentrate as an antidote for rivaroxaban. *J Thromb Haemost.* 2013;11:1111–1118.

58. Herrmann R, Thom J, Wood A, et al. Thrombin generation using the calibrated automated thrombinoscope to assess reversibility of dabigatran and rivaroxaban. *Thromb Haemost.* 2014;111:989–995.

59. Perzborn E, Heitmeier S, Laux V, Buchmuller A. Reversal of rivaroxaban-induced anticoagulation with prothrombin complex concentrate, activated prothrombin complex concentrate and recombinant activated factor VII in vitro. *Thromb Res.* 2014; 133:671–681.

60. Sin JH, Berger K, Lesch CA. Four-factor prothrombin complex concentrate for life-threatening bleeds or emergent surgery: a retrospective evaluation. *J Crit Care.* 2016;36:166–172.

61. Novoseven RT (coagulation factor VIIa-recombinant) [prescribing information]. Plainsboro, NJ: Novo Nordisk; 2014.

62. Hemphill JC III, Greenberg SM, Anderson CS, et al. Guidelines for the management of spontaneous intracerebral hemorrhage: a guideline for healthcare professionals from the American Heart Association/American Stroke Association. *Stroke.* 2015;46: 2032–2060.

63. Mayer SA, Brun NC, Begtrup K, et al. Efficacy and safety of recombinant activated factor VII for acute intracerebral hemorrhage. *N Engl J Med.* 2008;358:2127–2137.

64. Friedman PA, Rosenberg RD, Hauschka PV, Fitz-James A. A spectrum of partially carboxylated prothrombins in the plasmas of coumarin-treated patients. *Biochim Biophys Acta.* 1977;494:271–276.

65. Tsu LV, Dienes JE, Dager WE. Vitamin K dosing to reverse warfarin based on INR, route of administration, and home warfarin dose in the acute/critical care setting. *Ann Pharmacother.* 2012;46:1617–1626.

66. Raj G, Kumar R, McKinney WP. Time course of reversal of anticoagulant effect of warfarin by intravenous and subcutaneous phytonadione. *Arch Intern Med.* 1999;159:2721–2724.

67. Watson HG, Baglin T, Laidlaw SL, Makris M, Preston FE. A comparison of the efficacy and rate of response to oral and intravenous vitamin K in reversal of over-anticoagulation with warfarin. *Br J Haematol.* 2001;115:145–149.

68. Whitling AM, Bussey HI, Lyons RM. Comparing different routes and doses of phytonadione for reversing excessive anticoagulation. *Arch Intern Med.* 1998;158:2136–2140.

69. Mi YN, Ping NN, Xiao X, et al. The severe adverse reaction to vitamin k1 injection is anaphylactoid reaction but not anaphylaxis. *PLoS One.* 2014;9:e90199.

70. Naidech AM, Maas MB, Levasseur-Franklin KE, et al. Desmopressin improves platelet activity in acute intracerebral hemorrhage. *Stroke.* 2014;45:2451–2453.

71. Kapapa T, Rohrer S, Struve S, et al. Desmopressin acetate in intracranial haemorrhage. *Neurol Res Int.* 2014;2014:298767.

72. French KF, White J, Hoesch RE. Treatment of intracerebral hemorrhage with tranexamic acid after thrombolysis with tissue plasminogen activator. *Neurocrit Care.* 2012;17:107–111.

73. Goldstein JN, Marrero M, Masrur S, et al. Management of thrombolysis-associated symptomatic intracerebral hemorrhage. *Arch Neurol.* 2010;67:965–969.

74. Parkin TW, Kvale WF. Neutralization of the anticoagulant effects of heparin with protamine (salmine). *Am Heart J.* 1949;37:333–342.

75. Crowther MA, Berry LR, Monagle PT, Chan AK. Mechanisms responsible for the failure of protamine to inactivate low-molecular-weight heparin. *Br J Haematol.* 2002;116: 178–186.

76. Holst J, Lindblad B, Bergqvist D, et al. Protamine neutralization of intravenous and sub-cutaneous low-molecular-weight heparin (tinzaparin, Logiparin): an experimental investigation in healthy volunteers. *Blood Coagul Fibrinolysis.* 1994;5:795–803.
77. Schiele F, van Ryn J, Canada K, et al. A specific antidote for dabigatran: functional and structural characterization. *Blood.* 2013;121:3554–3562.
78. Glund S, Moschetti V, Norris S, et al. A randomised study in healthy volunteers to inves-tigate the safety, tolerability and pharmacokinetics of idarucizumab, a specific antidote to dabigatran. *Thromb Haemost.* 2015;113:943–951.
79. Glund S, Stangier J, Schmohl M, et al. Safety, tolerability, and efficacy of idarucizumab for the reversal of the anticoagulant effect of dabigatran in healthy male volunteers: a randomised, placebo-controlled, double-blind phase 1 trial. *Lancet.* 2015;386: 680–690.
80. Pollack CV Jr, Reilly PA, Eikelboom J, et al. Idarucizumab for dabigatran reversal. *N Engl J Med.* 2015;373:511–520.
81. Heidbuchel H, Verhamme P, Alings M, et al. EHRA practical guide on the use of new oral anticoagulants in patients with non-valvular atrial fibrillation: executive summary. *Eur Heart J.* 2013;34:2094–2106.
82. Lu G, DeGuzman FR, Hollenbach SJ, et al. A specific antidote for reversal of antico-agulation by direct and indirect inhibitors of coagulation factor Xa. *Nat Med.* 2013;19:446–451.
83. Siegal DM, Curnutte JT, Connolly SJ, et al. Andexanet alfa for the reversal of factor Xa inhibitor activity. *N Engl J Med.* 2015;373:2413–2424.
84. Ansell JE. Universal, class-specific and drug-specific reversal agents for the new oral anticoagulants. *J Thromb Thrombolysis.* 2016;41(2):248–252.
85. Husted S, Verheugt FW, Comuth WJ. Reversal strategies for NOACs: state of develop-ment, possible clinical applications and future perspectives. *Drug Saf.* 2016;39:5–13.
86. Mo Y, Yam FK. Recent advances in the development of specific antidotes for target-specific oral anticoagulants. *Pharmacotherapy.* 2015;35:198–207.
87. Ansell JE, Bakhru SH, Laulicht BE, et al. Use of PER977 to reverse the anticoagulant effect of edoxaban. *N Engl J Med.* 2014;371:2141–2142.
88. Juurlink DN, Gosselin S, Kielstein JT, et al. Extracorporeal treatment for salicylate poi-soning: systematic review and recommendations from the EXTRIP workgroup. *Ann Emerg Med.* 2015;66:165–181.
89. Parasrampuria DA, Marbury T, Matsushima N, et al. Pharmacokinetics, safety, and tol-erability of edoxaban in end-stage renal disease subjects undergoing haemodialysis. *Thromb Haemost.* 2015;113:719–727.
90. Stangier J, Clemens A. Pharmacology, pharmacokinetics, and pharmacodynamics of dabigatran etexilate, an oral direct thrombin inhibitor. *Clin Appl Thromb Hemost.* 2009; 15(suppl 1):9s–16s.
91. Stangier J, Rathgen K, Stahle H, Mazur D. Influence of renal impairment on the pharma-cokinetics and pharmacodynamics of oral dabigatran etexilate: an open-label, parallel-group, single-centre study. *Clin Pharmacokinet.* 2010;49:259–268.
92. Khadzhynov D, Wagner F, Formella S, et al. Effective elimination of dabigatran by haemodialysis: a phase I single-centre study in patients with end-stage renal disease. *Thromb Haemost.* 2013;109:596–605.
93. Chang DN, Dager WE, Chin AI. Removal of dabigatran by hemodialysis. *Am J Kidney Dis.* 2013;61:487–489.

94. Ross B, Miller MA, Ditch K, Tran M. Clinical experience of life-threatening dabigatran-related bleeding at a large, tertiary care, academic medical center: a case series. *J Med Toxicol.* 2014;10:223–228.

95. Kamboj J, Kottalgi M, Cirra VR, et al. Direct thrombin inhibitors: a case indicating benefit from 'plasmapheresis' in toxicity: a call for establishing "guidelines" in overdose and to find an "antidote"! *Am J Ther.* 2012;19:e182–e185.

96. Lam WW, Reyes MA, Seger JJ. Plasma exchange for urgent apixaban reversal in a case of hemorrhagic tamponade after pacemaker implantation. *Tex Heart Inst J.* 2015;42:377–380.

97. Ibrahim RB, Liu C, Cronin SM, et al. Drug removal by plasmapheresis: an evidence-based review. *Pharmacotherapy.* 2007;27:1529–1549.

98. Grzegorski T, Andrzejewska N, Kazmierski R. Reversal of antithrombotic treatment in intracranial hemorrhage—a review of current strategies and guidelines. *Neurol Neurochir Pol.* 2015;49:278–289.

99. Rivosecchi RM, Garavaglia J, Kane-Gill SL. An evaluation of intravenous vitamin K for warfarin reversal: are guideline recommendations being followed? *Hosp Pharm.* 2015;50:18–24.

100. Hickey M, Gatien M, Taljaard M, et al. Outcomes of urgent warfarin reversal with frozen plasma versus prothrombin complex concentrate in the emergency department. *Circulation.* 2013;128:360–364.

101. O'Shaughnessy DF, Atterbury C, Bolton Maggs P, et al. Guidelines for the use of fresh-frozen plasma, cryoprecipitate and cryosupernatant. *Br J Haematol.* 2004;126:11–28.

102. Broderick J, Connolly S, Feldmann E, et al. Guidelines for the management of sponta-neous intracerebral hemorrhage in adults: 2007 update: a guideline from the American Heart Association/American Stroke Association Stroke Council, High Blood Pressure Research Council, and the Quality of Care and Outcomes in Research Interdisciplinary Working Group. *Stroke.* 2007;38:2001–2023.

103. Wójcik C, Schymik ML, Cure EG. Activated prothrombin complex concentrate factor VIII inhibitor bypassing activity (FEIBA) for the reversal of warfarin-induced coagu-lopathy. *Int J Emerg Med.* 2009;2:217–225.

Pharmacotherapy for Cerebral Vasospasm Prophylaxis and Treatment in Subarachnoid Hemorrhage

5

Denise H. Rhoney, Kathryn Morbitzer,
and Jimmi Hatton-Kolpek

INTRODUCTION

Aneurysmal subarachnoid hemorrhage (aSAH) accounts for approximately 7% of all stroke cases and is associated with high morbidity and mortality, primarily affecting individuals aged 40 to 60 years.[1–3] Population-based studies show that the incidence varies from 6 to 20 per 100,000 population, with the highest rates reported in Finland and Japan.[4,5] Rupture of a secular aneurysm(s) accounts for 80% of all the cases.[6] The course of the disease can be prolonged and can be associated with serious neurological complications that compromise patient outcomes. Approximately 50% of patients will die, while 15% will be rendered severely disabled. Only one-fifth to one-third of patients who experience a ruptured intracranial aneurysm will go on to have a moderate or good recovery.[7] The greatest impact can be based in terms of productive life years lost and higher medical costs in both acute and follow-up periods.[8,9] In large part, this poor prognosis is related to the development of cerebral vasospasm. Although recent advancements have reduced the incidence of poor outcomes related to cerebral vasospasm, it still remains the leading cause of clinical deterioration and poor outcomes following aSAH.

Intracranial aneurysms were described beginning in ancient times, with Biumi being credited for first describing in 1778 a verified case of a ruptured intracranial aneurysm.[10] Delayed cerebral ischemia (DCI) was described in 1859 in a 30-year-old woman.[10] However, angiographic cerebral vasospasm was not first described until 1951 by Ecker and Riemenschneider.[11] Later, Fisher et al[12] published 50 cases of ruptured saccular aneurysms investigating the relationship between development of delayed cerebral ischemic deficits and the presence of cerebral vasospasm verified on angiography and was one of the first to use the term *delayed ischemic deficits*. In this publication, he noted that these deficits develop 3 to 13 days after aSAH and were reversible in 50% of the cases, with severe angiographic vasospasm required to result in DCI. Weir et al[13] further refined the clinical time course by measuring cerebral artery diameters in 293 patients with aneurysm and indicated vasospasm is present 3 to 12 days after aSAH, with the highest incidence around days 7 to 8. In up to 25% of patients, the delayed infarcts seen on computed tomography scans are not located in the vascular territory of the spastic artery or are found in patients who develop vasospasm.[14,15] The predictive value of radiographic vasospasm for DCI is only about 67%.[16] More recent studies using perfusion imaging methods now suggest that only severe vasospasm with at least a 50% luminal narrowing produces reductions in cerebral blood flow enough to cause symptomatic ischemia.[17]

Vasospasm constitutes a reduction in the caliber of the vessel. Following aSAH, this narrowing of the cerebral vessel lumen can have significant clinical manifestations, including intermittent neurological deficits that can potentially lead to cerebral infarction. Arterial vasospasm typically appears 3 to 4 days after rupture and reaches a peak in incidence and severity at 7 to 10 days and usually resolves 12 to 14 days after onset.[13] Cerebral vasospasm is radiographically present in up to 70% of patients and is clinically evident in 20% to 30%.[18,19] The consequence of vasospasm is disability in 25% to 50% of survivors, with only 30% to 45% returning to previous comparable jobs, and it is the cause of death in 10% to 23% of patients.[20,21]

RISK FACTORS

Studies have attempted to predict patients who are more likely to develop vasospasm after aSAH; however, no single risk factor or model can accurately predict every case of symptomatic vasospasm.[22,23] The strongest risk factor appears to be the volume of subarachnoid clot present, with patients with larger clot volumes at highest risk.[24] The Fisher grading scale has traditionally been used to grade the extent of the hemorrhage, but this scale has been modified to correct some of the initial limitations and has now shown to be more predictive for symptomatic vasospasm and prognosis. The modified scale criteria were as follows: grade 0, no aSAH or intraventricular hemorrhage (IVH); grade 1, focal or diffuse thin aSAH with no IVH; grade 2, focal or diffuse thin aSAH with

IVH; grade 3, focal or diffuse thick aSAH with no IVH; and grade 4, focal or diffuse thick aSAH with IVH.[25] This modification of the Fisher scale showed a stronger association of computed tomography (CT) findings with symptomatic vasospasm than the original scale.[25,26] In addition, the severity and duration of vasospasm is related to the thickness, density, location, and persistence of the subarachnoid blood.[27] Several other risk factors have also shown to be predictive of vasospasm, including clinical grade on admission, history of cigarette smoking, history of hypertension, and cocaine use.[28,29] Factors such as age, sex, aneurysm location, and treatment modality for aneurysm protection have been investigated, but definitive evidence linking them as strong risk factors is lacking.[23,30,31] Currently, investigators are assessing the role of genetic polymorphisms in predicting the risk of vasospasm and DCI. Recently, Gallek et al[32] reported differences in endothelin 1 (ET-1) cerebrospinal fluid exposure rates related to polymorphisms of the ET-1 gene in the aSAH population. These differences in genotypes may be a future way to inform clinical decision making and identifying patients at high risk for vasospasm.[32]

NOMENCLATURE

The term *cerebral vasospasm* is commonly used interchangeably to refer to both the clinical picture of delayed onset of ischemic neurological deficits associated with aSAH (symptomatic vasospasm) and the narrowing of cerebral vessels documented by angiography or other studies (angiographic or arterial vasospasm). Cerebral vasospasm can be defined as the delayed narrowing of the large arteries within the basal cisterns, which may be associated with clinical or radiographic signs of ischemia in the areas of the brain supplied by the spastic artery. *DCI* is an umbrella term in the literature that encompasses a number of clinical entities, including symptomatic vasospasm, delayed ischemic neurological deficit (DIND), and asymptomatic delayed cerebral infarction. Not all patients who develop vasospasm develop DCI. *DIND* is a much broader term that includes delayed neurologic deficits that occur with or without angiographic vasospasm. Ultimately, DCI is a clinical diagnosis of exclusion that may be hard to recognize in poor clinical grade aSAH patients. In 2010, a consensus statement by a multidisciplinary panel proposed new definitions for clinical deterioration caused by DCI and cerebral infarction after aSAH and was further supported by the 2011 Neurocritical Care Society consensus guidelines.[33,34] This group advocated for a separation of DCI from vasospasm after aSAH.

- DCI = the occurrence of focal neurological impairment (such as hemiparesis, aphasia, apraxia, or neglect) or a decrease of at least 2 points on the Glasgow Coma Scale (either the total scale or 1 component of the scale). This should last for at least 1 hour, not be apparent immediately after the aneurysm occlusion, and not be attributed to other causes.
- Cerebral infarction = the presence of cerebral infarction by CT or magnetic resonance imaging within 6 weeks after aSAH and not present between 24 and 48 hours after early occlusions and not attributable to other causes such as surgical clipping or endovascular treatment.

PATHOPHYSIOLOGY

The development of effective preventative and therapeutic interventions for cerebral vasospasm has been hindered by the lack of understanding of the underlying pathophysiological mechanisms. Cerebral vasospasm is a multifactorial process that involves different pathological changes that occur at different time points, resulting in early (acute) and delayed (chronic) vasospasm (Figure 5.1). Early vasospasm begins within 3 to 4 hours after aSAH while delayed vasospasm presents with gradual onset and presents us with the largest clinical challenge in management. As previously discussed, vasospasm generally refers to angiographic vasospasm, and for decades it was thought that angiographic vasospasm was the most important cause of DIND or DCI. However, this assumption has recently been called into question, especially with the publication of the Clazosentan to Overcome Neurological Ischemia and Infarct Occurring After Subarachnoid Hemorrhage (CONSCIOUS)study that showed clazosentan was effective in reducing moderate and severe angiographic vasospasm but had no impact on overall outcome.[35] This has led many to describe DIND now as a multifactorial process resulting not only from angiographic vasospasm but also from early brain injury and cortical spreading depression, which may induce spreading ischemia on a microvascular level.

Early brain injury has been used to describe the mechanisms of acute (first 72 hours) neurologic deterioration after aSAH and is the result of physiological derangements such as increased intracranial pressure, decreased cerebral blood flow, and global cerebral ischemia. These physiologic derangements will result in blood–brain barrier dysfunction, inflammation, and oxidative cascades that lead to neuronal cell death. For a more detailed discussion of these pathophysiological changes that occur with early brain injury, the reader should refer to recent comprehensive review articles.[36–38] In the acute phase, cerebral vasospasm occurs through calcium-dependent mechanisms. As a result of hemoglobin

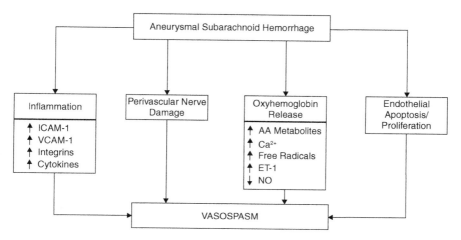

FIGURE 5.1. Pathophysiology of vasospasm.

exposure, there is an increase in intracellular calcium that drives myosin light chain kinase to phosphorylate the myosin light chains, which in turn will produce a transient contraction. Following aSAH, there is an overall increased calcium channel density with calcium influx and subsequent vasoconstriction. However, the mechanisms for the delayed vasospasm are largely due to calcium-independent mechanisms.[39]

Cerebral vasospasm is radiographically recognized as a reduction in the luminal wall of the intracranial arteries, but it has not been clearly established if this narrowing is a result of vasoconstriction alone or if it also involves structural changes within the luminal wall. Some emerging evidence suggests that delayed vasospasm may not be due to only vasoconstriction but also may involve vascular remodeling, resulting in a thickened hyperplastic arterial wall.[40,41] The main arteries affected by delayed vasospasm are the large intradural arteries of the circle of Willis. It is clear the prolonged exposure of these arteries to blood within the subarachnoid space is sufficient to cause vasospasm, and removal of the clot can lessen angiographic vasospasm.[42] Exposure to this blood is thought to catalyze immediate vascular constriction that can also lead to alterations in cerebral perfusion pressure and intracranial pressure and release of spasmogens from activated platelets within the clot. The major mediators for arterial wall vasospasm include (1) hemoglobin and oxidative stress, (2) increased expression of ET-1, (3) reduced levels of nitric oxide (NO), and (4) inflammation.[37]

Oxyhemoglobin is released from lysed red blood cells and is thought to be the primary spasmogenic agent leading to cerebral vasospasm through production of oxygen free radicals that induce oxidative stress through lipid peroxidation and formation of bilirubin oxidation products.[43] ET-1 is a 21–amino acid peptide and one of the most potent vasoconstrictors produced in endothelial cells on stimulation by ischemia. It has been suggested that ET-1 contributes to an imbalance in vasoconstriction and vasodilation during aSAH and can be found in high concentrations in the cerebrospinal fluid on day 5 postictus and corresponds with increased cerebral blood flow velocity.[44] Inhibition of smooth muscle relaxation of the cerebral arteries can contribute to vasospasm. Current data suggest depletion of cerebral NO through disappearance or dysfunction of NO synthase in cerebral vessels and due to the affinity for NO of the heme moiety in hemoglobin.[45] Blood-brain barrier breakdown due to aSAH has led to an increase in circulating leukocytes within the cerebrospinal fluid, which may contribute to vasospasm via promotion of free radicals and release of ET-1 and other vasoactive cytokines along with an increased expression of cell adhesion molecules.[46–48]

Angiographic vasospasm may be associated with DCI, but other pathophysiological factors may also play a role in the development of DCI such as microthrombosis, cortical spreading ischemia, microcirculatory constriction, and apoptosis.[37] Nimodipine is currently the only pharmacological agent that has demonstrated an improvement in outcome after aSAH and is indicated for use by the US Food and Drug Administration (FDA). In the clinical trials, nimodipine did not show a significant improvement in angiographic vasospasm, which led to other theories surrounding the benefit of this agent. It is proposed that nimodipine may slightly attenuate vasospasm but also inhibits cortical spreading ischemia and reduces microthrombi through its fibrinolytic activity.[37] For a more detailed overview of the various pathophysiological processes involved with the development of DIND, the reader should refer to a review by Macdonald.[37]

DIAGNOSTIC AND MONITORING APPROACHES

Noninvasive Approaches

Close clinical monitoring of vasospasm is one of the easiest and most important monitoring approaches. Frequent neurological examinations should be performed to establish each patient's baseline neurologic status and to detect any changes.[49] Cerebral vasospasm symptoms include exacerbating headache, neck stiffness, confusion, disorientation, drowsiness, and focal deficits, which are commonly fluctuating. Other causes for clinical decline, such as aneurysm rebleeding, hydrocephalus, electrolyte imbalance, hypoxia, seizures, and cardiopulmonary dysfunction and/or infection, should be immediately worked up and ruled out.[49]

The Glasgow Coma Scale is the most widely used scale to monitor patients clinically over time. However, some limitations need to be taken into account when assessing patients with aSAH for cerebral vasospasm. First, the scale incorporates the verbal response, which is not possible to assess in intubated patients. Second, the scale scores the best motor response, consequently failing to detect a side deficit.[50] Furthermore, while clinical examination can detect subtle changes in patients with low-grade aSAH, these same changes may not be apparent in a patient who is comatose. Therefore, clinical examination alone cannot be used to screen for vasospasm.

Invasive Approaches

To attribute a clinical worsening to cerebral vasospasm, an arterial narrowing has to be demonstrated. Several direct and indirect methods are commonly used in clinical practice.

Digital subtraction angiography is considered the gold standard for diagnosing cerebral vasospasm. This method provides a dynamic idea of circulation time and allows the study of all vascular compartments. However, digital subtraction angiography is not routinely used in the clinical setting for surveillance monitoring as it is costly and has a small but nonnegligible risk of neurologic complications. The serious complication rate is 1% to 2% and includes risk of the anesthetic regimen, puncture site complications, contrast nephropathy, allergic reactions, embolic or thrombotic strokes, perforation of the cerebral artery, and intracranial hemorrhage. The advantage of angiography is that it provides the opportunity to treat vasospasm by endovascular approaches, but the use of this invasive approach is not appropriate for surveillance monitoring of vasospasm.[31,49]

Transcranial Doppler (TCD) monitoring is a less invasive approach for monitoring cerebral vasospasm and is a current mainstay of vasospasm monitoring in patients with aSAH. TCD monitoring is an indirect measure of cerebral vasospasm as it measures cerebral blood flow velocity, which is inversely proportional to its diameter. When the proximal cerebral arteries narrow, the velocity of blood flow in that artery increases and can be detectable by TCD.[49,51]

The middle cerebral artery is the easiest artery to monitor with TCD and is the most described in the literature.[52–54] Absolute velocity of blood flow in the middle cerebral artery has demonstrated strong correlations with the lack or presence of vasospasm. An absolute velocity of less than 120 cm/s exhibits a low risk for cerebral vasospasm while an absolute velocity of greater than 200 cm/s is considered high risk. However, the absolute velocity has not been shown to correlate well in the intermediate range.[51] The Lindegaard ratio is another value commonly calculated using TCD measurements, which has also been shown to be predictive of vasospasm. The Lindegaard ratio is the middle cerebral artery velocity compared with the velocity in the proximal extracranial internal carotid artery. A value greater than 3 has been shown to be consistent with vasospasm.[55]

Several limitations exist with the use of TCDs for monitoring vasospasm. First, TCD measurements are susceptible to high interrater variability that is dependent on the operator. In addition, many patients may have dense temporal bone windows that will prohibit an accurate measurement of the blood flow velocity. Finally, TCD measurements are also inadequate to identify vasospasm of more distal arteries. Despite these limitations, monitoring via TCD measurements is commonly performed in patients with aSAH to evaluate trends and complement the clinical examination.[49,56]

Several techniques are currently used to detect alterations of cerebral perfusion. Imaging using methods of perfusion, such as CT, magnetic resonance imaging, and/or positron emission tomography, are used to screen and confirm cerebral vasospasm. These perfusion studies can be combined with noninvasive arteriography to acquire more complete information. CT angiography has correlated with conventional angiography for large artery narrowing and can be used as a screening tool. CT perfusion imaging provides a measure of tissue perfusion. Severe vasospasm is associated with absolute cerebral blood flows of less than 25 mL/100 g/min and mean transit times greater than 6.4 seconds or 20% higher than average.[57] The use of imaging methods for the diagnosis of cerebral vasospasm has several limitations, such as cumulative radiation exposure, higher cost, lower availability, and logistical problems associated with patient transport.[49]

Other invasive tools are used in the intensive care unit (ICU) to evaluate the presence of cerebral vasospasm, including electroencephalogram, brain tissue oxygen monitoring, and cerebral microdialysis.[33] Electroencephalography can be used for continuous bedside monitoring in patients with aSAH. Electroencephalography parameters evaluated include fast over slow activity, alpha variability, and the alpha/delta ratio. Relative decreased alpha variability precedes clinical diagnosis of vasospasm by 3 days.[58] Microdialysis consists of sampling parenchymal extracellular glucose, lactate, pyruvate, glutamate, glycerol concentrations, and other metabolic parameters by means of an intracerebral microcatheter probe. This provides a method to assess bedside comparisons of neurochemical changes with the patient's neurological examination. Lactate and glutamate have been shown to be sensitive markers of impending cerebral ischemia.[59] Brain tissue oxygenation, thermal diffusion cerebral blood flow, and near-infrared spectroscopy have also been used to monitor patients with aSAH, although the value of all of these approaches in detecting cerebral vasospasm is not currently known.[49]

PHARMACOTHERAPY APPROACHES FOR PREVENTION

For an overview of the pharmacotherapy approaches to vasospasm prevention please refer to Table 5.1

Calcium Channel Antagonists

The only pharmacologic intervention that reduces the incidence of DCI and risk of poor outcome after aSAH is the calcium channel antagonist, nimodipine.[60] Nimodipine is a dihydropyridine calcium channel blocker that exhibits cerebral vascular selectivity by preferentially dilating cerebral blood vessels to a greater degree than the peripheral and coronary vasculature.[61] Nimodipine has become the standard of care in the United States based on a clinical trial published in 1983 in which 13% of patients who were randomized to the placebo group had severe neurologic deficits compared with 1.7% of patients randomized to nimodipine.[62] A larger trial found reductions of 34% in ischemic stroke and 40% in poor outcome at 3 months in patients treated with nimodipine compared with placebo.[63] A subsequent meta-analysis that evaluated 9 prospective randomized trials including 1514 patients demonstrated significantly reduced incidence of delayed neurological deficits by 38% (odds ratio [OR], 0.62; 95% confidence interval [CI], 0.5–0.78) and cerebral infarcts by 48% (OR, 0.52; 95% CI, 0.41–0.66).[64] Originally, it was hypothesized that the benefit from nimodipine is related to a reduction in vasospasm, but clinical trials never found a reduction in vasospasm even while showing an overall improvement in outcome. In addition to being a calcium channel antagonist, nimodipine may exert its mechanism through a variety of different mechanisms. In vitro and in vivo data have shown that nimodipine has an effect on the whole vasculature by inhibition contractions due to noradrenaline and serotonin, as well as potassium membrane depolarization,[65] and it can also increase the fibrinolytic activity by decreasing the level of plasminogen activator inhibitor 1.[66]

Clinical trials that have shown the benefit of enteral nimodipine in patients with aSAH used a dose of 60 mg every 4 hours for 21 days. The most common

TABLE 5.1 Current Therapeutic Interventions for the Prevention and Treatment of Vasospasm

Preventative Interventions
Maintenance of euvolemia with crystalloids
Maintenance of normal or elevated systemic blood pressure
Prevention of hypomagnesemia and hyponatremia
Nimodipine 60 mg by mouth or nasogastric tube q4h for 21 days
Treatment Interventions
Maintain euvolemia with crystalloids
Induced hypertension with vasopressors (phenylephrine or norepinephrine) and/or hemodynamic augmentation with inotropes (dobutamine or milrinone) for symptomatic vasospasm
Endovascular approaches, including pharmacologic and balloon angioplasty

adverse effect is hypotension and is reported to occur in about 7.7% of patients. This can be a serious concern because hemodynamic lability is independently associated with death or severe disability after aSAH.[67] Avoiding blood pressure fluctuations is key in the management of these patients, so there have been suggested alterations in the dosing strategy of nimodipine (30 mg every 2 hours) in patients who experience hypotension, but this has not been evaluated in clinical trials. A recent retrospective study evaluated dosing practices of nimodipine in 270 patients following aSAH. They reported that 28.6% had the dosage reduced by 50% due to hypotension and 27.7% had the nimodipine discontinued. While this was a small study, they did find that dose reduction or discontinuation was associated with unfavorable outcomes on multivariate analysis.[68] Not only has nimodipine been shown to be effective, but it also is cost-effective as it increased patient life years at a very low incremental cost.[69] The 2 guidelines recommend that oral nimodipine (60 mg every 4 hours) should be given for 21 days after aSAH.[33,51]

The drug was approved as a 30-mg liquid-filled capsule, and until 2013, this was the only dosage formulation available in the United States. Since many patients following aSAH are unable to swallow the large capsules, many centers have pharmacy-compounded syringes or the nurses extract the liquid from the capsule at the bedside. Pharmacy-compounded syringes in which the nimodipine liquid is extracted from the capsules and stored in amber-colored syringes and then placed in light-protected bags at room temperature have been shown to be stable for up to 31 days.[70] Some serious drug errors have been reported when oral nimodipine is extracted at the bedside and is administered intravenously instead of through a nasogastric tube when patients are not able to swallow the capsule. The drug comes with instructions for making a hole in both ends of the capsule with a standard 18-gauge needle for removing the contents with a syringe and then administering through the nasogastric tube and flushing with 30 mL of normal saline.[71] Because these needles do not fit on an oral syringe, an intravenous syringe is used, which has resulted in intravenous administration. Intravenous administration can result in cardiac arrest, dramatic drops in blood pressure, or other cardiovascular adverse events. The FDA issued a drug safety communication in 2010 for which they reported 25 intravenous nimodipine prescribing or administration errors, where 4 patients died and 5 had near-death events.[72] In 2013, the FDA approved a new oral nimodipine solution in an effort to reduce drug errors because this dosage form eliminated the need for needle extraction of nimodipine from the capsules.[73] Recently, Oyler et al[74] conducted a simulation of both bedside gel extraction and pharmacy batch-compounded nimodipine to evaluate accuracy. Simulated bedside extraction provided lower yield than the pharmacy-compounded syringes, suggesting that there is no role for bedside extraction of nimodipine in clinical practice. There is also potential for drug interactions between nimodipine and strong inhibitors and inducers of CYP3A4. The clinical significance of these drug interactions is the possibility of significant hypotension when administered with CYP3A4 inhibitors and lack of effectiveness when coadministered with CYP3A4 inducers.

The future direction for delivery of nimodipine is currently being investigated in clinical trials. EG-1962 is a novel polymeric nimodipine microparticle that is administered directly into the cerebral ventricles and provides sustained drug exposure throughout 21 days. EG-1962 uses a programmable, biodegradable polymer-based development platform known as Precisa. This delivery system allows for targeted drug delivery to the site of injury to provide sustained drug exposure while avoiding systemic toxicities. This site-specific delivery of nimodipine microparticles reduces angiographic vasospasm after aSAH in dogs.[75] EG-1962 was evaluated in a phase I/II study, NEWTON (Nimodipine microparticles to Enhance recovery While reducing TOxicity after subarachNoid hemorrhage), for safety, tolerability, and pharmacokinetic properties.[76,77] In August 2015, EDGE Therapeutics announced that a single intraventricular injection of EG-1962 met its primary and secondary study end points.[78] This trial evaluated 6 dose cohorts (100, 200, 400, 600, 800, and 1200 mg). The primary end point was to establish the maximum tolerated dose, which has been determined to be 800 mg. Safety results show that no patients (0 of 54) experienced EG-1962–related hypotension, while 17% of patients

(3 of 18) treated with oral nimodipine experienced drug-related hypotension. The steady-state plasma concentration measured in patients treated with EG-1962 in the NEWTON trial was below 30 ng/mL, the level of plasma concentrations observed to cause systemic hypotension. The study was not powered for outcome, but an exploratory assessment of outcome based on the 90-day extended Glasgow Outcome Scale Extended (GOSE) revealed that 60% of patients treated with EG-1962 had favorable outcome (GOSE >5) compared with 28% of those treated with the current standard of care, oral nimodpine.[78]

Nicardipine is another calcium channel blocker that has been evaluated for prophylactic use after aSAH. Intravenous nicardipine (0.15 mg/kg/h for up to 14 days) was compared with placebo. In contrast to the results reported for nimodipine, nicardipine was associated with lower symptomatic vasospasm but was not associated with improvement in neurological outcome at 3 months. Hypotension is the major concern with the use of intravenous nicardipine and occurred in 34.5% of nicardipine-treated patients compared with 17.5% of placebo-treated patients. The potential positive effect on outcome may have been negated by the 3% incidence of life-threatening hypotension that developed.[79,80] Nonetheless, intravenous nicardipine may provide an alternative to nimodipine in times of drug shortage or when the oral route cannot be used. Lower doses of nicardipine (0.075 mg/kg/h) are better tolerated and equivalent to higher doses in the clinical trials.

Dantrolene

The dihydropyridine class of calcium channel blockers includes L-type specific calcium channel blockers and may only be partially effective since they affect only the influx of extracellular calcium and have no effect on ryanodine receptor-mediated intracellular calcium release. Dantrolene is an agent currently on the market and is a ryanodine receptor blocker that may be an emerging therapeutic intervention for improving outcomes after aSAH. Animal models suggest that it may have neuroprotective properties and inhibit cerebral vasoconstriction alone and exponentially when combined with nimodipine.[81–83] There are some safety concerns with dantrolene, especially with repeated doses, including exacerbation of hyponatremia and cerebral edema along with systemic hypotension and the "black-box warning" for liver toxicity. Two small human pilot studies suggest a single dose of intravenous dantrolene may attenuate cerebral vasospasm after aSAH.[84,85] Recently, a single-center, randomized, placebo-controlled trial evaluated the safety and feasibility of repeated dosing of intravenous dantrolene (1.25 mg/kg every 6 hours) over 7 days in 31 patients with aSAH.[86] They found a numerically higher number of adverse effects (venous irritation, liver toxicity) in the patients receiving intravenous dantrolene, but it did not reach statistical significance. The study was not powered for outcome efficacy, but proportionally fewer patients required angiography for clinical vasospasm.[86] The results of this study from both a safety and efficacy perspective need to be validated in a larger clinical trial.

Fasudil

Fasudil is a potent RhoA/Rho kinase inhibitor, which is thought to inhibit the action of free intracellular calcium along with inhibition of protein kinases A, G, and C and the myosin light chain directly. While typically thought to be a vasodilator, it may also inhibit cytokine release from leukocytes and antagonize ET-1. Fasudil has been studied after aSAH and shown beneficial effects on the development of cerebral vasospasm, DCI, and outcome, although these studies were limited to small sample sizes.[87] It has been compared with intravenous nimodipine and demonstrated improved outcome, but a large multicenter trial has not yet been conducted.[88] Fasudil is currently commonly used in Japan and China.

Statins

Statins have been widely used clinically for their cholesterol-lowering effects; however, the use of these agents has generated a lot of interest in the prevention of vasospasm after aSAH. This is due to their pleiotropic effects, which include anti-inflammatory properties, upregulation of endothelial nitric oxide synthase, antiadhesive effects on the endothelium, amelioration of glutamate-mediated excitotoxicity, and inhibition of platelet aggregation.[89,90] Based on strong experimental evidence, several studies examined the clinical effect of simvastatin and pravastatin for the prevention of vasospasm and DCI. The primary difference between these statins is that simvastatin has a higher affinity for hydroxymethylglutaryl coenzyme A reductase and is more lipophilic than pravastatin, so it has higher blood-brain barrier penetration.[91] Initially, at least 4 randomized controlled trials[92–95] and 6 observational studies[89,96–101] have been critically appraised in meta-analyses.[102–104] Sillberg et al[104] included 3 randomized controlled trials that included 158 patients and found a reduction in the incidence of vasospasm, DIND, and mortality with the statins compared with placebo. In the other meta-analysis of these same 3 randomized controlled trials along with the inclusion of 2 "pseudo"-randomized trials by Vergouwen et al,[103] more mixed results were reported.[102] Simvastatin 80 mg was used in 3 of the 4 randomized studies, and pravastatin 40 mg was used in the other study. There was no statistical difference in transcranial Doppler-detected vasospasm, incidence of DCI, or neurologic outcomes between statin treatment and placebo.[102,103] The results of these meta-analyses should be viewed cautiously as the definitions of DCI were inconsistent. Atorvastatin 40 mg/d for 21 days was studied in 142 patients to evaluate if this statin could reduce vasospasm-induced ischemia by measuring serum S100B (biomarker for cerebral ischemia) and ischemic lesion volume by CT. Atorvastatin reduced the incidence of cerebral vasospasm, severity of vasospasm, volume of ischemia, and serum S100B concentrations, but there were no differences in clinical outcomes at 1 year.[105]

STASH (Simvastatin in Aneurysmal Subarachnoid Hemorrhage), a phase III randomized trial in 803 patients that compared simvastatin 40 mg with placebo for up to 21 days, was recently published.[106] Despite demonstrating no safety concerns, this trial failed to show any short-term or long-term benefit in outcome, and the investigators concluded that simvastatin should not be routinely used during the acute stages. Several experimental and clinical studies suggest that sudden withdrawal of statins can suppress endothelial nitric oxide production, leading to higher risk of hemorrhage and vasospasm.[97,107] However, statin use prior to admission was not shown to improve functional outcomes or prevent DCI in a small number of patients with aSAH.[108] The current guidelines indicate that statins may be initiated in statin-naive patients for reducing DCI after aSAH but were published before the STASH results. The guidelines do mention continuing patients on statins if they were receiving them before presentation with aSAH.[33,51]

Magnesium

Magnesium, a noncompetitive calcium antagonist that is thought to result in smooth muscle relaxation and vessel dilation, has been used widely in obstetrics and cardiology. Magnesium may also have neuroprotective properties as it decreases glutamate release and reduces calcium entry into cells.[109,110] Hypomagnesemia occurs in more than 50% of patients with aSAH and is associated with poor outcome and a predictor of DCI.[111] Several clinical trials have investigated the effects of magnesium after aSAH with dosing ranges of 20 to 80 mmol with a target plasma concentration goal of 2 to 2.5 mmol, and it originally showed a trend toward improving clinical outcomes.[112–120] The first phase III randomized controlled trial enrolled 327 patients within 48 hours of aSAH to either magnesium 20 mmol (5 g) over 30 minutes followed by an infusion of 80 mmol (20 g)/d for up to 14 days posthemorrhage or placebo (0.9% sodium chloride). The magnesium infusion was adjusted to achieve magnesium concentration twice the patient's baseline up to a maximum of 2.5 mmol/L. There were no significant differences in 6-month outcomes or in the percentage of patients with clinical vasospasm.[119] MASH-2 (Magnesium for Aneurysmal Subarachnoid Hemorrhage) is another phase III randomized placebo-controlled trial in 1204 patients that did not find significant benefit of intravenous magnesium infusion on favorable outcome.[120] The investigators of this trial also completed a meta-analysis with 2407 patients and confirmed the lack of benefit of magnesium after aSAH.[120]

Magnesium was administered intravenously in these clinical trials, but this route of administration does not result in a significant increase in cerebrospinal fluid magnesium values even if serum magnesium level is increased by 50% or more.[121] Direct administration of magnesium into the basal cisterns may be a more effective approach, although currently, no ongoing clinical trials are investigating magnesium given via this route after aSAH.[122,123] Intravenous administration of magnesium is not currently recommended for treatment of aSAH, but hypomagnesemia should be avoided.[33,51]

Clearance of Subarachnoid Spaces

Because the breakdown by-product of the subarachnoid clot is believed to play a key role in the development of vasospasm and DCI, removal of the blood would appear to be a rational preventive strategy. Some evidence indicates that subarachnoid clot removal through the use of intracisternal injections of recombinant tissue plasminogen activator may reduce the risk of vasospasm.[124] The recombinant tissue plasminogen activator is generally administered at the time of aneurysm clipping, and since endovascular approaches to aneurysm stabilization are being used increasingly, this approach is not practical for all patients. In addition, the results appear to be inconclusive, and this approach can increase the risk of intracerebral hemorrhage. Currently, the use of intracisternal thrombolytics cannot be recommended.

Intraventricular administration of thrombolytic agents has been investigated as a method to prevent the development of vasospasm. A meta-analysis of 5 trials that included a total of 465 patients showed significant reductions in the development of vasospasm and DCI.[42] The results of this meta-analysis should be viewed cautiously as there were considerable differences in the study methodology of the trials included in the meta-analysis such that routine use cannot be currently recommended.

The use of lumbar drains is another approach for clearing subarachnoid blood and has been part of clinical practice despite the lack of supporting evidence. Retrospective data found that patients who were treated with a lumbar drain had a lower incidence of DCI, lower need for rescue therapy, and better outcome.[125,126] However, the Lumbar Drainage of cerebrospinal Fluid after

Aneurysmal Subarachnoid Hemorrhage: A Prospective, Randomized, Controlled Trial (LUMAS) study found that lumbar drainage reduced DCI but had no impact on overall outcome.[127] A current clinical trial is investigating the benefit of this approach (Outcome after Early Lumbar CSF-Drainage in Aneurysmal Subarachnoid Hemorrhage [EARLYDRAIN]).[128]

ET-1 Antagonist

ET-1 is a 21–amino acid peptide and one of the most potent vasoconstrictors produced in endothelial cells on stimulation by ischemia. It has been suggested that ET-1 contributes to an imbalance in vasoconstriction and vasodilation during aSAH and can be found in high concentrations in the cerebrospinal fluid on day 5 postictus and corresponds with increased cerebral blood flow velocity.[44] Binding of ET-1 to the ET-A receptor promotes angiographic vasospasm through smooth muscle proliferation and contraction.[129] The ETA receptor is located in vascular endothelial cells and is known to mediate the endothelium-dependent vasodilatory actions of endothelins. Clazosentan is a selective ETA receptor antagonist that decreases and reverses cerebral vasospasm in experimental aSAH; however, the results of the 3 large randomized controlled trials were not as expected. The CONSCIOUS-1 (Clazosentan to Overcome Neurological Ischemia and Infarct Occurring after Subarachnoid Hemorrhage) trial found significant dose-dependent effects on the angiographic incidence of vasospasm with a 65% reduction at the highest dose.[130] The phase III trial, CONSCIOUS-2, was designed to target patients at highest risk of vasospasm and DCI, such as those with substantial blood-clot thickness and who had undergone surgical clipping. The results of the CONSCIOUS-2 trial showed that clazosentan at 5 mg/h had no significant effect on mortality, vasospasm-related morbidity, or functional outcome. Pulmonary complications, anemia, and hypotension were more common in the patients who received clazosentan.[35] A similar study in patients who were treated with coiling (CONSCIOUS-3) was stopped early after 577 of the 1500 patients were enrolled.[131] The results of CONSCIOUS-3 demonstrated similar findings to CONSCIOUS-2 for the 5-mg/h dose; however, the 15-mg/h dose significantly reduced vasospasm-related morbidity and all-cause mortality but did not lead to improved outcome at week 12. The CONSCIOUS-2 and CONSCIOUS-3 trials have raised questions regarding the efficacy of ET-1 antagonists in preventing vasospasm, and the possibility remains that these agents may have clinical utility as part of a complex treatment regimen for aSAH. Animal models have suggested that outcomes are improved when clazosentan was administered in combination with additional intervention such as a fibrinolytic.[132]

Future Directions

In the future, there will be investigation of other modalities aimed at preventing DCI along with the establishment of combination therapy approaches. Some of the targets for future interventions include vasodilation, anticoagulation, antiplatelets, inhibition of apoptosis pathways, free radical neutralization, suppression of cortical spreading depolarization, and attenuation of inflammation.[133] Several of these modalities are currently under investigation, including the use of prostacyclin (vasodilator and inhibitor of platelet function),[134] sodium nitrite (increases local availability of NO),[135,136] and the use of hypercapnia (cerebral vasodilator).[137] In addition, genotypic variability may define the susceptibility of individual patients to both early brain injury and DIND caused by the aneurysm rupture so better identification of patient selection for various interventions is another avenue for the future.

PHARMACOTHERAPY APPROACHES FOR TREATMENT

For an overview of the pharmacotherapy approaches to vasospasm treatment please refer to Table 5.1

Hemodynamic Therapy

Triple-H therapy is commonly used for the treatment of cerebral vasospasm, despite the moderate quality of evidence supporting this intervention. Triple-H refers to the combination of hypervolemia (central venous pressures 10–12 mm Hg), induced hypertension (systolic blood pressure 180–220 mm Hg), and hemodilution (hematocrit 30%-35%).[138]

The rationale for triple-H therapy is based on the hemodynamic consequences of cerebral arterial vasospasm. As arterial narrowing increases, cerebrovascular resistance shifts from the penetrating arterioles to the major branches of the circle of Willis and the proximal conducting vessels. Once this shift occurs, the brain supplied by these narrowed branches loses its capacity for autoregulation, limiting cerebral blood flow. Therefore, the purpose of triple H-therapy is to maintain high circulating blood volume, increase cerebral perfusion pressures, and decrease blood viscosity, which will enhance cerebral blood flow in the face of vasoconstriction.[139] However, there is currently no definitive evidence from randomized controlled trials that triple-H therapy or its separate components improves cerebral blood flow or clinical outcome in patients with aSAH.[139–141] Prophylactic triple-H therapy to reduce the occurrence of delayed cerebral ischemia and death following aSAH has also been investigated. However, no evidence suggests that this approach is beneficial, and it has been associated with a higher risk of serious adverse effects and death; thus, this approach should be reserved to managing patients with symptomatic vasospasm.[142,143]

When used, aggressive triple-H therapy is implemented immediately following a diagnosis of symptomatic vasospasm. Usually, CT angiography is performed to document arterial vasoconstriction, and other tests are performed to exclude other causes of neurological symptoms, as discussed previously.[139] Even if an endovascular intervention is planned, aggressive efforts with triple-H therapy may still occur.

Recent literature suggests that induced hypertension may be the most important component of triple-H therapy.[31] Case series and observational studies have linked induced hypertension with neurologic improvement and increased cerebral blood flow, especially in patients with angiographic vasospasm or in brain regions that are hypoperfused.[33,144,145] The reasoning behind the administration of vasoactive agents is that it produces a sustained increase in systemic blood pressure, which results in improved cerebral perfusion pressure, cerebral blood flow, and cerebral tissue oxygenation. In several studies, induced hypertension was found to be more effective and safer at improving cerebral oxygenation than aggressive hypervolemia.[146–148] There are varying approaches in clinical practice as to defining the blood pressure targets. Some clinicians will target a percent increase from baseline blood pressure, whereas others will target an arbitrary number. Regardless of the approach, the blood pressure should be increased in a stepwise fashion guided by assessment of the neurological examination, neuromonitoring, or radiological evidence of improved perfusion.[33]

The most common agents used to induce hypertension are phenylephrine and norepinephrine, while dopamine is used sparingly.[33] No literature currently exists comparing the effect of different agents on cerebral blood flow. In a prospective case series, the use of high-dose phenylephrine had a good safety profile.[149] Vasopressin is an effective vasopressor agent but not routinely used in patients with aSAH because of its potential to exacerbate hyponatremia that can occur in these patients. However, vasopressin may be useful in situations where achieving blood pressure targets requires very high doses of vasopressors.[33] In 1 study, the addition of vasopressin (0.01–0.04 U/min) to maximal phenylephrine therapy (4–5 mcg/kg/min) in patients with clinically symptomatic vasospasm found that vasopressin was effective in reducing the phenylephrine dosage without reducing serum sodium concentrations or causing detrimental effects on cerebral perfusion or worsening vasospasm.[150]

An alternative to induced hypertension is augmentation of cardiac output with inotropes, such as milrinone or dobutamine, although this is generally considered if the response to induced hypertension is inadequate.[33] The rationale behind this treatment is that in addition to vasospasm, patients with aSAH may have reduced cardiac output because of "stunned myocardium." A major concern with routine use of these agents is the potential to lower blood pressure. Milrinone may be more potent than dobutamine in increasing cardiac output and is more effective in patients with normal vascular resistance and normal blood pressure yet reduced systolic function. Dobutamine may be a preferred option when vascular resistance or blood pressure is reduced.[151] Inotropic agents may be useful in patients who fail to respond to induced hypertension or have poor cardiac function. However, these agents should not be used prophylactically.[33,151]

It is common practice to target euvolemia and prevent hypovolemia in patients with aSAH as hypovolemia is associated with worse clinical outcomes.[33] Hypovolemia is a common complication following aSAH and is more prevalent 6 to 72 hours after aSAH for those patients who underwent surgical intervention.[152] Prophylactic hypervolemia has not been shown to improve cerebral blood flow or prevent symptomatic vasospasm and is associated with increased risk of cardiopulmonary complications because of the fluid overload.[33,142] In addition, hypervolemia has not been shown to offer any benefit over euvolemia when treating cerebral vasospasm. In a study of 16 patients with severe vasospasm documented with angiography, the impact of hypervolemia (1000 mL/d colloid plus 3740 mL/d crystalloid; mean central venous pressure increase from 5.4–7.4 cm H_2O), induced hypertension with phenylephrine (mean arterial pressure increase from 102–132 mm Hg), or enhanced cardiac output with dobutamine (mean cardiac index increased from 4.1–5 L/min/m²) was compared using cerebral blood flow as the outcome measurement. Improvements in cerebral blood flow were observed only in those patients who received phenylephrine or dobutamine.[153] Similar results were reported in an observational study of 45 patients, with induced hypertension increasing brain tissue oxygenation in 90% of patients with an 8% complication rate, while hypervolemia was only effective in 12% of patients but had a 53% complication rate.[148] Therefore, the role of hypervolemia as a single component of triple-H therapy does not appear to be supported by these small studies. The Neurocritical Care Society consensus recommendations suggest consideration of a saline bolus to increase cerebral blood flow in areas of ischemia as a prelude to other interventions, like induced hypertension.[33]

Volume status should be routinely monitored in patients with aSAH. Although a target central venous pressure of 8 mm Hg or higher has been recommended, it is important to understand the lack of reliability of central venous pressure in estimating intravascular. Goal-directed hemodynamic management using PiCCO has been successfully used in patients with aSAH.[154,155] The specific targets that have been suggested include the following:

- Cardiac index greater than 3.0 L/min/m²
- Global end-diastolic volume index equal to 700 to 900 mL/m²
- Extravascular lung water index less than 14 mL/kg

Larger randomized controlled trials are needed to validate the usefulness of goal-directed hemodynamic monitoring in patients with aSAH.

The choice of fluid for volume management in patients with aSAH is typically isotonic crystalloids.[33,51] However, some other fluid choices have been assessed in patients with aSAH. Hypertonic saline has not been part of the traditional regimen for triple-H therapy, although limited data suggest hypertonic saline may be an alternative fluid for use in patients with poor-grade aSAH.[156] A prospective study administered a 2-mL/kg infusion of 23.4% sodium chloride over 10 to 30 minutes to 44 patients with poor-grade aSAH. This study found that hypertonic saline increased systemic blood pressure, reduced intracranial pressure (ICP), and improved cerebral blood flow, cerebral oxygenation, and brain tissue pH with effects lasting 2 to 4 hours after administration.[156]

Albumin is another fluid currently being investigated as it may possess neuroprotective properties through several mechanisms that include increasing serum oncotic pressure, improving microcirculatory blood flow, decreasing the inflammatory response, and free radical scavenging properties.[157] A retrospective evaluation of high doses of 25% human albumin used to increase the central venous pressure above 8 mm Hg reported an association with improved outcomes and reduced costs in patients with aSAH.[158] A phase I dose escalation study evaluated the safety and efficacy of 25% albumin in doses of 0.625 g/kg/d, 1.25 g/kg/d, 1.875 g/kg/d, and 2.5 g/kg/d for up to 7 days. Doses up to 1.25 g/kg/d were well tolerated, but the study was stopped early once the dose reached 1.875 g/kg/d because of the development of pulmonary edema.[159] In addition, Albumin in Subarachnoid Hemorrhage (ALISAH) II, a phase III randomized placebo-controlled trial powered to test the efficacy of albumin, is planned. While albumin is included in many of the triple-H regimens evaluated in the literature, no studies exist comparing albumin to crystalloids. Despite limited data available regarding the use of albumin in patients with aSAH, a recent survey to health care providers of patients with aSAH reported almost half (45.9%) of the respondents commonly administer albumin to their patients with aSAH but also acknowledged the need for a randomized clinical trial.[160]

Hemodilution is the most controversial component of triple-H therapy. Although cerebral blood flow will increase with a decreasing hematocrit, this approach is also associated with decreased oxygen-carrying capacity and increased volume of ischemic areas of the brain. Higher hemoglobin values have been shown to be associated with decreased rates of cerebral infarction, poor outcome, and death after aSAH.[161] However, blood transfusions have been associated with increased rates of angiographic vasospasm, cerebral ischemia, and worse functional outcomes.[162] There are no convincing data to support an ideal hematocrit; thus, induced hemodilution to achieve a lower hemoglobin or hematocrit to improve blood rheology should be avoided. The current guidelines recommend maintaining hemoglobin concentrations of greater than 8 to 10 g/dL with packed red blood cells, although higher thresholds may be appropriate in patients at high risk of DCI.[33,51] Transfusion with packed red blood cells, however, is not without risk as a recent retrospective study reported transfusion with red blood cells was independently associated with increased mortality in patients with aSAH.[163]

Two systematic reviews have assessed the different components of triple-H therapy.[140,141] Hypervolemia did not appear to be superior to normovolemia and was associated with more adverse effects.[141] Hemodilution was not shown to be associated with a change in cerebral blood flow, and hypertension was associated with higher cerebral blood flow regardless of the volume status.[140,141] The current clinical guidelines recommend maintenance of euvolemia and induction of hypertension in patients with delayed cerebral ischemia, except in patients with elevated blood pressure at baseline or comorbid cardiac disease that would preclude its use.[33] In patients with preexisting cardiac disease and the elderly, the risk of complications with hypervolemic and/or hypertensive therapy is increased, with the risk of cardiac failure, pulmonary edema, cerebral edema, and elevated intracranial pressure.[149]

Endovascular Approaches

Endovascular approaches for the treatment of cerebral vasospasm are typically reserved for after failure of conventional therapy. Transluminal balloon angioplasty has been shown to be an effective approach to immediately produce dilation of the involved artery and increase distal cerebral blood flow in the proximal cerebral arteries with significant symptomatic vasospasm.[164] However, transluminal balloon angioplasty has several limitations, including only being a suitable treatment for vessels with a diameter of 2 mm or more and having the effectiveness of treatment being closely tied to the expertise of the operator. This intervention also has the potential for serious adverse events with a complication rate of about 5%. Potential complications include vessel rupture, thromboembolic complications, and delayed stenosis. However, the results of this intervention tend to be more durable than pharmacologic intervention.[165] While no randomized trials can confirm the clinical efficacy of this approach, clinical guidelines state that angioplasty is reasonable in symptomatic patients who do not respond to medical therapies.[33]

Rescue Therapy

Another method for treating cerebral vasospasm after failure of conventional therapy is targeted delivery of pharmacologic agents through intra-arterial, intraventricular, or intrathecal administration. With this method, it is important to evaluate the products directly administered into the central nervous system and assess the potential risk of the diluent and other excipients that are contained in the product.[166]

Papaverine is a vasodilator agent that preferentially vasodilates cerebral and coronary vascular smooth muscle. Intra-arterial injection of papaverine (150–600 mg) has been reported to be successful in treating cerebral vasospasm in published reports of clinical experience.[167–171] However, papaverine is no longer recommended for use as it has several significant safety concerns. These include the potential for the development of neurotoxicity because of altered mitochondrial cellular respiration with high exposure, increased intracranial pressure, hemiplegia, seizures, agitation, altered mental status, and hypotension.[172,173]

Nicardipine has been one of the most widely investigated vasodilators for the treatment of cerebral vasospasm. Nicardipine has shown promise when administered by intra-arterial, intrathecal, or intraventricular routes of administration.[174–178] Intra-arterial administration involves diluting intravenous nicardipine with 0.9% sodium chloride to a concentration of 0.1 mg/mL and administering in 1-mL aliquots through the microcatheter to a maximum of 5 mg per vessel. Nicardipine has been shown to be effective at inducing vasodilation and reducing mean peak systolic velocities on TCD from pretreatment for 4 days after the infusion. Overall neurologic improvement was reported in 42% of patients.[174]

Intraventricular administration of nicardipine is an attractive treatment option because it can be administered in the ICU and avoids transport of the patient to the angiography suite. However, evidence for this treatment approach is limited. One small case series reported on 8 patients in which nicardipine 4 mg was administered through the intraventricular catheter every 12 hours for 5 to

17 days. The drug was well tolerated, and 7 of the 8 patients had good functional outcomes.[177] There are several other more recent studies, 2 of which report a significant and sustained reduction in mean cerebral blood flow velocity after intraventricular nicardipine, although neither study was powered for clinical outcomes.[179,180]

Verapamil is another calcium channel antagonist that has been used via intra-arterial administration for treating cerebral vasospasm. The published data are from retrospective evaluations in which verapamil was administered at dosages of between 25 and 369 mg per vessel by continuous infusion.[165,181] Verapamil was effective in reversing vasospasm and demonstrated neurological improvement, but close hemodynamic monitoring is advised as common complications include hypotension and bradycardia.[165,181,182]

Sodium nitroprusside is another less commonly used vasodilating agent that has been administered by the intraventricular route. In a prospective study of 25 patients with aSAH, nitroprusside 4 mg/mL was given in escalating doses (8–30 mg) and frequency based on mean blood flow velocity on TCD. An improvement in blood flow velocity was reported, with complications including hypotension and vomiting.[183]

Milrinone is an agent that combines vasodilating and inotropic properties that is widely used to treat patients with acute heart failure, but intra-arterial milrinone has also been used to treat cerebral vasospasm.[184–186] Milrinone is a bipyridine inotropic vasodilator that inhibits peak III cyclic adenosine monophosphate phosphodiesterase isozyme. In a study of 22 patients evaluating the combination of intra-arterial milrinone (8 mg over 30 minutes repeated up to a maximum of 24 mg) with intravenous milrinone (0.5–1.5 mcg/kg/min) until day 14 after the initial bleed, milrinone was considered safe and effective for reversing cerebral vasospasm.[185]

Local administration of all the agents discussed provides a more targeted approach for treating cerebral vasospasm. However, most of the data for this approach are limited to small case series or case reports, making it difficult to provide definitive recommendations and resulting in significant practice variation.

PHARMACOKINETIC CONSIDERATIONS IN PHARMACOTHERAPY OPTIMIZATION

Despite studies of individual treatments showing promise, translating these reports into optimized clinical care remains difficult. Concomitant physiologic and pharmacologic changes over the course of critical illness have the potential

TABLE 5.2 Considerations in Pharmacokinetic Alterations

Absorption	Distribution	Metabolism	Elimination
• Formulation • PH • Concomitant therapies • Gastrointestinal transit time	Systemic • Protein binding • Hepatic and gastrointestinal transporters	Hepatic • Phase I CYP-450 enzymes • Phase II	Systemic • Renal • Biliary
	Central • Central nervous system transporter • Blood-brain barrier junction changes	Central • P450 enzymes	Central • External ventricular drains

to significantly affect treatment responses (Table 5.2). Progressive physiologic changes combined with treatment interventions can affect drug absorption, distribution, metabolism, or excretion.[187–190] Altered drug concentrations in the clinical setting of vasospasm are poorly defined so patient responses are typically measured using TCDs or other clinical correlates of patient cognitive status. Correlating clinical measures to drug-specific interventions for efficacy end points is difficult and often fails in sensitivity, specificity, and reproducibility of these results.[189] Critically ill patients with neurologic illness are a complex population with a number of factors impacting drug pharmacokinetic profiles that affect response.

Absorption Considerations

Physicochemical drug properties affect membrane penetration, and physiologic dynamics can also affect absorption. Altered gastrointestinal blood flow, concomitant enteral nutrition, concomitant pill burden, and enteric pH values may confound the amount of drug systemically available. Agents at risk for altered absorption include nimodipine, cilastazol, and clazosentan.[191,192] Preventative and treatment interventions targeting vasospasm with fluid volume management may alter gastrointestinal blood flow. Enteral nutrition via gastric or duodenal feeding tubes may lower nimodipine absorption because of binding or pH changes.[192] Similarly, stress ulcer prophylaxis and bowel regimens may lead to variability in nimodipine absorption.

Ideally, administer nimodipine without other medications at the same time. If administered via feeding tube, flush with water and hold the feeding for up to 60 minutes. Package labeling calls for administration on an empty stomach at least 1 hour before or 2 hours after meals. With dosing every 4 hours, this approach will affect nutritional intake significantly. If specialized nutritional products or new treatments are introduced affecting motility or pH during the 21-day course, systemic concentrations may change.

Distribution Considerations

Distribution of drugs can be affected systemically and within the central nervous system because of the endogenous response to release of inflammatory mediators.[190,193–196] The acute phase response includes a decline in serum albumin and an increase in acute phase proteins systemically. Drugs with significant protein binding, such as nimodipine, may transiently have higher unbound concentrations that fluctuate as these protein reservoirs normalize. This increase in unbound nimodipine presented to the blood-brain barrier may provide an opportunity for enhanced uptake, but it also is a likely factor contributing to systemic hypotension.

Metabolism Considerations

Most drugs are chemically altered endogenously to facilitate elimination. Although different methods of metabolism exist (phase I and phase II), most drug interactions occur during phase I oxidation by the cytochrome (CYP) P450 enzymes.[197–199] These enzymes are located in the liver, intestine, and brain tissues. The functional impact of CYP-P450 enzymes in brain tissues is poorly understood.

Drug substrates for specific subsets of the cytochrome P450 enzymes vary, and polymorphisms are reported in different populations. Polymorphic changes in genes for 2D6, 3A4, and 3A5 may affect drug substrates for these enzymes and alter their concentrations. Cytochrome P450 enzyme activity can be increased or decreased in the presence of different drugs. When concomitant substrates are administered, the potential for drug interactions increases. Attention should be paid to medications used prior to admission if continued during ICU stays. Standardized treatment guidelines include drugs subject to interactions via the cytochrome enzymes. Adding maintenance medications to the regimens may increase the risk of unexpected adverse effects, so careful review is recommended.

Although other cytochrome P450 enzymes can affect treatment responses, the CYP3A4 family is routinely examined for drug interaction risks. ICU drugs used in patients with vasospasm that are metabolized by this enzyme include some benzodiazepines, cilostazol, dantrolene, fentanyl, statins, nicardipine, and nimodipine.[200–202] These are substrates and can be affected by concomitant drugs acting to stimulate or inhibit the activity of this enzyme. In the ICU, azole antifungals, haloperidol, metronidazole, propofol, and serotonin modulators are agents that downregulate the activity of this enzyme. This downregulation may increase concentrations of substrate drugs. In contrast, ICU treatments that stimulate the enzyme will reduce the concentration of the substrate drug. Inducers of CYP3A4 used in the ICU include carbamazepine, dexamethasone, phenytoin, some antibiotics, and pentobarbital. It is important to examine the potential contribution of enzymatic metabolism to drug inactivation, generation of active or toxic metabolites, and also drug-drug interactions affecting treatment response.

Investigational treatments for vasospasm should include information about phase I and phase II metabolism and first-pass metabolism. When drugs have a "high first-pass metabolism" profile, liver blood flow dynamics affect the concentration of drug available for target delivery. Nimodipine has extensive first-pass metabolism along with CYP3A4 substrate properties. These properties combined with protein binding of more than 95% create significant confounding factors that may affect patient response. When clinical management also includes triple-H regimens, blood flow changes may further affect the amount of active nimodipine available to the target tissues.

Elimination Considerations

Renal clearance is higher than predicted in patients with subarachnoid hemorrhage.[203] Whether this augmented clearance is attributed to triple-H regimens or an endogenous response to central nervous system injury remains to be determined. The consequence of higher renal clearance may include lower systemic drug concentrations or variance in concentrations, particularly if fluid therapy and vasopressin are introduced in the treatment. Protein binding restricts glomerular filtration, so highly bound treatments may be less affected by this physiologic change. Although augmented renal clearance would not affect nimodipine, other treatments, including antibiotics and levetiracetam, may be affected.[1,2] It is unknown if this clinical phenomenon influences the response to magnesium as a potential treatment for vasospasm.

SUMMARY

Cerebral vasospasm is associated with significant morbidity and mortality following aSAH. Despite significant investigation, the pathophysiology of cerebral vasospasm and the development of early brain injury and DIND is poorly understood, which limits our ability to identify the most effective treatment target or combination of targets. Many clinical studies have evaluated pharmacologic interventions for both the prevention and treatment of cere-bral vasospasm. Overall, there is a paucity of evidence-based interventions that are used in clinical practice. Nimodipine remains the only proven method of preventing DCI. The mainstay intervention for treatment has been triple-H therapy, although the treatment combination remains controversial. Recent evidence suggests that induced hypertension is the component most beneficial for vasospasm treatment. aSAH is a very complex disease, with cerebral vaso-spasm representing only one of the many complications that can occur; there-fore, care of the patient by a multidisciplinary health care team in a dedicated neuroscience ICU is essential. Individualization of the pharmacotherapy plan is important for optimizing medication outcomes and overall patient outcomes.

References

1. Browning M, Shear DA, Bramlett HM, et al. Levetiracetam treatment in traumatic brain injury: operation brain trauma therapy. *J Neurotrauma*. 2016;33(6):581–594.
2. Hobbs AL, Shea KM, Roberts KM, Daley MJ. Implications of augmented renal clear-ance on drug dosing in critically ill patients: a focus on antibiotics. *Pharmacotherapy*. 2015;35:1063–1075.
3. Ingall T, Asplund K, Mahonen M, Bonita R. A multinational comparison of subarach-noid hemorrhage epidemiology in the WHO MONICA stroke study. *Stroke*. 2000; 31:1054–1061.
4. Sarti C, Tuomilehto J, Salomaa V, et al. Epidemiology of subarachnoid hemorrhage in Finland from 1983 to 1985. *Stroke*. 1991;22:848–853.
5. Schievink WI. Intracranial aneurysms. *N Engl J Med*. 1997;336:28–40.
6. van Gijn J, Rinkel GJ. Subarachnoid haemorrhage: diagnosis, causes and management. *Brain*. 2001;124:249–278.
7. Saveland H, Sonesson B, Ljunggren B, et al. Outcome evaluation following subarach-noid hemorrhage. *J Neurosurg*. 1986;64:191–196.
8. Dombovy ML, Drew-Cates J, Serdans R. Recovery and rehabilitation following sub-arachnoid haemorrhage: Part II. Long-term follow-up. *Brain Injury*. 1998;12:887–894.
9. Lee WC, Christensen MC, Joshi AV, Pashos CL. Long-term cost of stroke subtypes among Medicare beneficiaries. *Cerebrovasc Dis*. 2007;23:57–65.
10. Macdonald RL. Origins of the concept of vasospasm. *Stroke*. 2016;47:e11–e15.
11. Ecker A, Riemenschneider PA. Arteriographic demonstration of spasm of the intracra-nial arteries, with special reference to saccular arterial aneurysms. *J Neursurg*. 1951; 8:660–667.
12. Fisher CM, Roberson GH, Ojemann RG. Cerebral vasospasm with ruptured saccular aneurysm—the clinical manifestations. *Neurosurgery*. 1977;1:245–8.
13. Weir B, Grace M, Hansen J, Rothberg C. Time course of vasospasm in man. *J Neurosurg*. 1978;48:173–178.
14. Brown RJ, Kumar A, Dhar R, et al. The relationship between delayed infarcts and angio-graphic vasospasm after aneurysmal subarachnoid hemorrhage. *Neurosurgery*. 2013; 72:702–708.

15. Rabinstein AA, Weigand S, Atkinson JL, Wijdicks EF. Patterns of cerebral infarction in aneurysmal subarachnoid hemorrhage. *Stroke*. 2005;36:992–997.
16. Rabinstein AA, Friedman JA, Weigand SD, et al. Predictors of cerebral infarction in aneurysmal subarachnoid hemorrhage. *Stroke*. 2004;35:1862–1866.
17. Mir DI, Gupta A, Dunning A, et al. CT perfusion for detection of delayed cerebral ischemia in aneurysmal subarachnoid hemorrhage: a systematic review and meta-analysis. *AJNR*. 2014;35:866–871.
18. Kassell NF, Sasaki T, Colohan AR, Nazar G. Cerebral vasospasm following aneurysmal subarachnoid hemorrhage. *Stroke*. 1985;16:562–572.
19. Weir B, Macdonald RL, Stoodley M. Etiology of cerebral vasospasm. *Acta Neuroschi Suppl*. 1999;72:27–46.
20. Ropper AH, Zervas NT. Outcome 1 year after SAH from cerebral aneurysm: management morbidity, mortality, and functional status in 112 consecutive good-risk patients. *J Neursurg*. 1984;60:909–915.
21. Solenski NJ, Haley EC Jr, Kassell NF, et al. Medical complications of aneurysmal subarachnoid hemorrhage: a report of the Multicenter Cooperative Aneurysm Study. *Crit Care Med*. 1995;23:1007–1017.
22. Gonzalez NR, Boscardin WJ, Glenn T, et al. Vasospasm probability index: a combination of transcranial Doppler velocities, cerebral blood flow, and clinical risk factors to predict cerebral vasospasm after aneurysmal subarachnoid hemorrhage. *J Neursurg*. 2007;107:1101–1112.
23. Inagawa T. Risk for cerebral vasospasm following aneurysmal subarachnoid hemorrhage: a review of the literature. *World Neurosurg*. 2016;85:56–76.
24. Reilly C, Amidei C, Tolentino J, et al. Clot volume and clearance rate as independent predictors of vasospasm after aneurysmal subarachnoid hemorrhage. *J Neurosurg*. 2004;101:255–261.
25. Frontera JA, Claassen J, Schmidt JM, et al. Prediction of symptomatic vasospasm after subarachnoid hemorrhage: the modified fisher scale. *Neurosurgery*. 2006;59:21–27.
26. Kramer AH, Hehir M, Nathan B, et al. A comparison of 3 radiographic scales for the prediction of delayed ischemia and prognosis following subarachnoid hemorrhage. *J Neurosurg*. 2008;109:199–207.
27. Fisher CM, Kistler JP, Davis JM. Relation of cerebral vasospasm to subarachnoid hemorrhage visualized by computerized tomographic scanning. *Neurosurgery*. 1980;6:1–9.
28. Conway JE, Tamargo RJ. Cocaine use is an independent risk factor for cerebral vasospasm after aneurysmal subarachnoid hemorrhage. *Stroke*. 2001;32:2338–2343.
29. Harrod CG, Bendok BR, Batjer HH. Prediction of cerebral vasospasm in patients presenting with aneurysmal subarachnoid hemorrhage: a review. *Neurosurgery*. 2005;56:633–654.
30. Rabinstein AA, Pichelmann MA, Friedman JA, et al. Symptomatic vasospasm and outcomes following aneurysmal subarachnoid hemorrhage: a comparison between surgical repair and endovascular coil occlusion. *J Neurosurg*. 2003;98:319–325.
31. Lee Y, Zuckerman SL, Mocco J. Current controversies in the prediction, diagnosis, and management of cerebral vasospasm: where do we stand? *Neurol Res Int*. 2013;373458.
32. Gallek MJ, Alexander SA, Crago E, et al. Endothelin-1 gene polymorphisms influence cerebrospinal fluid endothelin-1 levels following aneurysmal subarachnoid hemorrhage. *Biol Res Nurs*. 2015;17:185–190.
33. Diringer MN, Bleck TP, Claude Hemphill J III, et al. Critical care management of patients following aneurysmal subarachnoid hemorrhage: recommendations from the

Neurocritical Care Society's Multidisciplinary Consensus Conference. *Neurocrit Care.* 2011;15:211–240.

34. Vergouwen MD, Vermeulen M, van Gijn J, et al. Definition of delayed cerebral ischemia after aneurysmal subarachnoid hemorrhage as an outcome event in clinical trials and observational studies: proposal of a multidisciplinary research group. *Stroke.* 2010; 41:2391–2395.

35. Macdonald RL, Higashida RT, Keller E, et al. Clazosentan, an endothelin receptor antagonist, in patients with aneurysmal subarachnoid haemorrhage undergoing surgical clipping: a randomised, double-blind, placebo-controlled phase 3 trial (CONSCIOUS-2). *Lancet Neurol.* 2011;10:618–625.

36. Sehba FA, Friedrich V. Early events after aneurysmal subarachnoid hemorrhage. *Acta Neurochir Suppl.* 2015;120:23–28.

37. Macdonald RL. Delayed neurological deterioration after subarachnoid haemorrhage. *Nat Rev Neurol.* 2014;10:44–58.

38. Sabri M, Lass E, Macdonald RL. Early brain injury: a common mechanism in subarachnoid hemorrhage and global cerebral ischemia. *Stroke Res Treat.* 2013;2013:394036.

39. Wellman GC, Nathan DJ, Saundry CM, et al. Ca2+sparks and their function in human cerebral arteries. *Stroke.* 2002;33:802–808.

40. Findlay JM, Weir BK, Kanamaru K, Espinosa F. Arterial wall changes in cerebral vasospasm. *Neurosurgery.* 1989;25:736–746.

41. Gibbons GH, Dzau VJ. The emerging concept of vascular remodeling. *N Engl J Med.* 1994;330:1431–1438.

42. Kramer AH, Fletcher JJ. Locally-administered intrathecal thrombolytics following aneurysmal subarachnoid hemorrhage: a systematic review and meta-analysis. *Neurocrit Care.* 2011;14:489–499.

43. Clark JF, Sharp FR. Bilirubin oxidation products (BOXes) and their role in cerebral vasospasm after subarachnoid hemorrhage. *J Cereb Blood Flow Metab.* 2006;26:1223–1233.

44. Kastner S, Oertel MF, Scharbrodt W, et al. Endothelin-1 in plasma, cisternal CSF and microdialysate following aneurysmal SAH. *Acta Neurochir.* 2005;147:1271–1279.

45. Pluta RM. Delayed cerebral vasospasm and nitric oxide: review, new hypothesis, and proposed treatment. *Pharmacol Ther.* 2005;105:23–56.

46. Fassbender K, Hodapp B, Rossol S, et al. Endothelin-1 in subarachnoid hemorrhage: an acute-phase reactant produced by cerebrospinal fluid leukocytes. *Stroke.* 2000; 31:2971–2975.

47. Fassbender K, Hodapp B, Rossol S, et al. Inflammatory cytokines in subarachnoid haemorrhage: association with abnormal blood flow velocities in basal cerebral arteries. *J Neurol Neurosurg Psych.* 2001;70:534–537.

48. Rothoerl RD, Ringel F. Molecular mechanisms of cerebral vasospasm following aneurysmal SAH. *Neurol Res.* 2007;29:636–642.

49. Bacigaluppi S, Zona G, Secci F, et al. Diagnosis of cerebral vasospasm and risk of delayed cerebral ischemia related to aneurysmal subarachnoid haemorrhage: an overview of available tools. *Neurosurg Rev.* 2015;38:603–618.

50. Rosen DS, Macdonald RL. Subarachnoid hemorrhage grading scales: a systematic review. *Neurocrit Care.* 2005;2:110–118.

51. Connolly ES Jr, Rabinstein AA, Carhuapoma JR, et al. Guidelines for the management of aneurysmal subarachnoid hemorrhage: a guideline for healthcare professionals from the American Heart Association/American Stroke Association. *Stroke.* 2012;43: 1711–1737.

52. McGirt MJ, Blessing RP, Goldstein LB. Transcranial Doppler monitoring and clinical decision-making after subarachnoid hemorrhage. *J Stroke Cerebrovasc Dis.* 2003; 12:88–92.

53. Vora YY, Suarez-Almazor M, Steinke DE, et al. Role of transcranial Doppler monitoring in the diagnosis of cerebral vasospasm after subarachnoid hemorrhage. *Neurosurgery.* 1999;44:1237–1248.

54. Sloan MA, Haley EC Jr, Kassell NF, et al. Sensitivity and specificity of transcranial Doppler ultrasonography in the diagnosis of vasospasm following subarachnoid hemorrhage. *Neurology.* 1989;39:1514–1518.

55. Lindegaard KF, Nornes H, Bakke SJ, et al. Cerebral vasospasm diagnosis by means of angiography and blood velocity measurements. *Acta Neurochir.* 1989;100:12–24.

56. Darwish RS, Ahn E, Amiridze NS. Role of transcranial Doppler in optimizing treatment of cerebral vasospasm in subarachnoid hemorrhage. *J Intensive Care Med.* 2008;23: 263–267.

57. Rabinstein AA, Lanzino G, Wijdicks EF. Multidisciplinary management and emerging therapeutic strategies in aneurysmal subarachnoid haemorrhage. *Lancet Neurol.* 2010;9:504–519.

58. Vespa PM, Nuwer MR, Juhasz C, et al. Early detection of vasospasm after acute subarachnoid hemorrhage using continuous EEG ICU monitoring. *Electroencephalogr Clin Neurophysiol.* 1997;103:607–615.

59. Nilsson OG, Brandt L, Ungerstedt U, and Saveland H. Bedside detection of brain ischemia using intracerebral microdialysis: subarachnoid hemorrhage and delayed ischemic deterioration. *Neurosurgery.* 1999;45:1176–1185.

60. Dorhout Mees SM, Rinkel GJ, Feigin VL, et al. Calcium antagonists for aneurysmal subarachnoid haemorrhage. *Cochrane Database Syst Rev.* 2007;3:CD000277.

61. Liu-Deryke X, Rhoney DH. Cerebral vasospasm after aneurysmal subarachnoid hemorrhage: an overview of pharmacologic management. *Pharmacotherapy.* 2006;26:182–203.

62. Allen GS, Ahn HS, Preziosi TJ, et al. Cerebral arterial spasm—a controlled trial of nimodipine in patients with subarachnoid hemorrhage. *N Engl J Med.* 1983;308:619–624.

63. Pickard JD, Murray GD, Illingworth R, et al. Effect of oral nimodipine on cerebral infarction and outcome after subarachnoid haemorrhage: British aneurysm nimodipine trial. *BMJ.* 1989;298:636–642.

64. Liu GJ, Luo J, Zhang LP, et al. Meta-analysis of the effectiveness and safety of prophylactic use of nimodipine in patients with an aneurysmal subarachnoid haemorrhage. *CNS Neurol Disord Drug Targets.* 2011;10:834–844.

65. Brandt L, Andersson KE, Edvinsson L, Ljunggren B. Effects of extracellular calcium and of calcium antagonists on the contractile responses of isolated human pial and mesenteric arteries. *J Cereb Blood Flow Metab.* 1981;1:339–347.

66. Roos Y, Rinkel GJE, Vermeulen M, et al. Antifibrinolytic therapy for aneurysmal subarachnoid haemorrhage: a major update of a cochrane review. *Stroke.* 2003;34:2308–2309.

67. Claassen J, Vu A, Kreiter KT, et al. Effect of acute physiologic derangements on outcome after subarachnoid hemorrhage. *Crit Care Med.* 2004;32:832–838.

68. Sandow N, Diesing D, Sarrafzadeh A, et al. Nimodipine dose reductions in the treatment of patients with aneurysmal subarachnoid hemorrhage. *Neurocrit Care.* 2016;25(1):29–39.

69. Karinen P, Koivukangas P, Ohinmaa A, et al. Cost-effectiveness analysis of nimodipine treatment after aneurysmal subarachnoid hemorrhage and surgery. *Neurosurgery.* 1999; 45:780–784.

70. Green AE, Banks S, Jay M, Hatton J. Stability of nimodipine solution in oral syringes. *AJHP*. 2004;61:1493–1496.

71. Nimodipine capsure (Nimotop) [package insert]. Bayer Corporation; 2000.

72. FDA Drug Safety Communication. Serious medication errors from intravenous administration of nimodipine oral capsules. 2010. www.fda.gov/Drugs/DrugSafety /PostmarketDrugSafetyInformationforPatientsandProviders/ucm220386.htm. Accessed December 20, 2016.

73. FDA News Release. FDA approves Nymalize—first nimodipine oral solution for use in certain brain hemorrhage patients. 2013. www.fda.gov/NewsEvents/Newsroom/Press Announcements/ucm352280.htm. Accessed December 20, 2016.

74. Oyler DR, Stump SE, Cook AM. Accuracy of nimodipine gel extraction. *Neurocrit Care*. 2015;22:89–92.

75. Cook DJ, Kan S, Ai J, et al. Cisternal sustained release dihydropyridines for subarachnoid hemorrhage. *Curr Neurovasc Res*. 2012;9:139–148.

76. Etminan N, Macdonald RL, Davis C, et al. Intrathecal application of the nimodipine slow-release microparticle system eg-1962 for prevention of delayed cerebral ischemia and improvement of outcome after aneurysmal subarachnoid hemorrhage. *Acta Neurochir Suppl*. 2015;120:281–286.

77. Hanggi D, Etminan N, Macdonald RL, et al. NEWTON: Nimodipine microparticles to enhance recovery while reducing toxicity after subarachnoid hemorrhage. *Neurocrit Care*. 2015;23:274–284.

78. Edge Therapeutics, Inc. Edge Therapeutics reports positive top-line phase 1/2 NEWTON trial results of EG-1962 in aneurysmal subarachnoid hemorrhage. 2015. www .edgetherapeutics.com/news/edge-therapeutics-reports-positive-top-line-phase-12 -newton-trial-results-of-eg-1962-in-aneurysmal-subarachnoid-hemorrhage. Accessed December 20, 2016.

79. Haley EC Jr, Kassell NF, Torner JC. A randomized trial of nicardipine in subarachnoid hemorrhage: angiographic and transcranial Doppler ultrasound results. A report of the Cooperative Aneurysm Study. *J Neurosurg*. 1993;78:548–553.

80. Haley EC Jr, Kassell NF, Torner JC. A randomized controlled trial of high-dose intravenous nicardipine in aneurysmal subarachnoid hemorrhage: a report of the Cooperative Aneurysm Study. *J Neurosurg*. 1993;78:537–547.

81. Muehlschlegel S, Sims JR. Dantrolene: mechanisms of neuroprotection and possible clinical applications in the neurointensive care unit. *Neurocrit Care*. 2009;10:103–115.

82. Frandsen A, Schousboe A. Dantrolene prevents glutamate cytotoxicity and Ca2+release from intracellular stores in cultured cerebral cortical neurons. *J Neurochem*. 1991; 56:1075–1078.

83. Salomone S, Soydan G, Moskowitz MA, Sims JR. Inhibition of cerebral vasoconstriction by dantrolene and nimodipine. *Neurocrit Care*. 2009;10:93–102.

84. Muehlschlegel S, Rordorf G, Bodock M, Sims JR. Dantrolene mediates vasorelaxation in cerebral vasoconstriction: a case series. *Neurocrit Care*. 2009;10:116–121.

85. Muehlschlegel S, Rordorf G, Sims J. Effects of a single dose of dantrolene in patients with cerebral vasospasm after subarachnoid hemorrhage: a prospective pilot study. *Stroke*. 2011;42:1301–1306.

86. Muehlschlegel S, Carandang R, Hall W, et al. Dantrolene for cerebral vasospasm after subarachnoid haemorrhage: a randomised double blind placebo-controlled safety trial. *J Neurol Neurosurg Psychiatry*. 2015;86:1029–1035.

87. Liu GJ, Wang ZJ, Wang YF, et al. Systematic assessment and meta-analysis of the efficacy and safety of fasudil in the treatment of cerebral vasospasm in patients with subarachnoid hemorrhage. *Eur J Clin Pharmacol.* 2012;68:131–139.

88. Zhao J, Zhou D, Guo J, et al. Efficacy and safety of fasudil in patients with subarachnoid hemorrhage: final results of a randomized trial of fasudil versus nimodipine. *Neurol Med Chir.* 2011;51:679–683.

89. McGirt MJ, Lynch JR, Parra A, et al. Simvastatin increases endothelial nitric oxide synthase and ameliorates cerebral vasospasm resulting from subarachnoid hemorrhage. *Stroke.* 2002;33:2950–2956.

90. O'Driscoll G, Green D, Taylor RR. Simvastatin, an HMG-coenzyme A reductase inhibitor, improves endothelial function within 1 month. *Circulation.* 1997; 95:1126–1131.

91. Thelen KM, Rentsch KM, Gutteck U, et al. Brain cholesterol synthesis in mice is affected by high dose of simvastatin but not of pravastatin. *J Pharmacol Exp Ther.* 2006;316:1146–1152.

92. Chou SH, Smith EE, Badjatia N, et al. A randomized, double-blind, placebo-controlled pilot study of simvastatin in aneurysmal subarachnoid hemorrhage. *Stroke.* 2008;39: 2891–2893.

93. Lynch JR, Wang H, McGirt MJ, et al. Simvastatin reduces vasospasm after aneurysmal subarachnoid hemorrhage: results of a pilot randomized clinical trial. *Stroke.* 2005;36:2024–2026.

94. Vergouwen MD, Meijers JC, Geskus RB, et al. Biologic effects of simvastatin in patients with aneurysmal subarachnoid hemorrhage: a double-blind, placebo-controlled randomized trial. *J Cereb Blood Flow Metab.* 2009;29:1444–1453.

95. Tseng MY, Czosnyka M, Richards H, et al. Effects of acute treatment with pravastatin on cerebral vasospasm, autoregulation, and delayed ischemic deficits after aneurysmal subarachnoid hemorrhage: a phase II randomized placebo-controlled trial. *Stroke.* 2005; 36:1627–1632.

96. Singhal AB, Topcuoglu MA, Dorer DJ, et al. SSRI and statin use increases the risk for vasospasm after subarachnoid hemorrhage. *Neurology.* 2005;64:1008–1013.

97. Moskowitz SI, Ahrens C, Provencio JJ, et al. Prehemorrhage statin use and the risk of vasospasm after aneurysmal subarachnoid hemorrhage. *Surg Neurol.* 2009;71:311–318.

98. McGirt MJ, Garces Ambrossi GL, Huang J, Tamargo RJ. Simvastatin for the prevention of symptomatic cerebral vasospasm following aneurysmal subarachnoid hemorrhage: a single-institution prospective cohort study. *J Neurosurg.* 2009;110:968–974.

99. Kramer AH, Gurka MJ, Nathan B, et al. Statin use was not associated with less vasospasm or improved outcome after subarachnoid hemorrhage. *Neurosurgery.* 2008;62:422–430.

100. Kerz T, Victor A, Beyer C, et al. A case control study of statin and magnesium administration in patients after aneurysmal subarachnoid hemorrhage: incidence of delayed cerebral ischemia and mortality. *Neurol Res.* 2008;30:893–897.

101. Kern M, Lam MM, Knuckey NW, Lind CR. Statins may not protect against vasospasm in subarachnoid haemorrhage. *J Clin Neurosci.* 2009;16:527–530.

102. Kramer AH, Fletcher JJ. Statins in the management of patients with aneurysmal subarachnoid hemorrhage: a systematic review and meta-analysis. *Neurocrit Care.* 2010;12:285–296.

103. Vergouwen MD, de Haan RJ, Vermeulen M, Roos YB. Effect of statin treatment on vasospasm, delayed cerebral ischemia, and functional outcome in patients with aneurysmal subarachnoid hemorrhage: a systematic review and meta-analysis update. *Stroke.* 2010;41:e47–e52.

104. Sillberg VA, Wells GA, Perry JJ. Do statins improve outcomes and reduce the incidence of vasospasm after aneurysmal subarachnoid hemorrhage: a meta-analysis. *Stroke.* 2008;39:2622–2626.

105. Sanchez-Pena P, Nouet A, Clarencon F, et al. Atorvastatin decreases computed tomography and S100-assessed brain ischemia after subarachnoid aneurysmal hemorrhage: a comparative study. *Crit Care Med.* 2012;40:594–602.

106. Kirkpatrick PJ, Turner CL, Smith C, et al. Simvastatin in aneurysmal subarachnoid haemorrhage (STASH): a multicentre randomised phase 3 trial. *Lancet Neurol.* 2014; 13:666–675.

107. Risselada R, Straatman H, van Kooten F, et al. Withdrawal of statins and risk of subarachnoid hemorrhage. *Stroke.* 2009;40:2887–2892.

108. Lizza BD, Kosteva A, Maas MB, et al. Preadmission statin use does not improve functional outcomes or prevent delayed ischemic events in patients with spontaneous subarachnoid hemorrhage. *Pharmacotherapy.* 2014;34:811–817.

109. Macdonald RL, Curry DJ, Aihara Y, et al. Magnesium and experimental vasospasm. *J Neurosurgery.* 2004;100:106–110.

110. Pyne GJ, Cadoux-Hudson TA, Clark JF. Magnesium protection against in vitro cerebral vasospasm after subarachnoid haemorrhage. *Br J Neurosurg.* 2001;15:409–415.

111. van den Bergh WM, Algra A, van der Sprenkel JW, et al. Hypomagnesemia after aneurysmal subarachnoid hemorrhage. *Neurosurgery.* 2003;52:276–282.

112. van den Bergh WM, Albrecht KW, Berkelbach van der Sprenkel JW, Rinkel GJ. Magnesium therapy after aneurysmal subarachnoid haemorrhage a dose-finding study for long term treatment. *Acta Neurochir.* 2003;145:195–199.

113. van den Bergh WM, Algra A, van Kooten F, et al. Magnesium sulfate in aneurysmal subarachnoid hemorrhage: a randomized controlled trial. *Stroke.* 2005;36:1011–1015.

114. Bradford CM, Finfer S, O'Connor A, et al. A randomised controlled trial of induced hypermagnesaemia following aneurysmal subarachnoid haemorrhage. *Crit Care Resusc.* 2013;15:119–125.

115. Muroi C, Terzic A, Fortunati M, et al. Magnesium sulfate in the management of patients with aneurysmal subarachnoid hemorrhage: a randomized, placebo-controlled, dose-adapted trial. *Surg Neurol.* 2008;69:33–39.

116. Veyna RS, Seyfried D, Burke DG, et al. Magnesium sulfate therapy after aneurysmal subarachnoid hemorrhage. *J Neurosurg.* 2002;96:510–514.

117. Westermaier T, Stetter C, Vince GH, et al. Prophylactic intravenous magnesium sulfate for treatment of aneurysmal subarachnoid hemorrhage: a randomized, placebo-controlled, clinical study. *Crit Care Med.* 2010;38:1284–1290.

118. Wong GK, Boet R, Poon WS, et al. Intravenous magnesium sulphate for aneurysmal subarachnoid hemorrhage: an updated systemic review and meta-analysis. *Crit Care.* 2011;15:R52.

119. Wong GK, Poon WS, Chan MT, et al. Intravenous magnesium sulphate for aneurysmal subarachnoid hemorrhage (IMASH): a randomized, double-blinded, placebo-controlled, multicenter phase III trial. *Stroke.* 2010;41:921–926.

120. Dorhout Mees SM, Algra A, Vandertop WP, et al. Magnesium for aneurysmal subarachnoid haemorrhage (MASH-2): a randomised placebo-controlled trial. *Lancet.* 2012;380:44–49.

121. Brewer RP, Parra A, Borel CO, et al. Intravenous magnesium sulfate does not increase ventricular CSF ionized magnesium concentration of patients with intracranial hypertension. *Clin Neuropharmacol.* 2001;24:341–345.

122. Mori K, Miyazaki M, Hara Y, et al. Novel vasodilatory effect of intracisternal injection of magnesium sulfate solution on spastic cerebral arteries in the canine two-hemorrhage model of subarachnoid hemorrhage. *J Neurosurg.* 2009;110:73–78.

123. Mori K, Yamamoto T, Nakao Y, et al. Initial clinical experience of vasodilatory effect of intra-cisternal infusion of magnesium sulfate for the treatment of cerebral vasospasm after aneurysmal subarachnoid hemorrhage. *Neurol Med Chir.* 2009;49:139–145.

124. Amin-Hanjani S, Ogilvy CS, Barker FG II. Does intracisternal thrombolysis prevent vasospasm after aneurysmal subarachnoid hemorrhage? A meta-analysis. *Neurosurgery.* 2004;54:326–335.

125. Klimo P Jr, Kestle JR, MacDonald JD, et al. Marked reduction of cerebral vasospasm with lumbar drainage of cerebrospinal fluid after subarachnoid hemorrhage. *J Neurosurg.* 2004;100:215–224.

126. Kwon OY, Kim YJ, Kim YJ, et al. The utility and benefits of external lumbar CSF drainage after endovascular coiling on aneurysmal subarachnoid hemorrhage. *J Korean Neurosurg Soc.* 2008;43:281–287.

127. Al-Tamimi YZ, Bhargava D, Feltbower RG, et al. Lumbar drainage of cerebrospinal fluid after aneurysmal subarachnoid hemorrhage: a prospective, randomized, controlled trial (LUMAS). *Stroke.* 2012;43:677–682.

128. Bardutzky J, Witsch J, Juttler E, et al. EARLYDRAIN-outcome after early lumbar CSF-drainage in aneurysmal subarachnoid hemorrhage: study protocol for a randomized controlled trial. *Trials.* 2011;12:203.

129. Chow M, Dumont AS, Kassell NF. Endothelin receptor antagonists and cerebral vasospasm: an update. *Neurosurgery.* 2002;51:1333–1342.

130. Macdonald RL, Kassell NF, Mayer S, et al. Clazosentan to overcome neurological ischemia and infarction occurring after subarachnoid hemorrhage (CONSCIOUS-1): randomized, double-blind, placebo-controlled phase 2 dose-finding trial. *Stroke.* 2008;39: 3015–3021.

131. Macdonald RL, Higashida RT, Keller E, et al. Randomized trial of clazosentan in patients with aneurysmal subarachnoid hemorrhage undergoing endovascular coiling. *Stroke.* 2012;43:1463–1469.

132. Pisapia JM, Xu X, Kelly J, et al. Microthrombosis after experimental subarachnoid hemorrhage: time course and effect of red blood cell-bound thrombin-activated pro-urokinase and clazosentan. *Exp Neurol.* 2012;233:357–363.

133. Serrone JC, Maekawa H, Tjahjadi M, Hernesniemi J. Aneurysmal subarachnoid hemorrhage: pathobiology, current treatment and future directions. *Expert Rev Neurother.* 2015;15:367–380.

134. Rasmussen R, Juhler M, Wetterslev J. Effects of continuous prostacyclin infusion on regional blood flow and cerebral vasospasm following subarachnoid haemorrhage: statistical analysis plan for a randomized controlled trial. *Trials.* 2014;15:228.

135. Oldfield EH, Loomba JJ, Monteith SJ, et al. Safety and pharmacokinetics of sodium nitrite in patients with subarachnoid hemorrhage: a phase IIa study. *J Neurosurg.* 2013;119:634–641.

136. National Library of Medicine. Intravenous nitrite infusion for reversal of cerebral vasospasm after subarachnoid hemorrhage. https://clinicaltrials.gov/ct2/show/NCT02176837. Accessed December 20, 2016.

137. Westermaier T, Stetter C, Kunze E, et al. Controlled transient hypercapnia: a novel approach for the treatment of delayed cerebral ischemia after subarachnoid hemorrhage? *J Neurosurg.* 2014;121:1056–1062.

138. Rhoney DH, McAllen K, Liu-DeRyke X. Current and future treatment considerations in the management of aneurysmal subarachnoid hemorrhage. *J Pharm Pract.* 2010; 23:408–424.

139. Lee KH, Lukovits T, Friedman JA. "Triple-H" therapy for cerebral vasospasm following subarachnoid hemorrhage. *Neurocrit Care.* 2006;4:68–76.

140. Dankbaar JW, Slooter AJ, Rinkel GJ, Schaaf IC. Effect of different components of triple-H therapy on cerebral perfusion in patients with aneurysmal subarachnoid haemorrhage: a systematic review. *Crit Care.* 2010;14:R23.

141. Treggiari MM, Deem S. Which H is the most important in triple-H therapy for cerebral vasospasm? *Cur Opin Crit Care.* 2009;15:83–86.

142. Lennihan L, Mayer SA, Fink ME, et al. Effect of hypervolemic therapy on cerebral blood flow after subarachnoid hemorrhage: a randomized controlled trial. *Stroke.* 2000;31:383–391.

143. Egge A, Waterloo K, Sjoholm H, et al. Prophylactic hyperdynamic postoperative fluid therapy after aneurysmal subarachnoid hemorrhage: a clinical, prospective, randomized, controlled study. *Neurosurgery.* 2001;49:593–606.

144. Kassell NF, Peerless SJ, Durward QJ, et al. Treatment of ischemic deficits from vasospasm with intravascular volume expansion and induced arterial hypertension. *Neurosurgery.* 1982;11:337–343.

145. Touho H, Karasawa J, Ohnishi H, et al. Evaluation of therapeutically induced hypertension in patients with delayed cerebral vasospasm by xenon-enhanced computed tomography. *Neurol Med Chir.* 1992;32:671–678.

146. Muench E, Horn P, Bauhuf C, et al. Effects of hypervolemia and hypertension on regional cerebral blood flow, intracranial pressure, and brain tissue oxygenation after subarachnoid hemorrhage. *Crit Care Med.* 2007;35:1844–1852.

147. Frontera JA, Fernandez A, Schmidt JM, et al. Clinical response to hypertensive hypervolemic therapy and outcome after subarachnoid hemorrhage. *Neurosurgery.* 2010;66: 35–41.

148. Raabe A, Beck J, Keller M, et al. Relative importance of hypertension compared with hypervolemia for increasing cerebral oxygenation in patients with cerebral vasospasm after subarachnoid hemorrhage. *J Neurosurg.* 2005;103:974–981.

149. Miller JA, Dacey RG Jr, Diringer MN. Safety of hypertensive hypervolemic therapy with phenylephrine in the treatment of delayed ischemic deficits after subarachnoid hemorrhage. *Stroke.* 1995;26:2260–2266.

150. Muehlschlegel S, Dunser MW, Gabrielli A, et al. Arginine vasopressin as a supplementary vasopressor in refractory hypertensive, hypervolemic, hemodilutional therapy in subarachnoid hemorrhage. *Neurocrit Care.* 2007;6:3–10.

151. Naidech A, Du Y, Kreiter KT, et al. Dobutamine versus milrinone after subarachnoid hemorrhage. *Neurosurgery.* 2005;56:21–67.

152. Nakagawa A, Su CC, Sato K, et al. Evaluation of changes in circulating blood volume during acute and very acute stages of subarachnoid hemorrhage: implications for the management of hypovolemia. *J Neurosurg.* 2002;97:268–271.

153. Joseph M, Ziadi S, Nates J, et al. Increases in cardiac output can reverse flow deficits from vasospasm independent of blood pressure: a study using xenon computed tomographic measurement of cerebral blood flow. *Neurosurgery.* 2003;53:1044–1052.

154. LeTourneau JL, Pinney J, Phillips CR. Extravascular lung water predicts progression to acute lung injury in patients with increased risk. *Crit Care Med.* 2012;40:847–854.

155. Mutoh T, Kazumata K, Ajiki M, et al. Goal-directed fluid management by bedside transpulmonary hemodynamic monitoring after subarachnoid hemorrhage. *Stroke.* 2007;38:3218–3224.

156. Al-Rawi PG, Tseng MY, Richards HK, et al. Hypertonic saline in patients with poor-grade subarachnoid hemorrhage improves cerebral blood flow, brain tissue oxygen, and pH. *Stroke.* 2010;41:122–128.

157. Horstick G, Lauterbach M, Kempf T, et al. Early albumin infusion improves global and local hemodynamics and reduces inflammatory response in hemorrhagic shock. *Crit Care Med.* 2002;30:851–855.

158. Suarez JI, Shannon L, Zaidat OO, et al. Effect of human albumin administration on clinical outcome and hospital cost in patients with subarachnoid hemorrhage. *J Neurosurg.* 2004;100:585–590.

159. Suarez JI, Martin RH, Calvillo E, et al. The Albumin in Subarachnoid Hemorrhage (ALISAH) multicenter pilot clinical trial: safety and neurologic outcomes. *Stroke.* 2012;43:683–690.

160. Suarez JI, Martin RH, Calvillo E, et al. Human albumin administration in subarachnoid hemorrhage: results of an international survey. *Neurocrit Care.* 2014;20:277–286.

161. Naidech AM, Jovanovic B, Wartenberg KE, et al. Higher hemoglobin is associated with improved outcome after subarachnoid hemorrhage. *Crit Care Med.* 2007;35:2383–2289.

162. Smith MJ, Le Roux PD, Elliott JP, Winn HR. Blood transfusion and increased risk for vasospasm and poor outcome after subarachnoid hemorrhage. *J Neurosurg.* 2004;101:1–7.

163. Festic E, Rabinstein AA, Freeman WD, et al. Blood transfusion is an important predictor of hospital mortality among patients with aneurysmal subarachnoid hemorrhage. *Neurocrit Care.* 2013;18:209–215.

164. Firlik AD, Kaufmann AM, Jungreis CA, Yonas H. Effect of transluminal angioplasty on cerebral blood flow in the management of symptomatic vasospasm following aneurysmal subarachnoid hemorrhage. *J Neurosurg.* 1997;86:830–839.

165. Pierot L, Aggour M, Moret J. Vasospasm after aneurysmal subarachnoid hemorrhage: recent advances in endovascular management. *Curr Opin Crit Care.* 2010;16:110–116.

166. Cook AM, Mieure KD, Owen RD, et al. Intracerebroventricular administration of drugs. *Pharmacotherapy.* 2009;29:832–845.

167. Clouston JE, Numaguchi Y, Zoarski GH, et al. Intraarterial papaverine infusion for cerebral vasospasm after subarachnoid hemorrhage. *AJNR.* 1995;16:27–38.

168. Firlik KS, Kaufmann AM, Firlik AD, et al. Intra-arterial papaverine for the treatment of cerebral vasospasm following aneurysmal subarachnoid hemorrhage. *Surg Neurol.* 1999;51:66–74.

169. Kassell NF, Helm G, Simmons N, et al. Treatment of cerebral vasospasm with intra-arterial papaverine. *J Neurosurg.* 1992;77:848–852.

170. Little N, Morgan MK, Grinnell V, Sorby W. Intra-arterial papaverine in the management of cerebral vasospasm following subarachnoid haemorrhage. *J Clin Neurosci.* 1994;1:42–46.

171. Liu JK, Tenner MS, Gottfried ON, et al. Efficacy of multiple intraarterial papaverine infusions for improvement in cerebral circulation time in patients with recurrent cerebral vasospasm. *J Neurosurg.* 2004;100:414–421.

172. Smith WS, Dowd CF, Johnston SC, et al. Neurotoxicity of intra-arterial papaverine preserved with chlorobutanol used for the treatment of cerebral vasospasm after aneurysmal subarachnoid hemorrhage. *Stroke.* 2004;35:2518–2522.

173. Carhuapoma JR, Qureshi AI, Tamargo RJ, et al. Intra-arterial papaverine-induced seizures: case report and review of the literature. *Surg Neurol.* 2001;56:159–163.
174. Badjatia N, Topcuoglu MA, Pryor JC, et al. Preliminary experience with intra-arterial nicardipine as a treatment for cerebral vasospasm. *AJNR.* 2004;25:819–826.
175. Ehtisham A, Taylor S, Bayless L, et al. Use of intrathecal nicardipine for aneurysmal subarachnoid hemorrhage-induced cerebral vasospasm. *South Med J.* 2009;102:150–153.
176. Linfante I, Delgado-Mederos R, Andreone V, et al. Angiographic and hemodynamic effect of high concentration of intra-arterial nicardipine in cerebral vasospasm. *Neurosurgery.* 2008;63:1080–1087.
177. Goodson K, Lapointe M, Monroe T, Chalela JA. Intraventricular nicardipine for refractory cerebral vasospasm after subarachnoid hemorrhage. *Neurocrit Care.* 2008;8:247–252.
178. Tejada JG, Taylor RA, Ugurel MS, et al. Safety and feasibility of intra-arterial nicardipine for the treatment of subarachnoid hemorrhage-associated vasospasm: initial clinical experience with high-dose infusions. *AJNR.* 2007;28:844–848.
179. Webb A, Kolenda J, Martin K, et al. The effect of intraventricular administration of nicardipine on mean cerebral blood flow velocity measured by transcranial Doppler in the treatment of vasospasm following aneurysmal subarachnoid hemorrhage. *Neurocrit Care.* 2010;12:159–164.
180. Lu N, Jackson D, Luke S, et al. Intraventricular nicardipine for aneurysmal subarachnoid hemorrhage related vasospasm: assessment of 90 days outcome. *Neurocrit Care.* 2012;16:368–375.
181. Keuskamp J, Murali R, Chao KH. High-dose intraarterial verapamil in the treatment of cerebral vasospasm after aneurysmal subarachnoid hemorrhage. *J Neurosurg.* 2008;108: 458–463.
182. Feng L, Fitzsimmons BF, Young WL, et al. Intraarterially administered verapamil as adjunct therapy for cerebral vasospasm: safety and 2-year experience. *AJNR.* 2002; 23:1284–1290.
183. Agrawal A, Patir R, Kato Y, et al. Role of intraventricular sodium nitroprusside in vasospasm secondary to aneurysmal subarachnoid haemorrhage: a 5-year prospective study with review of the literature. *Minim Invasive Neurosurg.* 2009;52:5–8.
184. Arakawa Y, Kikuta K, Hojo M, et al. Milrinone for the treatment of cerebral vasospasm after subarachnoid hemorrhage: report of seven cases. *Neurosurgery.* 2001;48:723–730.
185. Fraticelli AT, Cholley BP, Losser MR, et al. Milrinone for the treatment of cerebral vasospasm after aneurysmal subarachnoid hemorrhage. *Stroke.* 2008;39:893–898.
186. Schmidt U, Bittner E, Pivi S, Marota JJ. Hemodynamic management and outcome of patients treated for cerebral vasospasm with intraarterial nicardipine and/or milrinone. *Anesth Analg.* 2010;110:895–902.
187. Diringer MN, Dhar R, Scalfani M, et al. Effect of high-dose simvastatin on cerebral blood flow and static autoregulation in subarachnoid hemorrhage. *Neurocrit Care.* 2016;25(1):56–63.
188. Neuvonen PJ. Towards safer and more predictable drug treatment—reflections from studies of the First BCPT Prize awardee. *Basic Clin Pharmacol Toxicol.* 2012;110:207–218.
189. Pluta RM, Butman JA, Schatlo B, et al. Subarachnoid hemorrhage and the distribution of drugs delivered into the cerebrospinal fluid: laboratory investigation. *J Neurosurg.* 2009;111:1001–1007.
190. Theken KN, Deng Y, Kannon MA, et al. Activation of the acute inflammatory response alters cytochrome P450 expression and eicosanoid metabolism. *Drug Metab Dispos.* 2011;39:22–29.

191. Kimura H, Okamura Y, Chiba Y, et al. Cilostazol administration with combination enteral and parenteral nutrition therapy remarkably improves outcome after subarachnoid hemorrhage. *Acta Neurochir Suppl.* 2015;120:147–152.

192. Rong WL, Xiao X, Zhao JL, et al. Different doses of clazosentan for aneurismal subarachnoid hemorrhage: a meta-analysis of randomized controlled trials [published online January 7, 2016]. *Am J Ther.*

193. Hermann DM, Kilic E, Spudich A, et al. Role of drug efflux carriers in the healthy and diseased brain. *Ann Neurol.* 2006;60:489–498.

194. Rambeck B, Jurgens UH, May TW, et al. Comparison of brain extracellular fluid, brain tissue, cerebrospinal fluid, and serum concentrations of antiepileptic drugs measured intraoperatively in patients with intractable epilepsy. *Epilepsia.* 2006;47:681–694.

195. Shannon RJ, Carpenter KL, Guilfoyle MR, et al. Cerebral microdialysis in clinical studies of drugs: pharmacokinetic applications. *J Pharmacokinet Pharmacodyn.* 2013;40:343–358.

196. Kishore S, Ko N, Soares BP, et al. Perfusion-CT assessment of blood-brain barrier permeability in patients with aneurysmal subarachnoid hemorrhage. *J Neuroradiol.* 2012; 39:317–325.

197. Brown HS, Galetin A, Hallifax D, Houston JB. Prediction of in vivo drug-drug interactions from in vitro data: factors affecting prototypic drug-drug interactions involving CYP2C9, CYP2D6 and CYP3A4. *Clin Pharmacokinet.* 2006;45:1035–1050.

198. Yiannakopoulou E. Pharmacogenomics of phase II metabolizing enzymes and drug transporters: clinical implications. *Pharmacogenomics J.* 2013;13:105–109.

199. Zhou S, Yung Chan S, Cher Goh B, et al. Mechanism-based inhibition of cytochrome P450 3A4 by therapeutic drugs. *Clin Pharmacokinet.* 2005;44:279–304.

200. Elsby R, Hilgendorf C, Fenner K. Understanding the critical disposition pathways of statins to assess drug-drug interaction risk during drug development: it's not just about OATP1B1. *Clin Pharmacol Ther.* 2012;92:584–598.

201. Su SH, Xu W, Hai J, et al. Effects of statins-use for patients with aneurysmal subarachnoid hemorrhage: a meta-analysis of randomized controlled trials. *Sci Rep.* 2014;4:4573.

202. Zhou YT, Yu LS, Zeng S, et al. Pharmacokinetic drug-drug interactions between 1,4-dihydropyridine calcium channel blockers and statins: factors determining interaction strength and relevant clinical risk management. *Ther Clin Risk Manag.* 2014;10:17–26.

203. May CC, Arora S, Parli SE, et al. Augmented renal clearance in patients with subarachnoid hemorrhage. *Neurocrit Care.* 2015;23:374–379.

Pharmacotherapy of Acute Spinal Cord Injury

Kathleen A. Bledsoe, Christopher Morrison, and Ted Sindlinger

INTRODUCTION

Acute spinal cord injury (ASCI) is responsible for significant morbidity and mortality and results in health care costs in excess of $6 billion annually in the United States. The age of patients who have ASCI has increased over the past 40 years, with the average now at 42 years of age with males comprising approximately 80% of cases. Motor vehicle collisions are the most common cause of ASCI, followed closely by falls and then acts of violence and sports-related injuries. An estimated 300,000 individuals live with spinal cord injury in the United States.[1]

The treatment of spinal cord injury includes initial stabilization of the injury to prevent further injury, mitigation of acute pathophysiological effects of the injury, and then prevention of longer term complications from the injury. While there has been significant research devoted to the treatment of ASCI, there has yet to be a definitive therapy to reverse the effects of the injury and improve functional recovery. Much of the medication therapy is designed to treat symptoms associated with the injury, which may indirectly improve long-term functionality and improve quality of life. Even with the vast medication therapies that have been used to treat symptoms such as pain, spasticity, depression, and autonomic dysreflexia, there remains a paucity of clear, evidence-based literature to guide therapy. This chapter will present medication therapies commonly used in the treatment of ACSI and the various complications encountered in this patient population and will discuss potential future therapies for treatment of the acute injury geared toward improving functional outcomes.

INITIAL MANAGEMENT

Early management of patients with ASCI should focus on immediate immobilization of the spine to prevent any further damage and assessment of need of other supportive therapies. Cardiopulmonary support may be required immediately for those patients with high-level injuries. Consideration of definitive spine stabilization, typically through surgical intervention, should occur early in care, and patients should be transported to level I trauma centers equipped to treat these types of injuries. A thorough neurological assessment is important to determine level of function, including both motor and sensory function. Imaging is also useful to assess the level of injury and help determine the need for surgical intervention. Appropriate management during the first few hours to days after injury optimizes the potential for improved neurological recovery.

Steroid Therapy for Neuroprotection

Damage to the spinal cord occurs with the initial trauma. Further injury can occur over the course of hours to days secondary to edema and cytotoxic pathways. High-dose steroids were once proposed to be effective in mitigating these secondary effects and improving motor and sensory function after ASCI. Methylprednisolone was originally studied in the mid-1980s as a potential treatment for ASCI in the National Acute Spinal Cord Injury Study I (NASCIS I), but relatively low doses did not demonstrate a benefit in functional recovery for this patient population.[2] Based on animal data that became available after that original trial, the authors suggested the doses studied were below therapeutic targets. In 1990, the same authors performed a second randomized, controlled study (NASCIS II) that evaluated a significantly higher dose of methylprednisolone given within 12 hours of injury to determine if steroids had an effect on patient recovery.[3] In this study, patients received methylprednisolone (MP) 30 mg/kg as a bolus followed by 5.4 mg/kg/h for 23 hours. The study also included a naloxone treatment arm and a placebo arm. The results of the trial were stratified to time of drug administration (<8 h and 8–12 h after injury) and severity of injury (complete or incomplete). Overall, there was no significant difference in neurologic scores between groups at 6 weeks for all patients; however, there was a significant improvement in some points of motor function and tactile sensation in the MP group treated within 8 hours. Six months after injury, all MP patients demonstrated improvement in sensory function, and MP treated within 8 hours demonstrated improvement in motor and sensory function. The other groups did not demonstrate significant improvement.[3] The results of this trial were published widely in the lay press at that time, and the excitement of a potential treatment option for such a devastating injury was eagerly accepted. High-dose MP became the standard of care at the time, and no further placebo-controlled trials were subsequently performed.

In 1997, the same author group published the results of a third NASCIS trial (NASCIS III). In this study, the authors compared the administration of high-dose MP for 24 hours or 48 hours. Patients were treated within 8 hours of injury, and there were preplanned subgroups evaluated during early and late initiation of treatment as well as complete or incomplete injury. The results of this trial suggested that patients who were treated later, between 3 and 8 hours after injury, benefited from longer duration of MP treatment (48 hours). In patients treated in less than 3 hours, there was no difference in the 24-hour or 48-hour administration of MP. Based on the trial, the "gold standard" of treatment became high-dose MP for 24 hours if treatment was initiated within 3 hours of injury and 48 hours if initiated within 3 to 8 hours of injury.[4]

A separate publication just 2 years after the NASCIS II paper was published reported the results in the patient groups 1 year after injury. In the analysis, the benefit in sensory improvement seen in the MP group was lost at the 1-year point.[5] The 1-year results of the NASCIS III trial also failed to demonstrate a sustained benefit in improved functional recovery.[6] Other studies were also done in the years following the publications of the NASCIS trials and were unsuccessful in replicating the beneficial results. Adverse effects of the use high-dose MP, most commonly infection, were the only consistent finding among studies. Skepticism of the benefits of the treatment was widespread by the early 2000s, although many centers continued to use high-dose MP for the treatment of ASCI. Survey studies of medical directors and emergency medicine physicians at the time indicated that many of those who continued to use MP treatment did so out of uncertainty of the benefit and fear of legal ramifications for not providing this "gold-standard" treatment.[7,8] In 2002, the American Association of Neurological Surgeons (AANS) and the Congress of Neurological Surgeons (CNS) included the use of MP as an option in their first publication of *Guidelines for the Management of Acute Cervical Spine and Spinal Cord Injuries* but noted that evidence of harm was more consistent than evidence of clinical benefit.[9]

In 2006, a publication by Sayer and colleagues[7] systematically critiqued the methodologies and results of the NASCIS II and NASCIS III trials. The analysis raised many questions about the integrity of the study designs as well as the results. The key findings of the NASCIS II trial with respect to the time windows that were identified as significant were determined after the study was completed. In addition, data presented as significant were based on a very small subset of all patients enrolled in the trial, excluding about 70% of overall patients. The data demonstrating benefit with MP were only in patients with incomplete injury, which comprised an even smaller subset of patients. There were also inconsistencies with the results that have been described as "statistical artifacts," and with these, the results cannot reasonably support the authors' conclusions. For example, the placebo group treated within 8 hours had worse outcomes compared with the MP group, yielding the conclusion of the benefit of MP. However, those patients also did worse than the placebo group treated beyond 8 hours. In fact, the patients treated after 8 hours with placebo did as well as those treated under 8 hours with MP. There were similar concerns with the NASCIS III study methods and results being flawed. As with the NASCIS II, the time windows were arbitrary and unclear as to when they were determined. In both studies, other flaws included the lack of standardization of care across the various medical centers, the lack of minimal impairment for inclusion in the studies, and the lack of sustained benefit at the 1-year mark.

The Consortium for Spinal Cord Medicine and the Paralyzed Veterans of America published guidelines for the early management of ASCI in 2008 that stated that there was no definitive clinical evidence to recommend steroids as a neuroprotective agent.[10] In 2012, the AANS/CNS, with their second edition of the ASCI guidelines, stated that the use of MP for ASCI is not recommended.[11] With this final declaration, the use of high-dose steroids for treatment of ASCI should no longer be considered.

EARLY COMPLICATIONS AND TREATMENT IN ASCI

Shock States

The 2 shock states related to ASCI include neurogenic and spinal shock. Neurogenic shock can be defined as the disruption of autonomic pathways that results in hypotension and bradycardia. This usually occurs in patients with spinal injury above the T6 vertebrae. Injuries above this level result in increased vasodilation, decreased cardiac contractility, and an increase in unopposed vagal tone. Spinal shock can be defined as the reflex loss below the area of ACSI. Reflexes may return gradually as reflex arcs below the area of injury return, resulting in the occurrence of spasticity and autonomic dysreflexia in some patients with ASCI.[12,13] There has been a recently postulated 4-phase classification to spinal shock: areflexia (days 0–1), initial reflex return (days 1–3), early hyperreflexia (days 4–28), and late hyperreflexia (days 30–365).[12]

Due to the complications of neurogenic shock in patients with ASCI, the use of vasopressors and inotropes may be necessary. A mean arterial pressure (MAP) goal has been studied, and it is recommended in the 2008 practice guideline from the Consortium for Spinal Cord Medicine, titled *Early Acute Management in Adults with Spinal Cord Injury* (SCI).[10] In the 2013 American Association of Neurological Surgeons (AANS) published *Guidelines for the Management of Acute Cervical Spine and Spinal Cord Injuries*, a recommended MAP goal of 85 to 90 mm Hg for the first 7 days after SCI is safe and may improve spinal cord perfusion and neurological outcome.[14] A recent study in 2015 had results that are mostly consistent with the above guidelines for management of MAP in acute SCI with a suggestion that average MAP may only relate to neurological outcome in the first 2 to 3 days after injury. It is also stated by the authors that duration of time below treatment threshold may be of greater relevance to neurological recovery.[15]

Blood Pressure Augmentation

The first step to promote blood pressure augmentation is the assessment and optimization of fluid status.[16] Hypotension in patients with ASCI may be fluid resistant, and the fluid overloading may result in pulmonary edema.[12] The choice of pharmacological agent, either vasopressor or inotrope, depends on the level of SCI and clinical symptoms.[10] SCIs above T6 usually have both a hypotension and a bradycardic component, while in lower levels of injury, hypotension alone is due to peripheral dilation.[10] Based on these finding, it is important to know where the receptors for cardiovascular regulation are located in the body and the effect of stimulating or blocking these receptors has on blood pressure and heart rate (Table 6.1).[17] With knowledge of the receptors effects, the choice of pharmacological agent can be chosen based on which receptors need to be targeted to provide blood pressure augmentation to stabilize the cardiovascular system.[17] The drugs of choice used in ASCI are dopamine and norepinephrine. Both these agents have α and β activity, resulting in increased peripheral vasoconstriction and heart contractility for patients with T6 or above injury. For patients with lower injuries,

TABLE 6.1 Cardiovascular Agents Used in Acute Spinal Cord Injury

Medication Dosing

Intravenous Infusions Vasopressors/Inotropes	Dosing Range, mcg/kg/min	Receptor Activity	Response
Dopamine	1–20	Dopamine, α, β	Vasoconstriction, ↑HR, ↑ contractility
Norepinephrine	0.02–3	$\alpha \gg \beta_1$	Vasoconstriction, ↑HR, ↑ contractility
Phenylephrine	0.5–9	Pure α	Vasoconstriction, ↑BP
Epinephrine	0.01–3	$\alpha > \beta$	Vasoconstriction, ↑HR, ↑ contractility
Dobutamine	2–20	$\beta_1\beta_2 \gg \alpha_1\alpha_2$	↑HR, ↑ contractility, vasodilation, ↓BP

Topical or Oral Vasoconstrictors	Dosing Range	Typical Frequency
Midodrine	2.5–10 mg	3 times daily
Droxidopa	100–600 mg	3 times daily
Vasodilators		
Nitroglycerin topical	0.5–2 in.	q12h as needed
Nifedipine, immediate release	10–20 mg	May repeat dose 20 minutes after first dose
Hydralazine	10–75 mg	q4h–q6h as needed
Captopril	25 mg	Once, escalate to other therapy if suboptimal response
Miscellaneous		
Fludrocortisone	0.1–0.3 mg	Daily

Source: Reference 17, 19.

Note: BP, blood pressure; HR, heart rate.

the drug of choice is phenylephrine due to its singular α receptor activity that improves peripheral vasoconstriction.[10,16,18] Other agents that may be considered for use are epinephrine or dobutamine in patients with profound bradycardia.[16,18] The use of vasopressors or inotropes requires the patient to have central-line access for administration and continuous monitoring of cardiovascular parameters.[16] Adjunctive therapy with midodrine, an oral α_1 agonist, or fludrocortisone, an oral corticosteroid that promotes increased reabsorption of sodium and loss of potassium from renal distal tubules resulting in water retention, may be used to assist with blood pressure augmentation and long-term issues with orthostatic hypotension.[13,19] A newer agent with possible benefit in this patient population is droxidopa, an oral α- and β-agonist that is metabolized to norepinephrine by the enzyme dopadecarboxylase, thereby increasing blood pressure by inducing peripheral arteria and venous vasoconstriction.[19]

TABLE 6.2 Summary of Triggers for Autonomic Dysreflexia Based on Body System

Body System	Common Triggers
Urinary	Bladder distension, urinary tract infection, renal stone(s), urinary catheter blocks
Gastrointestinal	Bowel overdistension (impaction, constipation), hemorrhoids, acute abdominal pain, digital rectal stimulation, gastric ulcer, anal fissure, gastroesophageal reflux
Skin	Pressure sores, burns, insect bites, blisters, extreme external temperatures, dressing changes, tight shoelaces, contact with hard or sharp objects
Reproductive	Menstruation, pregnancy, sexual intercourse, ejaculation
Respiratory	Pulmonary infarction or emboli, vigorous coughing

Source: References 20.

Autonomic Dysreflexia

Autonomic dysreflexia (AD) is secondary complication of SCI at T6 or above that can be life threatening and usually occurs 6 months or later after injury but can occur sooner. The most common signs associated with an AD episode include hypertension, defined as blood pressure elevated greater than 20 mm Hg or 20% increase from baseline, cardiac arrhythmias, bradycardia or tachycardia, piloerection, and sweating.[13,20,21] Common symptoms associated with episodes of AD include headache, skin flushing superior to the level of SCI, nasal and/or conjunctival congestion, and cold extremities inferior to SCI.[13,20] The recognition of AD by patients with SCI and caregivers is relatively low. One study showed that 41% of patients with SCI had never heard of this complication, and 22% of patients with SCI had reported signs and symptoms of AD that also were not recognized as AD.[20] A number of body systems have been found to have triggers that potentiate episodes of AD, including urinary, gastrointestinal, skin, reproductive, and respiratory, in addition to other types of triggers. Common triggers include bladder or bowel distention and have been reported in up to 85% of cases of severe AD (Table 6.2).[20]

An acute SCI of T6 or above can have a complete or partial effect on the patient's sympathetic control of heart rate, contractility, and blood flow.[20] Due to the decentralized regulation of systemic vascular resistance and blood pressure control, this can result in decreased resting blood pressure, episodes of orthostatic hypertension, and abnormal daily fluctuations in blood pressure.[13,20] The fluctuations in the cardiovascular system due to AD in patients with SCI can be life threatening, leading to stroke, intracranial hemorrhage, seizures, pulmonary edema, myocardial infarction, and ultimately death.[13,20,21]

Nonpharmacological therapy suggestions for prevention of AD episodes include the following examples: ensure voiding of bladder and bowel, limit overstimulation, and wear loose-fitting clothes or shoes. Pharmacological therapy is targeted at the active sign and symptoms of the AD episode. Hypertensive episodes related to AD are usually transient, and as such, a short-acting antihypertensive agent is most appropriate.[13,20,21] Agents used include topical nitroglycerin (applied above the level of SCI), calcium channel blockers such as immediate-release nifedipine or intravenous infusions of nicardipine or clevidipine, and hydralazine due to their direct smooth muscle relaxation proprieties of the vascular system resulting in vasodilation. Topical nitroglycerin forms free radical nitric oxide, which in smooth muscle activates guanylate cyclase, which increases guanosine 3',5'-monophosphate, leading to dephosphorylation of myosin light chains and smooth muscle relaxation, producing a vasodilator effect on the peripheral veins and arteries with more prominent effects on the veins. Also, topical nitroglycerine reduces cardiac oxygen demand by decreasing preload and dilating coronary arteries, which improves collateral flow to ischemic regions. Nifedipine mechanism of action is via inhibition of calcium ions from entering the "slow channels" or select voltage-sensitive areas of vascular smooth muscle and myocardium during depolarization, producing a relaxation of coronary vascular smooth muscle and coronary vasodilation. It also reduces peripheral vascular resistance, producing a reduction in arterial blood pressure. Hydralazine produces a direct vasodilation of arterioles (with little effect on veins) with decreased systemic resistance. Another option is captopril, a competitive inhibitor of angiotensin-converting enzyme that prevents conversion of angiotensin I to angiotensin II, a potent vasoconstrictor, resulting in vasodilation.[13,20]

ONGOING TREATMENT CONSIDERATIONS

Neuropathic Pain

Pain associated with SCI is a frequent complication commonly occurring within the first 6 months of injury and can be refractory to pharmacologic management.[22] Modulation of the pain after SCI is a more realistic goal than being pain free. Pain may lead to a decreased quality of life and adversely affect recovery and activities of daily living, such as sleep. Pain can be categorized into 2 types: nociceptive or neuropathic. Nociceptive pain originates from the musculoskeletal system or visceral organs, with musculoskeletal pain being the most common manifesting from the initial trauma, spasms, abnormal or over-use of skeletal muscle, or inflammation. Neuropathic pain involves the central and peripheral nervous systems.

Neuropathic pain can be debilitating and difficult to treat since the severity of pain does not always correlate with the degree and location of the trauma.[23] The mechanisms contributing to central neuropathic pain are diverse and complex. There are a number of limitations to consider when trying to decide on appropriate pharmacologic treatment of this type of pain, including the lack of head-to-head randomized controlled trials focusing on central or peripheral pain in SCI, extrapolation of postherpetic neuralgia trial data to patients with SCI, poor study design and lack of power, and the short duration of these trials, usually 3 months, when pain associated with SCI can last much longer. Incorporating all of these limitations into management along with the heterogeneity of different neuropathic pain conditions emphasizes the need for individualized treatment.[24]

Medications affecting the reuptake of serotonin and norepinephrine have been included in a large number of trials for the treatment of various peripheral neuropathies. Depression is a comorbidity commonly affecting these patients, which can also be treated with this class of medications. Tricyclic antidepressants, including nortriptyline and amitriptyline, show beneficial effects 2 to 3 months after starting treatment but should be started at low doses due to the risk of anticholinergic effects, such as urinary retention. One randomized controlled trial that compared amitriptyline, gabapentin (an anticonvulsant medication also indicated for the treatment of neuropathic pain), and placebo demonstrated a benefit with amitriptyline compared with placebo but no difference between amitriptyline and gabapentin.[22] The use of amitriptyline could be considered in patients with neuropathic pain and depression.[25]

Selective serotonin norepinephrine reuptake inhibitors, venlafaxine and duloxetine, have been approved to treat neuropathic pain and major depressive disorder. Data support the use of venlafaxine for diabetic neuropathy and other polyneuropathy syndromes, while 1 trial involving duloxetine demonstrated a benefit up to 1 year in patients with painful diabetic peripheral neuropathy. Neither agent has been studied for central neuropathic pain.[26]

Several anticonvulsant medications have been studied in patients with SCI, including lamotrigine, valproic acid, and levetiracetam. Lamotrigine and valproic acid act on voltage-gated sodium channels that are thought to decrease neuronal firing. Valproic acid has the added effect of increasing gamma-aminobutyric acid (GABA) concentrations in the central nervous system. Clinical trials to evaluate improvement in overall pain in patients with SCI did not demonstrate a benefit with lamotrigine. However, a subgroup of patients with incomplete SCI reported a reduction in their at- or below-level neuropathic pain with lamotrigine.[22] A double-blind crossover study compared valproic acid with placebo in patients with SCI.[27] There was no significant improvement in pain control in the valproic acid group, but there was a trend toward better improvement scores while using the Danish version of the McGill Pain Questionnaire after 3 weeks of valproic acid treatment. Levetiracetam's exact mechanism of action is unclear. It has some activity on voltage-gated N-type calcium channels and also opposes negative modulators of GABA receptors. A double-blind crossover trial evaluated the improvement in daily pain scores while patients received levetiracetam or placebo.[28] The study measured at- and below-level pain relief, allodynia, or spasms. No significant differences were seen in either primary or secondary outcomes.

A robust amount of data supports the use of gabapentin and pregabalin in patients with various polyneuropathies. A trial evaluating pregabalin demonstrated a benefit in central neuropathic pain associated with SCI in a flexible-dose study.[29] Participants were allowed to continue other pain medications if previously stable on those medications for 1 month except gabapentin. The study also showed an improvement in sleep and less anxiety during the 12-week period with somnolence and dizziness as the main adverse effects. These medications work on neuropathic pain by binding to voltage-gated calcium channels at the $\alpha2\delta$ subunit preventing excitatory neurotransmitter release.

Tramadol and opioids have shown to be beneficial in various neuropathic pain conditions. Tramadol, a weak opioid mu-receptor agonist and inhibitor of serotonin norepinephrine reuptake, provides relief to a lesser extent than opioids. Tramadol has a relatively quick onset of action, but factors such as patient age, renal or hepatic dysfunction, and drug interactions, which can lead to serotonin syndrome, should be taken into account prior to initiating this medication. Tramadol can also lower the seizure threshold. Opioids are effective for pain control in SCI, but the long-term risk of abuse, constipation, and oversedation should be taken into consideration when being prescribed. These should be reserved for intractable pain associated with SCI.[22,30]

In clinical practice, most patients require more than 1 medication for management of pain associated with SCI. All of the agents studied in the discussed trials provided only partial pain relief, which emphasizes the need for multimodal therapy, although few studies have been published looking at multimodal therapy for either peripheral neuropathy or central neuropathic pain in SCI. Management of pain is also dependent on the tolerability of side effects. A randomized controlled crossover trial evaluated the efficacy of morphine, gabapentin, or the combination on pain intensity, quality of life, mood, and side effects in patients with painful diabetic neuropathy or postherpetic neuralgia.[31] Patients on combination therapy had overall improved pain scores and mood but were limited by the side effect of constipation at higher doses. A multicenter Italian study evaluated the use of controlled-release oxycodone and pregabalin in patients with various types of neuropathic pain.[32] This was the first trial to study the use of these 2 agents and enrolled significantly more patients than other trials evaluating neuropathic pain. The results demonstrated that most patients had improved pain control, supporting the idea of multimodal therapy for neuropathic pain. Further studies in this area are needed.

Spasticity

Spasticity is a common problem in SCI. It can cause pain, resulting in a decrease in sleep and participation in activities of daily living during rehabilitation. It occurs secondarily following complete or incomplete SCI and is characterized by hypertonicity, hyperreflexia, and clonus.[33] The belief that management of spasticity is based on achieving a balance between the detrimental effects on an individual's quality of life and harmful dose-dependent pharmacologic effects of antispasmodics is more definitive than the various definitions and methods to evaluate spasticity.[34,35] Spasticity is classified as an upper motor neuron syndrome, and the proposed mechanism of spasticity is due to an interaction between interneurons and motor neurons. Spasticity tends to be more diffuse in patients with SCI, with a greater incidence of spasticity in upper motor neuron injury and upper-level spinal injury compared with lower motor neuron and lower-level spinal injury. Management of spasticity takes a multimodal approach incorporating both physical rehabilitation and pharmacologic intervention. The approach to management and therapy is based on whether the spasticity is generalized or local. Initially, systemic pharmacologic agents are used based on the severity and onset of the spasms, time since injury, adverse effects of the medications, and cognitive status of the patient. It is important to note that a reduction in spasticity does not always correlate with better outcomes.

Baclofen is the antispasmodic of choice in patients with SCI. It may be effective in reducing flexor spasms and does not have evidence of the development of patient tolerance, making it an optimal choice for long-term utilization.[34] Baclofen acts on $GABA_B$ receptors presynaptically and postsynaptically in laminae I to IV of the spinal cord, inhibiting monosynaptic and polysynaptic spinal reflexes. $GABA_B$ receptors are abundant in the superficial dorsal horn and laminae I and II. When baclofen binds to presynaptic $GABA_B$ receptors, a decrease in the influx of calcium occurs, causing a decrease in the release of excitatory neurotransmitters and leading to a decrease in α motor neuron activity in the spinal cord. As baclofen binds to postsynaptic receptors, an outflow of potassium occurs, resulting in a hyperpolarized state and leading to a decrease in action potential transmission. Baclofen is limited by its adverse effects, including sedation, ataxia, and drowsiness, which can affect rehabilitation effort and outcomes.

An alternative approach to minimize systemic toxicities of baclofen is through the use of intrathecal baclofen in conjunction with oral baclofen.[33,34] Intrathecal baclofen has demonstrated efficacy to improve the management of spasticity in SCI since the first trial in 1985.[36] Indications for use in the management of spasticity associated with SCI are not well defined and include oral antispasmodic intolerance to severe spasticity. The benefit of intrathecal baclofen is the ability to deliver the drug directly into the cerebrospinal fluid (CSF), bypassing the blood-brain barrier via an implantable pump. Oral baclofen is minimally absorbed, and at higher concentrations, patients are more likely to experience more adverse effects rather than increased clinical benefit. Intrathecal baclofen is delivered directly into the CSF, resulting in fewer systemic adverse effects, but the long-term ramifications of this method are not well studied.[33]

Benzodiazepines, specifically diazepam and clonazepam, are options for patients with hyperactive reflexes, severe spasms, and nighttime spasms in SCI. Diazepam is the most commonly used agent to treat spasticity, causing a reduction in monosynaptic and polysynaptic reflexes by working on $GABA_A$ receptors on the postsynaptic membrane.[34] When diazepam binds to postsynaptic $GABA_A$ receptors, chloride ions flow into the postsynaptic membrane, hyperpolarizing the membrane and preventing action potential transmission. The main adverse effect with all benzodiazepines is sedation.

Tizanidine has been shown to reduce muscle spasms in SCI, but a demonstrated improvement in functional recovery is still lacking. Strength is not decreased when using tizanidine, although weakness has been reported. It is a centrally acting α_2-adrenergic agonist that decreases the release of glycine and other excitatory neurotransmitters in spinal interneurons.[33,34] This prevents further activation of motor neurons in the spinal cord, which leads to reduced spasms. The adverse effects of this medication include dose–dependent hypotension, drowsiness, and sedation.

Botulinum neurotoxin is produced from the anaerobic bacteria, *Clostridium botulinum*. There is evidence to support its use in generalized spasticity secondary to SCI, but it is not commonly used in practice. The benefit has been demonstrated in patients with focal spasticity with reductions in muscle tone and pain and an improvement in range of motion, function, and walking ability.[33] The botulinum toxin can be injected into specific muscle areas with little adverse effects. The botulinum toxin improves spasticity by inhibiting acetylcholine release from presynaptic nerve terminals at the neuromuscular junction, leading to a decrease in muscle contraction. Muscle weakness can accompany botulinum administration, but it is usually dose dependent.

Neurogenic Bowel Management

Neurogenic bowel is a syndrome commonly affecting patients with SCI and their quality of life. It can significantly affect the morbidity of patients and is a priority among individuals with SCI. Neurogenic bowel is defined as colonic dysfunction resulting from the lack of central nervous system control. Bowel problems occur in up to 62% of patients with SCI.[37] These patients can experience issues including fecal urgency, constipation, abdominal distention, and hemorrhoids. Constipation is more common in patients with complete lesions, a history of urinary outlet surgery, or iatrogenic causes. Abdominal pain is typically due to constipation or abdominal distention and can be exacerbated by food. It usually improves after a bowel movement or passing flatus. The management of neurogenic bowel depends on the level of the SCI.[38]

The presentation of neurogenic bowel depends on whether the injury was above the conus medullaris, otherwise known as upper motor neuron (UMN) bowel syndrome, or at the conus medullaris or cauda equina, resulting in a lower motor neuron (LMN) bowel syndrome.[37] The UMN bowel syndrome usually occurs above an injury level of T12 on the spinal cord and is characterized by increased colonic and anal sphincter tones. In patients with UMN bowel syndrome, the spinal cord is still able to communicate with the colon, allowing for preserved reflex coordination and stool propulsion, but there is loss of voluntary control of the external anal sphincter, causing it to remain tight, leading to stool retention and constipation. Tone of the colon wall is increased. Stool expulsion occurs from the introduction of a stimulus with an irritant such as a suppository or digital stimulation. Those with injury above the level of T6 will generate abdominal pressure through the intercostal and diaphragmatic contractions.[38] This increased abdominal pressure can lead to a reflexive vaso-constrictive response that may result in symptoms of AD. This autonomic response can be blunted with the administration of lidocaine to the intersphinc-teric anal area before anoscopy, sigmoidoscopy, or bowel movement.[39]

LMN bowel syndrome is characterized by loss of peristalsis and slow stool propulsion, causing constipation. It is caused by injury at the level of S2 to S4.

Patients retain voluntary control of part or all of their abdominal muscles but have no spinal cord–mediated peristalsis. The external anal sphincter is denervated, and the levator ani muscles lack tone, leading to a reduction in the rectal angle. The result is constipation and/or incontinence and increased time required for defecation.[37–39] Those with an incomplete SCI may retain the sensation of fullness and the bowel evacuation or may behave similarly to a patient with complete SCI requiring a bowel regimen for management of constipation.

Management of neurogenic bowel dysfunction can be cumbersome and time-intensive for patients with SCI. Those with LMN bowel syndrome may require manual evacuation to prevent further stool incontinence. Implementation of bowel programs is integral to improve morbidity and prevent complications requiring surgical intervention. Bowel programs allow for bowel training, predictable defecation, and continence of stool. However, bowel regimens may produce variable results. More than 20% of patients with SCI report difficulty with bowel evacuation with prolonged efforts, up to 3 hours, yielding insufficient results.[40] Optimal results are obtained using a multimodal approach. Bowel programs can comprise anal and/or abdominal massage, digital stimulation, suppositories/enemas, laxatives, fiber, and manual evacuation. Fiber and bulking agents such as bran, wheat husk, and psyllium work in the colon and increase bulk and fluid retention, leading to stool softness.[40] This aids in intestinal transit through the gastrointestinal tract by increasing the intraluminal water content and overall volume of stool. The use of fiber for bowel management in patients with SCI has been studied and was found to decrease colonic transit time. However, the results of one case series involving 11 patients with SCI demonstrated the opposite effect when fiber was added to the bowel regimen.[41] Despite the variable data, fiber is generally recommended to be added to the bowel regimen in patients with SCI since it is well tolerated with minimal adverse effects such as occasional bloating or flatulence.

Suppositories are an important component and commonly used in bowel programs for patients with SCI. Bisacodyl and glycerin are the most commonly used suppositories. Bisacodyl suppositories are available in a hydrogenated vegetable oil base (HVB) or a polyethylene glycol base (PGB). Bisacodyl acts as a contact laxative by increasing spasmodic propulsive peristaltic activity. The PGB bisacodyl suppository has demonstrated a beneficial effect on decreasing bowel care time and time to defecation compared with the HVB bisacodyl suppository in a prospective randomized double-blind trial involving 15 patients.[40] The PGB suppository does not depend on body heat to melt and disperse the medication after being administered. The effectiveness of the PGB bisacodyl suppositories was also demonstrated in a 35-year-old man with a 10-year history of T2 complete stable paraplegia that resulted from a spinal cord arteriovenous malformation.[42] There was a reduction in stool flow time of 31 minutes with HVB vs 21 minutes with PGB suppositories. Although most studies to date have been of small sample size and case reports, the consensus is that the use of PGB bisacodyl suppositories is preferred due to the decreased time to defecation, decreased nursing time, and decreased overall time for bowel care. Glycerin suppositories stimulate rectal contraction through hyperosmotic action and irritation. They are a less potent chemical stimulus used during the transition from bisacodyl to digital stimulation. Glycerin usually produces a bowel movement in 15 to 30 minutes and can be used in a daily alternating fashion with bisacodyl, but more glycerin may be needed to produce an effect in combination with digital stimulation.[38–40,43]

Laxatives are an important component of bowel regimens in patients with SCI and can be grouped into 3 categories: anthraquinone-containing substances, electrolyte salt-containing substances, and hyperosmolar laxatives. Anthraquinone-containing substances, such as senna, work by enhancing the intestinal motility by generating increased propulsive activity and by exerting a direct effect on the myenteric plexus. Senna is best for UMN-level injuries and works in 6 to 12 hours but requires colonic bacteria to be absorbed.[39] Side effects are usually dose dependent and can result in abdominal cramping, electrolyte imbalance, and diarrhea. Some patients may develop a decreased responsiveness to anthraquinone-based substances over time with daily use known as a cathartic colon. The mechanism of this process is unknown but may be due to the direct effects of these laxatives on the myenteric plexus, resulting in damage.[39,40]

Salt-containing substances with magnesium, sodium, or potassium are the most common laxatives used. They act by drawing water into the small intestine, which stimulates motility. Milk of Magnesia has the beneficial effect of releasing cholecystokinin-stimulating motility. Other commonly used products include Fleet's Phosphosoda and magnesium citrate.

Hyperosmolar laxatives, including lactulose, sorbitol, and polyethylene glycol, also act osmotically to draw fluid intraluminally. Polyethylene glycol solutions are the most effective of this group and have a minimal effect on mucosal irritation and electrolyte imbalance. Lactulose and sorbitol have a higher incidence of abdominal cramping.

Enemas work on the colonic mucosa and stimulate the distal colon and rectum. They have the benefit of a rapid onset of action, inducing evacuation in

2 to 6 hours. However, the results can be unpredictable, also causing abdominal pain/cramping, dehydration, and electrolyte imbalances. Enemas should be reserved for when bowel management fails due to the risk of developing enema-dependent bowel based on long-term use. Other complications of enema use are bowel perforation, rectoanal trauma, and AD.[39]

Managing bowel function in the hospital and at home can be challenging due to the time and effort required for a bowel program. A multimodal approach, including conservative and pharmacologic management along with mechanical methods at routine intervals, has shown to be most effective in decreasing constipation and fecal incontinence and improving quality of life. A survey distributed to 1334 individuals with SCI in the United Kingdom reiterated the common interventions, including eating a regular diet, the use of laxatives, and mechanical methods, with manual evacuation being the most common intervention.[44] Although the optimal diet has not been defined, it is one of the most important components in a bowel management program for patients with SCI. If conservative management fails, then pharmacologic management should be tailored to the individual to improve quality of life, minimize adverse effects, and reduce the risk of gastrointestinal complications.[45,46]

Venous Thromboembolism Prevention and Treatment

Venous thromboembolism (VTE) can frequently occur in patients recovering from SCI. VTE is a significant cause of morbidity and mortality in patients with SCI, with the age of the patient and the presence of factors increasing the risk of developing a clot. The incidence of deep vein thrombosis (DVT) ranges from 9% to 90% and pulmonary embolism (PE) is 16%. The mortality associated with PE is estimated to be as high as 5%, depending on the study population, screening tool, demographics, use of mechanical and/or pharmacologic prophylaxis, and associated injury.[47–50] The development of a DVT is thought to be linked to the presence of 1 or more aspects of Virchow's triad of intimal vessel injury, stasis, and hypercoagulability from direct vessel injury, paralysis, and hypoperfusion.[51] The literature has cited numerous risk factors related to the development of VTEs in patients with SCI, but a universal tool has still not been developed to stratify patients based on various risk factors. Advanced age and immobility are some of the generally recognized risk factors associated with the development of VTEs, while paralysis is a considerable risk factor with a higher rate of DVTs.

Literature supports the use of various methods to prevent VTE formation in patients with SCI despite methodological problems encountered in most studies. Early administration of VTE prophylaxis (within 72 hours from the onset of injury) and a 3-month duration of treatment are optimal. Patients with incomplete injury and mobility in the lower extremities may require a shorter duration of prophylaxis. The use of low-dose heparin (LDH), typically 5000 units given 2 or 3 times daily, by itself has been shown to reduce the incidence of DVT by 20% to 40%.[51,52] Adjusted-dose heparin and warfarin are not supported as prophylaxis options in patients with SCI. LDH compared with adjusted-dose heparin with a targeted activated partial thromboplastin time (aPTT) 1.5 times the normal value resulted in a lower incidence of thromboembolic events in the adjusted-dose group but a higher incidence of bleeding.[53] LDH is the preferred regimen over adjusted-dose heparin and is recommended to be used in combination with other modalities.

Studies suggest that the use of both mechanical and pharmacologic measures decreases the incidence of VTE in SCI. A study conducted by Merli and colleagues[54] demonstrated a benefit in patients receiving LDH and electrical stimulation over those receiving placebo or LDH alone. The incidence of DVT in the dual-treatment group was approximately 7%, while the incidence in the heparin-alone and placebo group was 50%. A nonrandomized pilot study including 21 patients with SCI demonstrated a notable incidence of DVT of 5% compared with the placebo group. Pneumatic compression stockings in combination with LDH is currently recommended as a prophylactic treatment strategy by the Joint Section on Disorders of the Spine and Peripheral Nerves of the AANS and the CNS.[55]

Low-molecular-weight heparin (LMWH) attracted attention in the 1990s as a possible alternative to LDH associated with lower rates of DVT and PE. Enoxaparin was evaluated in high-risk trauma patients for the prevention of DVT, demonstrating safety and efficacy using a dose of 30 mg twice a day.[56] In 1994, a study concluded that LMWH should be the agent of choice for DVT prophylaxis in trauma patients over LDH. The lower incidence of DVT and proximal DVT was statistically significant at 31% and 6%, respectively.[57] Dalteparin and fondaparinux have been recently studied for DVT prophylaxis in trauma patients. Dalteparin was found to be noninferior compared with enoxaparin for VTE prophylaxis in patients with SCI, but a larger well-powered study should be conducted to validate these results.[58] A pilot study used fondaparinux, an alternative in a patient with heparin-induced thrombocytopenia, for DVT prophylaxis in trauma patients, resulting in a 1.2% incidence of DVT with no evidence of bleeding, leading the authors to conclude that it offers protection against DVTs.[58] Best medical management with LDH plus intermittent pneumatic compression stockings compared with enoxaparin was evaluated in the acute period after SCI. There was a lower incidence of

DVT in the best medical management group compared with enoxaparin, although it was not statistically significant. The incidence of PE was statistically significant in favor of enoxaparin, with no cases of fatal PE in either group.[59] The American College of Chest Physicians (ACCP) currently recommends LMWH for DVT prophylaxis in patients with multiple trauma, which includes ASCI.[60]

The high risk of developing a VTE after SCI validates the need for mechanical and pharmacologic prophylaxis in these high-risk patients. The duration of chemoprophylaxis should last 3 months, continuing through the period of highest risk of thromboembolic events. The ACCP recommends continuing DVT prophylaxis until discharge. Vena cava filters are only recommended when patients are not candidates for pharmacologic prophylaxis and/or medical devices.[60] When LMWH is used for VTE prophylaxis, mechanical prophylaxis should be used in combination.

Stress Ulcer Prophylaxis

Stress ulcers and gastrointestinal ulcerations are common in the trauma patient population. There is a paucity of data regarding this issue specific to the ASCI patient population, but these patients are often included in larger trials of trauma patients. Much of the evidence that is used to support the practice of providing stress ulcer prophylaxis (SUP) to the ASCI patient population is extrapolated from the larger trauma patient population. It has been suggested that all patients with SCI are at risk of gastrointestinal bleeding, especially those with cervical cord injuries. However, there is conflicting evidence regarding the need for drug therapy for SUP in ASCI, with methodological issues clouding much of the data interpretation from the available studies. In the 1970s, gastrointestinal hemorrhage associated with ASCI was estimated to be between 5% and 22%.[61] However, a more recent retrospective analysis found an incidence of only 0.05% to 2.3% of stress-induced bleeding in trauma patients, of which ACSI was a subset of included patients.[62]

The cause of gastrointestinal bleeding associated with stress ulcers in ASCI is thought to be multifactorial with unopposed vagal tone, mucosal ischemia, and direct stress from the accident itself the main contributors to damage of the gastric mucosa. Damage to the gastric mucosa manifests in the first 4 weeks from injury, with the period of greatest risk between the fourth and tenth days after injury. Two independent risk factors associated with the highest risk of bleeding in patients with ASCI are mechanical ventilation and coagulopathy in the intensive care unit. According to a survey of 119 level I trauma centers, 86% commonly prescribe SUP to trauma patients, including ASCI, while in the intensive care unit. However, upon discharge from the intensive care unit, there is a lack of consensus about whether patients should be continued on SUP while still in the hospital. Most practitioners believe the risk of clinical bleeding to be too low to warrant continuation of any agent since these agents are not without consequence.[61–67]

There are no adequately powered studies evaluating the drug of choice for SUP in patients with ASCI. The current literature available includes trauma patients in the collective of all critically ill patients, with insufficient numbers to draw a conclusion. Data have not demonstrated proton pump inhibitors (PPIs) to be superior to histamine-2 antagonists (H_2RAs) or sucralfate. In addition, there is controversy regarding the use of PPIs for SUP and the development of infection. Gastric acid plays an important role in bactericidal action at a pH less than 4. Increasing the gastric pH above this level may allow for the colonization of pathologic organisms, which could lead to higher rates of *Clostridium difficile* infection and pneumonia. A recent retrospective review at the University Hospital Aachen found that PPIs were an independent risk factor for *C difficile* infection with a significantly increased risk of mortality.[68]

There is evidence supporting the development of ventilator-associated pneumonia when using drugs that increased the gastric pH. A randomized controlled trial compared an antacid, ranitidine, and sucralfate in intubated patients for the prevention of gastrointestinal bleeding and early and late-onset pneumonia. The findings demonstrated that all agents increased the incidence of pneumonia, but the ranitidine and antacid groups had a higher incidence of late-onset pneumonia.[69] A meta-analysis looking at H_2RAs compared with placebo supported the association between SUP with increasing rates of pneumonia.[70] PPIs have also been linked to increasing the risk of developing community acquired pneumonia. No significant differences have been demonstrated with the use of PPIs or H_2RAs in rates of pneumonia in the critically ill and overall mortality.[71,72]

SUP use is still the subject of ongoing debate in intensive care units but is necessary in specific patient populations with independent risk factors. It is unclear if ASCI itself is an independent risk factor, but often patients with ASCI meet other criteria for the use of SUP. There is still a lack of evidence to support which agent should be used in critically ill patients, but H_2RAs are thought to be effective with a more favorable side effect profile. Ultimately, the duration of SUP is determined by the need for mechanical ventilation or the presence of a coagulopathy while in the critical care setting and should be reevaluated and discontinued if appropriate when transitioning to acute care.

Urinary Tract Infections

More than half of patients with SCI will experience a urinary tract infection (UTI) within the first year after injury. It is one of the most common secondary medical complications in ASCI during the acute care phase or during rehabilitation. However, the diagnosis is complicated due to the lack of specificity of signs and symptoms. Reliance on makers such as pyuria and leukocytes in the urine to make the diagnosis is necessary but contradicts the current recommendation for diagnosis from the Infectious Disease Society of America (IDSA) guidelines. After SCI, patients may be left with structural or physiological changes that can increase the risk of developing a UTI. Patients may experience vesicoureteral reflux, large postvoid residuals, detrusor-sphincter dyssynergia, or outlet obstruction after trauma. The development of UTIs in patients with SCI will be highly dependent on the method by which these complications are managed. However, despite the method of urinary drainage, antimicrobial prophylaxis is not currently indicated in SCI.[73–76]

The use of antimicrobial prophylaxis in patients with SCI is not supported by the IDSA because of concern about the promotion and development of bacterial resistance. There are also limited data to support the benefit of use. A randomized controlled study evaluated the incidence of clinical infection with the use of trimethoprim-sulfamethoxazole compared with placebo and found no significant difference between groups.[77] Studies conducted in the 1980s and 1990s had methodological problems with too few subjects, varied definitions of UTI, and questionable study durations. In 1992, a consensus statement from the National Institute on Disability and Rehabilitation Research concluded that there was not sufficient evidence to support the use of antimicrobial prophylaxis in patients with SCI.[78] A later meta-analysis of 15 controlled trials evaluating antimicrobial prophylaxis in patients with SCI concluded there was no difference in the reduction of symptomatic infection with the use of prophylaxis, but it was associated with a 2-fold increase in the proportion of antimicrobial-resistant bacteria cultures from patients.[73] The potential for adverse effects and the development of resistance outweigh the use of antimicrobial prophylaxis in patients with SCI.

Treatment of Depression

Depression following SCI is a common psychological issue encountered and was previously accepted and expected in all patients as a universal response. However, current literature suggests it occurs less frequently than once thought, ranging from 20% to 45% of all patients.[79,80] Initial feelings of depression or despair are common and often oscillate with feelings of optimism or hope. These oscillations may lead practitioners and caregivers to fear the patient is either depressed or in denial, but it has been found that these feelings are common and not indicative of underlying pathology. Allowing the patient to maintain hope is healthy and can lead to better outcomes in rehabilitation. The notion that all patients will experience depression is not accurate, and patients should only be treated for depression if clinically indicated. The diagnosis of depression should be made using the criteria set forth in the *Diagnostic and Statistical Manual of Mental Disorders*.[10]

When depression is present, the sequelae of depressive symptoms can lead to lower functional independence, less social integration, increased expenditures, and longer rehabilitation stays with decreased quality of life. When initiating treatment for depression in patients with SCI, it is important to consider patient-specific variables when assessing the risks and benefits of the psychopharmacologic agents. Pain often occurs concurrently with depression, suggesting depressive symptoms are determinants of physical pathology. In patients with SCI, pain overlaps with depression 30% to 60% of the time, and pain has been shown to attenuate the response to depression treatment. The choice of antidepressant should be made based on comorbidities, such as pain, for which newer agents such as the serotonin norepinephrine inhibitors have been approved.[81,82] A study evaluating chronic neuropathic pain in patients with SCI showed a direct correlation between depression severity and pain scores.[83] It is also important to allow for an adequate trial of the antidepressant, usually lasting 1 to 2 months. If the agent is effective, continuation of treatment for up to 1 year for a major depression is recommended. When a patient does experiences a major depressive episode, there is a 50% chance of recurrence and up to a 90% chance of recurrence after 2 episodes. Lifelong therapy should be considered in this particular population.[84,85]

FUTURE DIRECTIONS IN TREATMENT

Continued focus on the treatment of ASCI includes ongoing studies to identify agents to provide neuroprotective or regenerative effects in the acute setting. The goal is to find a treatment strategy that improves neurological recovery and functional outcome. It is theorized that successful disruption of the mechanisms that cause secondary injury will prevent additional edema, ischemia, and cytotoxity that contribute to worse outcomes. Efforts to target reduction in neurotransmitter accumulation, decreased ionic derangements, and decreased lipid peroxidase with various agents are a few of the more promising pharmacological studies under way. While many investigational drugs have been tried, none have yet to be successful. There seems to be a difference between what can be achieved through bench research and animal models and that which translates to clinical effect in human studies. There are several investigation studies under way currently for which the results are eagerly anticipated. Stem cell research is also thought to be a promising therapy for ASCI. Limited data are available on these interventions currently, but ongoing efforts to support research in this area continue.

Riluzole

The Riluzole in Spinal Cord Injury Study is currently in phase II/III of investigation. It is an international multicenter, randomized, placebo-controlled, double-blinded trial designed to evaluate the effect of riluzole on change in motor function 6 months after injury. It will also include neurologic and sensory recover, function outcomes, and quality of life. Riluzole is approved by the US Food and Drug Administration for the treatment of amyotrophic lateralizing sclerosis, and although its exact mechanism of action is unknown, it is thought to have an attenuating effect on excitatory neurotransmitter pathways. Animal models of ASCI have demonstrated improvement in axonal conduction and neurobehavioral outcomes and decreases in inflammation and apoptosis with riluzole.[86] Its inhibitory effects on some of the damaging excitatory neurotransmitters and pathways may provide some protection from these secondary mechanisms of injury in the ASCI patient population.[87]

Minocycline

Minocycline, a tetracycline antibiotic, is thought to have neuroprotective properties through its selective effects on M1 microglia. Inhibition of M1 microglia, which is a proinflammatory immune cell, may result in decreased excitotoxicity, inhibition of metalloproteinases, neutralization of free radicals, regulation of calcium, and mitochondrial stabilization. The specific targets of minocycline in the central nervous system, and its favorable safety and tolerability profile makes it an ideal agent for potentially providing benefit in the ASCI patient population. A phase III clinical trial is currently under way that is investigating the combined effects of minocycline and spinal perfusion augmentation in ASCI.[86,88]

Stem Cell Therapy

Cell-based therapies are thought to have potential benefit for many neurological-based diseases. The ability of the cells to differentiate may offer opportunities for regrowth and restructure of neuronal cell-based injuries that have not been afforded by any other mechanism. Stem cells obtained from bone marrow, either directly or by way of mobilization therapy with granulocyte colony-stimulating factor, have been studied in animal models and clinical trials. Bone marrow–derived mononuclear cells (BM-MNCs) have been studied most commonly. They are relatively easily obtained from bone marrow harvest procedures and can be readily isolated for use. They are thought to promote repair and regeneration of nervous system cells both peripherally and centrally. They may also promote axonal growth and remyelination, although evidence to support this is less conclusive. For these reasons, BM-MNCs have been theorized to have a potential benefit in the treatment of ASCI. A small number of clinical trials with BM-MNCs have demonstrated some improvement in neurological rating scores, although how this translates to functional improvement has yet to be determined.[89–91]

CONCLUSION

ASCI remains a complicated disease process with no established treatment to reverse the effects of the damage inflicted at the time of injury. Studies continue to focus on interventions that may limit secondary injury caused by edema and cytotoxic pathways, thereby allowing for improved neurological recovery. Other considerations in patients with ASCI can have a significant impact on care in the immediate postinjury setting. Immediate considerations include hemodynamic compromise and cardiac support. In the long-term setting, one must be cognitive of other issues such as pain, depression, SUP, VTE prevention, and bowel and bladder concerns. While definitive treatments for improving neurological function have not been forthcoming, many pharmacological interventions can be made to improve the quality of life in this patient population.

References

1. National Spinal Cord Injury Statistical Center. *Facts and Figures at a Glance.* Birmingham: University of Alabama at Birmingham; 2015.
2. Bracken MB, Collins WF, Freeman DF, et al. Efficacy of methylprednisolone in acute spinal cord injury. *JAMA.* 1984;251(1):45–52.
3. Bracken MB, Shepard M, Collins WF, et al. A randomized, controlled trial of methylprednisolone or naloxone in the treatment of acute spinal cord injury. *N Engl J Med.* 1990;322(20):1405–1411.
4. Bracken, MB, Shepard MJ, Holford TR, et al. Administration of methylprednisolone for 24 or 48 hours or tirilazad mesylate for 48 hours in the treatment of acute spinal cord injury. *JAMA.* 1997;277(20):1597–1604.

5. Bracken MB, Shepard M, Collins WF, et al. Methylprednisolone or naloxone treatment after acute spinal cord injury: 1 year follow-up data. *J Neurosurg.* 1992;76(1):23–31.

6. Bracken MB, Shepard MJ, Holford TR, et al. Methylprednisolone or tirilazad mesylate administration after acute spinal cord injury: 1-year follow up. Results of the third National Acute Spinal Cord Injury randomized controlled trial. *J Neurosurg.* 1998;89(5):699–706.

7. Sayer FT, Kronvall E, Nilsson OG. Methylprednisolone treatment in acute spinal cord injury: the myth challenged through a structured analysis of published literature. *Spine J.* 2006;6(3):335–343.

8. Vellman WP, Allison PH, Lammertse DP. Administration of corticosteroids for acute spinal cord injury. *Spine.* 2003;28(9):941–947.

9. Hadley MN, Walters BC, Grabb PA, et al. Guidelines for the management of acute cervical spine and spinal cord injuries. *Neurosurgery.* 2002;50(3)(suppl):S1–S199.

10. Consortium for Spinal Cord Medicine/Paralyzed Veterans of America. Early acute management in adults with spinal cord injury: a clinical practice guideline for health-care providers. *J Spinal Cord Med.* 2008;31(4):403–479.

11. Hurlbert RJ, Hadley MN, Walters BC, et al. Pharmacological therapy for acute spinal cord injury. *Neurosurgery.* 2013;72(suppl 2):93–105.

12. Bonner S, Smith C. Initial management of acute spinal cord injury. *Cont Educ Anaesth Crit Care Pain.* 2013;13(6):224–231.

13. Phillips AA, Krassioukov AV. Contemporary cardiovascular concerns after spinal cord injury: mechanisms, maladaptations, and management. *J Neurotrauma.* 2015;32(24):1927–1942.

14. Ryken TC, Hurlbert RJ, Hadley MN, et al. The acute cardiopulmonary management of patients with cervical spinal cord injuries. *Neurosurgery.* 2013;72(suppl 2):84–92.

15. Hawryluk G, Whetstone W, Saigal R, et al. Mean arterial blood pressure correlates with neurological recover after human spinal cord injury: analysis of high frequency physiological data. *J Neurotrauma.* 2015;32(24):1958–1967.

16. Stein DM, Roddy V, Marx J, et al. Emergency neurological life support: traumatic spine injury. *Neurocrit Care.* 2012;17(suppl 1):S102–S111.

17. Maclaren R, Dasta JF. Use of vasopressors and inotropes in the pharmacotherapy of shock. In: DiPiro JT, Talbert RL, Yee GC, Matzke GR, Wells BG, Posey L, eds. *Pharmacotherapy: A Pathophysiologic Approach.* 9th ed. New York, NY: McGraw-Hill; 2014.

18. Inoue T, Manley GT, Patel N, Whetstone WD. Medical and surgical management after spinal cord injury: vasopressor usage, early surgerys, and complications. *J Neurotrauma.* 2014;31(3):284–291.

19. Lexicomp Online. Lexi-Drugs. Hudson, OH: Lexi-Comp; 2015.

20. Furlan JC. Autonomic dysreflexia: a clinical emergency. *J Trauma Acute Care Surg.* 2013;75(3):496–500.

21. Wan D, Krassioukov AV. Life-threatening outcomes associated with autonomic dysreflexia: a clinical review. *J Spinal Cord Med.* 2014;37(1):2–10.

22. Teasell RW, Mehta S, Aubut JA, et al. A systematic review of pharmacological treatments of pain following spinal cord injury. *Arch Phys Med Rehabil.* 2010;91(5):816–831.

23. Wrigley PJ, Siddall PJ. Pain following spinal cord injury. In: McMahon SB, Koltzenburg M, Tracey I, Turk DC, eds. *Wall and Melzack's Textbook of Pain.* 6th ed. Philadelphia, PA: Elsevier; 2013.

24. Dworkin RH, O'Connor AB, Audette J, et al. Recommendations for the pharmacologic management of neuropathic pain: an overview and literature update. *Mayo Clin Proc.* 2010;85(3):S3–S14.

25. Attal N, Cruccu G, Baron R, et al. EFNS guidelines on the pharmacological treatment of neuropathic pain: 2010 revision. *Eur J Neurol.* 2010;17(9):1113–1123.

26. Raskin J, Smith TR, Wong K, et al. Duloxetine versus routine care in the long-term management of diabetic peripheral neuropathic pain. *J Palliat Med.* 2006;9(1):29–40.

27. Drewes AM, Andreasen A, Poulsen LH. Valproate for treatment of chronic central pain after spinal cord injury: a double-blind cross-over study. *Paraplegia.* 1994; 32(8):565–569.

28. Finnerup NB, Grydehoj J, Bing J, et al. Levetiracetam in spinal cord injury pain: a randomized controlled trial. *Spinal Cord.* 2009;47(12):861–867.

29. Siddall PJ, Cousins MJ, Otte A, et al. Pregabalin in central neuropathic pain associated with spinal cord injury. *Neurology.* 2006;67(10):1792–1800.

30. Kwon BK, Tetzlaff W, Grauer JN, et al. Pathophysiology and pharmacologic treatment of acute spinal cord injury. *Spine J.* 2004;4(4):451–465.

31. Gilron I, Bailey JM, Tu D, et al. Morphine, gabapentin, or their combination for neuropathic pain. *N Engl J Med.* 2005;352(13):1324–1334.

32. Gatti A, Sabato AF, Occhioni R, et al. Controlled-release oxycodone and pregabalin in the treatment of neuropathic pain: results of a multicenter Italian study. *Eur Neurol.* 2009;61(3):129–137.

33. Rabchevsky AG, Kitzman PH. Latest approaches for the treatment of spasticity and autonomic dysreflexia in chronic spinal cord injury. *Neurotherapeutics.* 2011;8(2):274–282.

34. Adams MM, Hicks AL. Spasticity after spinal cord injury. *Spinal Cord.* 2005; 43(10):577–586.

35. Priebe MM, Sherwood AM, Thornby JI, et al. Clinical assessment of spasticity in spinal cord injury: a multidimensional problem. *Arch Phys Med Rehabil.* 1996;77(7):713–716.

36. Loubser PG, Akman NM. Effects of intrathecal baclofen on chronic spinal cord injury pain. *J Pain Symptom Manage.* 1996;12(4):241–247.

37. Krassioukov A, Eng JJ, Claxton G, et al; The SCIRE Research Team. Neurogenic bowel management after spinal cord injury: a systematic review of the evidence. *Spinal Cord.* 2010;48(10):718–733.

38. Ebert E. Gastrointestinal involvement in spinal cord injury: a clinical perspective. *J Gastrointest Liver Dis.* 2012;1(21):75–82.

39. Stiens SA, Bergman SB, Goetz, LL. Neurogenic bowel dysfunction after spinal cord injury: clinical evaluation and rehabilitative management. *Arch Phys Med Rehabil.* 1997;78(3)(suppl):S86–S102.

40. House JG, Stiens SA. Pharmacologically initiated defecation for persons with spinal cord injury: effectiveness of three agents. *Arch Phys Med Rehabil.* 1997;78:1062–1065.

41. Cameron KJ, Nyulasi IB, Collier GR, Brown DJ. Assessment of the effect of increased dietary fibre intake on bowel function in patients with spinal cord injury. *Spinal Cord.* 1996;34:277–283.

42. Stiens SA. Reduction in bowel program duration with polyethylene glycol based bisacodyl suppositories. *Arch Phys Med Rehabil.* 1995;76(7):674–677.

43. Yi Z, Jie C, Wenyi Z, et al. Comparison of efficacies of vegetable oil based and polyethylene glycol based bisacodyl suppositories in treating patients with neurogenic bowel dysfunction after spinal cord injury: a meta-analysis. *Turk J Gastroenterol.* 2014; 25(5):488–492.

44. Coggrave M, Norton C, Wilson-Barnett J. Management of neurogenic bowel dysfunction in the community after spinal cord injury: a postal survey in the United Kingdom. *Spinal Cord.* 2009;47(4):323–333.

45. Rosman AS, Chaparala G, Monga A, et al. Intramuscular neostigmine and glycopyrrolate safely accelerated bowel evacuation in patients with spinal cord injury and defecatory disorders. *Dig Dis Sci*. 2008;53(10):2710–2713.

46. Korsten MA, Rosman AS, Ng A, et al. Infusion of neostigmine-glycopyrrolate for bowel evacuation in persons with spinal cord injury. *Am J Gastroenterol*. 2005;100(7):1560–1565.

47. Christie S, Thibault-Halman G, Casha S. Acute pharmacological DVT prophylaxis after spinal cord injury. *J Neurotrauma*. 2011;28(8):1509–1514.

48. Slavik RS, Chan E, Gorman SK, et al. Dalteparin versus enoxaparin for venous thromboembolism prophylaxis in acute spinal cord injury and major orthopedic trauma patients: 'DETECT' Trial. *J Trauma*. 2007;62(5):1075–1081.

49. Teasell RW, Hsieh TJ, Aubut JAL, et al. Venous thromboembolism following spinal cord injury. *Arch Phys Med Rehabil*. 2009;90(2):232–245.

50. Maung AA, Schuster KM, Kaplan LJ, et al. Risk of venous thromboembolism after spinal cord injury: not all levels are the same. *J Trauma*. 2011;71(5):1241–1245.

51. Toker S, Hak DJ, Morgan SJ. Deep vein thrombosis prophylaxis in trauma patients. *Thrombosis*. 2011;2011:505373.

52. Deep venous thrombosis and thromboembolism in patients with cervical spinal cord injuries. In: Guidelines for the management of acute cervical spine and spinal cord injuries. *Neurosurgery*. 2002;50(3)(suppl):S73–SS0.

53. Green D, Lee MY, Ito VY, et al. Fixed- vs adjusted-dose heparin in the prophylaxis of thromboembolism in spinal cord injury. *JAMA*. 1988;260(9):1255–1258.

54. Merli GJ, Herbison GJ, Ditunno JF, et al. Deep vein thrombosis: prophylaxis in acute spinal cord injured patients. *Arch Phys Med Rehabil*. 1988;69(9):661–664.

55. Dhall SS, Hadley MN, Aarabi B, et al. Deep venous thrombosis and thromboembolism in patients with cervical spinal cord injuries. *Neurosurgery*. 2013;72(suppl 2):244–254.

56. Knudson MM, Lewis FR, Clinton A, et al. Prevention of venous thromboembolism in trauma patients. *J Trauma*. 1994;37(3):480–487.

57. Geerts WH, Jay RM, Code KI, et al. A comparison of low-dose heparin with low-molecular-weight heparin as prophylaxis against venous thromboembolism after major trauma. *N Engl J Med*. 1996;335(10):701–707.

58. Lu JP, Knudson MM, Bir N, et al. Fondaparinux for prevention of venous thromboembolism in high-risk trauma patients: a pilot study. *J Am Coll Surg*. 2009;209(5):589–594.

59. Spinal Cord Injury Thromboprophylaxis Investigators. Prevention of the venous thromboembolism in the acute treatment phase after spinal cord injury: a randomized, multicenter trial comparing low-dose heparin plus intermittent pneumatic compression with enoxaparin. *J Trauma*. 2003;54(6):1116–1126.

60. Gould MK, Garcia DA, Wren SM, et al. Prevention of VTE in nonorthopedic surgical patients. *Chest*. 2012;141(2)(suppl):e227S-e277S.

61. Anwar F, Al-Khayer A, El-Mahrouki H, and Purcell M. Gastrointestinal bleeding in spinal injuries patient: is prophylaxis essential? *BJMP*. 2013;6(1):a607.

62. Barletta JF, Erstad BL, Fortune JB. Stress ulcer prophylaxis in trauma patients. *Crit Care*. 2002;6(6):526–530.

63. Gardner TB, Robertson DJ. Stress ulcer prophylaxis in non-critically ill patients: less may be more. *Am J Gastroenterol*. 2006;101(10):2206–2208.

64. American Society of Health-System Pharmacists. ASHP Therapeutic Guidelines on Stress Ulcer Prophylaxis. *Am J Health Syst Pharm*. 1999;56(4):347–379.

65. Janicki T, Steward S. Stress-ulcer prophylaxis for general medicine patients: a review of the evidence. *J Hosp Med*. 2007;2(2):86–92.

66. Grube RR, May DB. Stress ulcer prophylaxis in hospitalized patients not in intensive care units. *Am J Health Syst Pharm.* 2007;64(13):1396–1400.

67. Bez C, Perrottet N, Zingg T, et al. Stress ulcer prophylaxis in non-critically ill patients: a prospective evaluation of current practice in a general surgery department. *J Eval Clin Pract.* 2013;19(2):374–378.

68. Buendgens L, Bruensing J, Matthes M, et al. Administration of proton pump inhibitors in critically ill medical patients is associated with increased risk of developing *Clostridum difficile*–associated diarrhea. *J Crit Care.* 2014;29(4):696.e11-5.

69. Prod'hom G, Leuenberger P, Koerfer J, et al. Nosocomial pneumonia in mechanically ventilated patients receiving antacid, ranitidine, or sucralfate as prophylaxis for stress ulcer. *Ann Intern Med.* 1994;120(8):653–662.

70. Cook DJ, Reeve BK, Guyatt GH, et al. Stress ulcer prophylaxis in critically ill patients: resolving discordant meta-analyses. *JAMA.* 1996;275(4):308–314.

71. Mohebbi L, Hesch K. Stress ulcer prophylaxis in the intensive care unit. *Proc (Bayl Univ Med Cent).* 2009;22(4):373–376.

72. Plummer MP, Blaser AR, Deane AM. Stress ulceration: prevalence, pathology and association with adverse outcomes. *Crit Care.* 2014;18(2):213.

73. Morton SC, Shekelle PG, Adams JL, et al. Antimicrobial prophylaxis for urinary tract infection in persons with spinal cord dysfunction. *Arch Phys Med Rehabil.* 2002;83(1):129–138.

74. Cardenas DD, Hooton TM. Urinary tract infection in persons with spinal cord injury. *Arch Phys Med Rehabil.* 1995;76(3):272–280.

75. Nicolle LE, Bradley S, Colgan R, et al. Infectious Disease Society of America guidelines for the diagnosis and treatment of asymptomatic bacteriuria in adults. *Clin Infect Dis.* 2005;40(5):643–654.

76. Hooton TM, Bradley SF, Cardenas DD, et al. Diagnosis, prevention, and treatment of catheter-associated urinary tract infection in adults: 2009 international clinical practice guidelines from the Infectious Disease Society of America. *Clin Infect Dis.* 2010;50(5):625–663.

77. Maynard FM, Diokno AC. Urinary infection and complications during clean intermittent catheterization following spinal cord injury. *J Urol.* 1984;132(5):943–946.

78. The prevention and management of urinary tract infections among people with spinal cord injuries: National Institute on Disability and Rehabilitation Research Consensus Statement: January 27–29, 1992. *J Am Paraplegia Soc.* 1992;15(3):194–204.

79. Craig AR, Hancock KM, Dickson HG. A longitudinal investigation into anxiety and depression in the first 2 years following a spinal cord injury. *Paraplegia.* 1994;32(10):675–679.

80. Elliott TR, Kennedy P. Treatment of depression following spinal cord injury: an evidence-based review. *Rehabil Psychol.* 2004;49(2):134–139.

81. Kalpakjian CZ, Bombardier CH, Schomer K, et al. Measuring depression in persons with spinal cord injury: a systematic review. *J Spinal Cord Med.* 2009;32(1):6–24.

82. Cuff L, Fann JR, Bombardier CH, et al. Depression, pain intensity, and interference in acute spinal cord injury. *Top Spinal Cord Inj Rehabil.* 2014;20(1):32–39.

83. Rintala DH, Holmes SA, Courtade D, et al. Comparison of the effectiveness of amitriptyline and gabapentin on chronic neuropathic pain in persons with spinal cord injury. *Arch Phys Med Rehabil.* 2007;88(12):1547–1560.

84. Campbell LC, Clauw DJ, Keefe FJ. Persistent pain and depression: a biopsychosocial perspective. *Biol Psychiatry.* 2003;54(3):399–409.

85. Cardenas DD, Warms CA, Turner JA, et al. Efficacy of amitriptyline for relief of pain in spinal cord injury: results of a randomized controlled trial. *Pain.* 2002;96(3):365–373.

86. Siddiqui AM, Khazaei M, Fehlings MG. Translating mechanisms of neuroprotection, regeneration, and repair to treatment of spinal cord injury. *Prog Brain Res.* 2015;218:15–54.

87. Fehlings MG, Nakashima H, Naqoshi N, et al. Rationale, design and critical end points for the Riluzole in Acute Spinal Cord Injury Study (RISCIS): a randomized, double-blinded, placebo controlled parallel multi-center trial. *Spinal Cord.* 2016;54(1):8–15.

88. Kobayashi K, Imagama S, Ohgomori T, et al. Minocycline selectively inhibits M1 polarization of microglia. *Cell Death Dis.* 2013;4:e525.

89. Kumar AA, Kumar SR, Narayanan R, et al. Autologous bone marrow derived mononuclear cell therapy for spinal cord injury: a phase I/II clinical safety and primary efficacy data. *Exp Clin Transplant.* 2009;7(4):241–248.

90. Aghayan HR, Arjmand B, Yaghoubi M, et al. Clinical outcome of autologous mononuclear cells transplantation for spinal cord injury: a systematic review and meta-analysis. *Med J Islam Repub Iran.* 2014;28:112.

91. Sahni V, Kessler JA. Stem cell therapies for spinal cord injury. *Nat Rev Neurol.* 2010;6(7):363–372.

Hemodynamic Management

Teresa A. Allison
and Amber Castle

INTRODUCTION

Effective hemodynamic management is essential in the care of neurocritically ill patients as both hypertension and hypotension can significantly affect patient outcomes. Hypertension may increase the risk of cardiovascular events, rebleeding, and hematoma expansion. Hypotension can compromise cerebral perfusion, leading to ischemia and infarction. The goal blood pressure varies by condition and must be individualized considering patient-specific factors. Fortunately, a variety of pharmacologic therapies are available to help achieve hemodynamic goals. This chapter reviews the hemodynamic management of neurocritically ill patients with hypertension or shock.

HYPERTENSIVE EMERGENCY OVERVIEW

Hypertension affects approximately 80 million people in the United States and is a significant cause of cerebral, cardiovascular, and renal events.[1,2] Hypertension is defined as elevations in blood pressures above 140 mm Hg systolic blood pressure (SBP) or 90 mm Hg diastolic blood pressure (DBP) (demonstrated on 2 readings taken 5 minutes apart within 24 hours of symptom onset). Approximately 1% to 2% of patients with hypertension will present with a hypertensive emergency at some time in their lives.[3] Hypertensive emergency is defined by acute severely elevated blood pressure (typically a SBP >180 mm Hg and/or DBP >120 mm Hg) associated with target end-organ damage. Hypertensive urgency is characterized by a similarly elevated blood pressure and no target end-organ damage.[4]

Each year, approximately 795,000 people experience a new or recurrent stroke, and approximately 77% of patients who have a first stroke have a history of hypertension.[2] In 2011, stroke accounted for 1 out of every 20 deaths in the United States. A linear relationship between blood pressure and stroke mortality has been observed. In patients with treated hypertension, a 1-mm Hg increase in SBP increases stroke deaths by 2%.[5] Therefore, control of hypertension is particularly important in this population.

In addition, hypertension is a significant complication of the acute stroke period. Elevated blood pressure (>140/90 mm Hg) occurs in approximately 75% of patients with an acute ischemic stroke (AIS) and greater than 80% of patients with an intracerebral hemorrhage (ICH). Hypertension in this setting is independently associated with poor functional outcomes.[6] Possible mechanisms for the acute hypertensive response observed after stroke include (1) undiagnosed or inadequately treated hypertension; (2) other causes such as pain, dehydration, or stress response; (3) Cushing response to the mass effect of cerebral edema; (4) shifting of the autoregulatory curve to a higher level in patients with chronic hypertension; (5) neuroendocrine response with activation of the sympathetic nervous system and the renin-angiotensin axis; and (6) direct injury to areas involved with cardiovascular function.[7] Acute hypertensive responses after stroke are typically transient, lasting for a few hours to days. In two-thirds of untreated patients, spontaneous decreases in blood pressure were observed within 10 days after stroke onset.[8]

Patients with an acute elevation in blood pressure and neurological abnormalities require a thorough initial neurological examination to diagnose and differentiate stroke subtypes. Optimization of blood pressure remains challenging in acute stroke management secondary to differences in the underlying pathophysiology of stroke subtypes, an incomplete understanding of the cause of elevated blood pressure, and the clinical effects of blood pressure lowering. Currently, guidelines predominantly consist of expert opinion based on observational studies and small clinical trials. Consequently, a consensus on the management of transient elevations of blood pressure and how aggressively to lower blood pressure in the acute stroke period is lacking. At this time, recommendations are to modestly lower the blood pressure to avoid secondary end-organ damage while maintaining adequate cerebral perfusion.

CEREBROVASCULAR PATHOPHYSIOLOGY IN HYPERTENSION

The pathophysiology of hypertensive emergencies varies depending on the organ systems involved. An understanding of cerebral perfusion is vital in the management of all hypertensive emergencies, especially those involving the brain. The brain uses approximately 20% of the total body oxygen consumption and receives 15% of the total cardiac output. Due to a limited ability to store oxygen and glucose, maintaining a constant cerebral blood flow (CBF) is imperative to ensure adequate oxygen and glucose delivery. According to Ohm's law, CBF is directly related to cerebral perfusion pressure (CPP) and indirectly related to cerebral vascular resistance (CVR), which is mathematically expressed as CBF = CPP/CVR. Cerebral perfusion pressure is a calculated value from the mean arterial pressure (MAP) and intracranial pressure (ICP) in the equation CPP = MAP - ICP. A normal ICP is considered 0 to 5 mm Hg, and as such, CPP generally equates to MAP unless the patient is experiencing elevations in ICP.

To maintain a constant CBF autoregulation produces vasoconstriction in arteries in response to increases in blood pressure and vasodilation in response to decreases in blood pressure. In normotensive patients, autoregulation maintains a constant CBF of 50 mL/100 g/min over a MAP range of 60 to 150 mm Hg during normal circumstances. However, in hypertensive patients, autoregulation is shifted to the right (increased MAP range) or upward (increased SBP and/or DBP range).[9] When CPP reductions lead to a decrease in CBF, the brain initially increases oxygen extraction. If the pressure falls below the lower limits of autoregulation, this compensatory mechanism will be inadequate to prevent ischemia or infarction. On the contrary, when the CPP exceeds the upper limit, cerebral vessels can no longer vasoconstrict effectively, and "breakthrough" vasodilation leads to cerebral edema and/or hemorrhage.

Acute Ischemic Stroke

AIS accounts for 80% of all strokes, while ICHs, including subarachnoid hemorrhages (SAHs), account for the other 20%. As mentioned previously, most patients who present with an ischemic stroke have an SBP greater than 140 mm Hg. Admission blood pressure (BP) and outcomes after ischemic stroke have been shown to follow a U-shaped relationship, with both low and high BP extremes associated with poor outcome.[10] For every 10 mm Hg of SBP below 150 mm Hg, the risk of early death increases by 3.6% and the risk of late death and dependency increases by 17.9%. Conversely, for every 10-mm Hg increase in SBP above 150 mm Hg, the risk of early death increases by 3.8%. Poor outcome because of increased BP is thought to be due to worsening cerebral edema, whereas poor outcome because of low BP may be due to cerebral hypoperfusion and cardiac events.[6]

In patients presenting with AIS and hypertension, it would seem logical to acutely lower the blood pressure. However, this can reduce cerebral blood flow to vulnerable regions. Ischemic stroke is the result of an occluded artery with ensuing moderate (penumbra) or severe (core) reduction in regional blood flow. The penumbra zone is viable but underperfused tissue where high blood pressure, along with collateral blood flow, is crucial.[11] In effect, lowering the BP can potentially increase the infarction. Conversely, elevated BP may cause further neurologic damage by exacerbating cerebral edema or lead to hemorrhagic transformation of the stroke.

Many questions remain regarding the optimal blood pressure management after ischemic stroke. In the absence of strong evidence supporting a specific target, BP ranges should be individualized based on the need for thrombolytics and patient-specific comorbidities. American Heart Association (AHA)/American Stroke Association (ASA) guidelines for AIS recommend a goal BP of less than 185/110 mm Hg in patients receiving thrombolytics and maintained less than 180/105 mm Hg to reduce the risk of hemorrhagic transformation. In patients not eligible for thrombolytic therapy, the recommendation is not to lower BP within the first 24 hours of ischemic stroke unless the BP is greater than 220/120 mm Hg or there is a concomitant medical condition that would benefit from lowering the BP to avoid cerebral hypoperfusion.[12]

Intracerebral Hemorrhage

Elevated BP is very common in the acute phase of ICH, with approximately 80% of patients presenting with an SBP greater than 140 mm Hg. Hypertension in ICH is associated with worse outcomes. First-day MAPs greater than 145 mm Hg are associated with worse 28-day survival rates, while an increased risk of morbidity and mortality has been shown with increasing SBP above 140 mm Hg.[13,14] Elevated BP after ICH is also associated with greater hematoma expansion as well as development of perihematomal cerebral edema. Whether hypertension is a marker of or contributor to active hematoma growth has yet to be determined. However, hematoma expansion is a major determinant of morbidity and mortality. For each 1-mL increase in absolute ICH volume, patients were 7% more likely to have a worse outcome.[15] Intensive BP lowering during the acute period of ICH has been shown to reduce hematoma expansion. The Intensive Blood Pressure Reduction in Acute Cerebral Hemorrhage Trial (INTERACT), which randomized patients within 6 hours of ICH onset to either intensive (SBP <140 mm Hg) or guideline (SBP <180 mm Hg) treatment, showed a 36% relative risk reduction of hematoma growth of 33% or more in the intensive treatment group.[16]

In contrast to AIS, the goal for BP reduction in ICH is to attenuate ongoing bleeding and reduce the risk of hematoma expansion. Two factors appear to make this safe in ICH. First, unlike in ischemic stroke, only 1 study of ICH demonstrated a poor outcome at an SBP less than 140 mm Hg.[10] Second, there does not appear to be a reduction in the cerebral blood flow within the peri-hematomal region when the SBP is lowered below 140 mm Hg during the acute ICH period measured by computed tomography (CT) perfusion.

Current evidence suggests that early intensive BP lowering is safe and that surviving patients show modestly better functional recovery, with a favorable trend seen toward a reduction in morbidity and mortality. In INTERACT II, there was a nonstatistically significant trend for reduction in the risk of death or major disability in patients randomized to less than 140 mm Hg.[17] In a pre-specified secondary end point, an ordinal analysis of 90-day modified Rankin Scale (mRS) scores showed that a favorable outcome was more likely in this group. However, trials conducted to date indicate that it is difficult to achieve a target of less than 140 mm Hg within 3 hours of ICH, the high-risk period for hematoma expansion. This may explain the failure of the INTERACT II trial to show definitive efficacy. In both INTERACT trials, the median time from symptom onset to initiation of intravenous BP treatment was 4 hours. Currently, the safe limit for lowering BP and how fast it can be lowered is undetermined. The AHA/ASA 2015 guidelines state for ICH patients presenting with SBP 150 to 220 mm Hg and without contraindication to acute BP treatment, acute lowering to SBP less than 140 mm Hg is safe (Class I; Level of Evidence A). For ICH patients presenting with SBP more than 220 mm Hg, aggressive treatment of BP and frequent monitoring should be considered (Class IIb; Level of Evidence C).[18]

Aneurysmal Subarachnoid Hemorrhage

The role of hypertension in aneurysmal subarachnoid hemorrhage (aSAH) is less well studied compared with ICH and AIS. Saccular aneurysms are formed at bifurcations and acute hypertensive episodes may facilitate rupture of the aneurysm. Recent guidelines indicate hypertension as a risk factor for the development of aSAH based on Class I Level B evidence.[19] A systematic review showed that the risk of aSAH is approximately 2.8 times in patients with hypertension.[20]

To prevent rebleeding after an aSAH, the AHA/ASA guidelines recommend controlling acute hypertension with a titratable agent until the aneurysm has been obliterated. During this time, prevention of rebleeding must be balanced with prevention of ischemic stroke and maintenance of cerebral perfusion pressure (Class 1; Level B evidence). Specific parameters for BP have not been defined. However, maintaining a SBP less than 160 mm Hg is considered reasonable.[19]

Conversely, BP augmentation to improve cerebral perfusion is recommended for patients with aSAH for the management of cerebral vasospasm and delayed cerebral ischemia unless the BP is already elevated at baseline or the patient has a cardiovascular contraindication.[19] Traditionally, BP augmentation has been part of triple-H therapy, which consists of hemodilution, hypervolemia, and hypertension. Literature now suggests patients should be managed with euvolemia and induced hypertension. Randomized trials with induced hypertension have not been conducted, but it is recommended based on the rapid improvement observed and subsequent worsening with premature discontinuation in many patients. The mechanism of its benefit is unknown. It has been proposed that increases in MAP may increase cerebral blood flow in the setting of autoregulation dysfunction or it may be a direct transluminal pressure effect that leads to arterial vasodilation.

ANTIHYPERTENSIVE THERAPIES

The management of acute BP lowering requires individualization based on the underlying disease states, as described above, to prevent further or new neurological damage. Most patients will require intermittent or continuous intravenous therapy during the acute period of BP control. Several different agents exist for use, all of which can successfully reduce arterial BP, when used correctly.

Minimizing cerebral effects in these patients is of utmost importance. Agent-specific effects on CBF, ICP, and CPP, as well as effects on other organs, must be considered when selecting therapy. Additional characteristics of the ideal agent for the management of hypertensive emergencies should include a rapid onset and offset of action, a predictable and easily managed dose-response relationship, and a lack of side effects and drug interactions, and be convenient. Individual classes and agents will be reviewed to assist in selection of the most appropriate agent.

Direct Vasodilators

Agents that directly vasodilate the peripheral vasculature and decrease systemic vascular resistance (SVR) include hydralazine, nitroprusside, and nitroglycerin. Depending on the agent, dilation of cerebral vascular beds with these agents likely leads to an increase in cerebral blood volume and ICP with a resulting decrease in MAP and CPP. It is uncertain if these agents act with equivalent efficacy on vascular smooth muscle within injured and normal brain regions. These agents can potentially cause a "cerebral steal phenomenon" by selectively dilating vascular smooth muscle in areas of normal brain regions, shunting blood away from injured areas, which would result in additional ischemic injury.

Hydralazine

Hydralazine is predominantly a direct arteriolar vasodilator, with minimum venous vasodilation. Hydralazine acts by interfering with vascular smooth muscle calcium transport and has also been shown to produce nitric oxide.[21] The resulting vasodilation produces a rapid decrease in BP, with diastolic pressure reduced more than systolic. The reduction in peripheral vascular resistance seen with hydralazine leads to reflex tachycardia and an increased cardiac output. Hydralazine may be administered in doses of 5 to 20 mg as a slow intravenous injection or 10 to 50 mg intramuscularly. The circulating half-life of hydralazine is 1.5 to 3 hours, but the half-life of its effect on BP is about 100 hours. Following administration, the onset of action is 10 to 15 minutes, often with precipitous falls in BP, which can last up to 12 hours.[22,23]

In patients with neurological injury and defective or absent cerebral autoregulation, the administration of hydralazine resulted in increased ICP. Despite the increase in ICP, the CBF remained stable or slightly increased.[24,25] In addition, hydralazine administration causes reflex stimulation of the sympathetic nervous system and an increase in ICP. Coadministration of β- receptor antagonists can be used to blunt these effects.

Because of its prolonged and unpredictable antihypertensive effects, the inability to titrate the drug's hypotensive response effectively, and its negative effects on the cerebrovasculature, hydralazine is best avoided in the management of neurologically injured patients with hypertensive crises.

Sodium Nitroprusside

Sodium nitroprusside (nitroprusside) is a potent arterial and venous vasodilator, which results in a reduction in vascular resistance and a corresponding reduction in preload and afterload, with little or no effect on cardiac output. Patients with heart failure and low cardiac output often experience an increase in cardiac output secondary to afterload reduction. Nitroprusside acts through production of endothelial–dependent relaxing factor, nitric oxide. It is one of the most commonly used parenteral agents due to an onset of action within seconds, a duration of action of 1 to 2 minutes after termination, and a plasma half-life of 3 to 4 minutes. Doses range from 0.5 to 10 mcg/kg/min. There are several limitations to the use of nitroprusside, including tachyphylaxis, need for arterial pressure monitoring, and need for a special delivery system secondary to photosensitivity. The most concerning limitation surrounding the use of nitroprusside is the potential accumulation of toxic metabolites, cyanide and thiocyanate, which can be seen with high doses, prolonged use, and end-organ failure.[26,27]

Nitroprusside is a nonselective vasodilator of cerebral vessels, which may lead to an increase in cerebral blood flow and ICP. Decreased MAP or increased ICP may lead to decreased CPP and further ischemic complications. In addition, in patients with elevated ICP, nitroprusside administration inhibits the normal vasoconstrictive response to hypocapnia.[28,29]

Nitroprusside is recognized in the latest ischemic stroke guidelines as one of the first-line agents for the management of hypertensive crises. However, in patients with altered intracranial compliance or disturbances in autoregulation, careful monitoring of CBF, CPP, and ICP is required. Combined with the limitations surrounding its use, significant expense, and the negative effects on the cerebrovasculature, selection of an alternative agent is suggested.

Nitroglycerin

At low doses, nitroglycerin is a potent venodilator causing a reduction in preload. It has little effect on arteriolar resistance and systemic arterial pressure. At higher doses, nitroglycerin vasodilates arterial smooth muscle, which reduces systemic BP and activates sympathetic reflexes. Nitroglycerin is not an effective antihypertensive agent and has an unpredictable dose response. However, it is an effective antianginal agent. By diminishing preload, it decreases left ventricular diastolic volume and pressure and myocardial wall tension, leading to a reduction in myocardial oxygen consumption. These changes favor redistribution of coronary blood flow to the subendocardium, which is more vulnerable to ischemia. In addition, it favors redistribution of coronary blood flow by dilating both epicardial coronary vessels with stenosis and their collaterals. As such, nitroglycerin is used predominantly in patients experiencing a hypertensive crisis associated with acute coronary syndrome or acute pulmonary edema.[1] The mechanism of vasodilation is via nitric oxide. Nitroglycerin is administered via intravenous continuous infusion at 5 to 100 mcg/min secondary to an onset of action of 1 to 2 minutes and a duration of action of 3 to 5 minutes after discontinuation.

Nitroglycerin vasodilates large intracranial arteries, but increased capacitance is thought to account for increases in CBF and cerebral volume in patients with normal or injured brains. This results in an elevation in ICP, which is more prominent in patients with altered intracranial compliance.[30–32] As nitroglycerin is a poor antihypertensive and can elevate ICP, it should be used with caution and requires frequent neurological monitoring. In patients requiring rapid BP reduction or without acute coronary syndrome or pulmonary edema, selection of an alternative agent is suggested.

Beta-Adrenergic Receptor Antagonists

β-Receptor antagonists can be categorized based on their β-receptor selectivity as well as their effects on the α_1-receptor. Intravenous β-receptor antagonists, which are used for BP reduction, include esmolol and labetalol. The initial antihypertensive effect is the result of the negative chronotropic and inotropic effects, which lead to a reduction in heart rate, stroke volume, and cardiac output. A decrease in vasomotor tone and SVR was reported with longer term therapy.

Esmolol

Esmolol is a β-1 selective adrenergic antagonist, which produces a reduction in heart rate, resulting in a reduction in cardiac output and arterial BP. It lacks membrane-stabilizing properties as well as intrinsic sympathomimetic activity. Esmolol is hydrophilic and rapidly metabolized by red blood cell and liver esterases; the clearance of the drug is independent of the liver or kidney.

Esmolol is very useful in acute settings on account of its rapid onset of action (60 seconds), short duration of action (10–20 minutes), and ease of reversibility. The typical dose is as an intravenous bolus of a 0.5- to 1-mL/kg loading dose over 1 minute followed by a continuous intravenous infusion of 50 to 300 mcg/min. As its physiologic effect is predominantly on heart rate, it is primarily used for the management of supraventricular tachycardia. It is not routinely used for hypertensive crisis due to the risk of developing severe bradycardia before lowering of BP occurs.

Labetalol

Labetalol is a combined selective α_1- and nonselective β-receptor antagonist with an α to β blocking ratio of 1:7 after intravenous administration. Arterial BP is lowered by reduction of SVR without significant alterations in heart rate or cardiac output. The onset of action is 5 to 15 minutes with precipitous drops in BP occurring predominantly with larger bolus doses. The duration of action is 3 to 6 hours. Labetalol may be administered as a 10- to 20-mg slow intravenous push every 10 to 15 minutes until the desired BP is achieved. Alternatively, it can be administered as an intravenous continuous infusion between 1 and 6 mg/min.

Data on the cerebrovascular effects of labetalol in patients with neurological injuries are lacking, but it has been used extensively for BP management in these patients. Available literature suggests there is no change in global and regional CBF, cerebral metabolism, and cerebral autoregulation. No worsening of neurological deficits has been reported after its administration. CBF, in healthy hypertensive patients, did not change once BP was controlled on labetalol.[33] Compared with nitroprusside, labetalol improved CPP and ICP in postoperative neurosurgical patients with refractory hypertension.[34]

Precipitous drops in BP and bradycardia can occur with labetalol administration. In addition, it has a slower onset and offset of action compared with other agents, as well as an absence of a predictable dose-response relationship, making it more difficult to titrate and control. Despite this, labetalol is used in a wide variety of hypertensive emergencies. This combined with its lack of effect on the cerebrovasculature has led to its routine use for the management of hypertensive crises in patients with neurological injuries.

Calcium Channel Antagonists

Three classes of calcium channel blockers exist based on chemical structure: dihydropyridines (nicardipine, clevidipine, amlodipine, nifedipine), benzothiazepines (diltiazem), and phenylalkylamines (verapamil), of which the dihydropyridines are chiefly used for BP management. Dihydropyridines inhibit the transmembrane influx of calcium ions into cardiac and smooth muscle, resulting in vasodilation of the peripheral vasculature and a decrease in SVR without a reduction in cardiac output or a negative inotropic effect.

Nicardipine

Nicardipine, a second-generation dihydropyridine, has obtained acceptance as a parenteral antihypertensive agent for several reasons, including ease of use, ease of titration, predictable dose response, and few side effects compared with other agents such as nitroprusside. Nicardipine is initially dosed at 5 mg/h and titrated by 1 to 2.5 mg/h every 5 to 15 minutes until goal response has been achieved or to a maximum dose of 15 mg/h. When administered intravenously, BP reductions occur as quickly as 2.5 minutes after initiation of the infusion and typically occur within 10 to 15 minutes. The duration of action is typically up to 4 hours after discontinuation of the infusion.

While nicardipine lowers BP, it increases CBF with little effect on ICP. In addition, it has been shown to decrease MAP and CPP, but the CPP remained within the critical level of autoregulation. Nicardipine is highly lipophilic and readily crosses the blood-brain barrier. Experimental animal studies have demonstrated a neuroprotective effect of nicardipine in hypertension-induced brain injury.[35,36] Recent work suggests it may have anti-neuroinflammatory effects on microglial cells.[37] More research will be required to determine if these observations can be applied clinically.

Due to the relatively rapid onset of action, ease of use, and potential for neuroprotection, nicardipine has become the parenteral antihypertensive of choice in many neurointensive care units. When a continuous infusion is required, the AHA/ASA acute ischemic stroke guidelines recommend nicardipine as a first-line agent.[12]

Clevidipine

Clevidipine, a third-generation dihydropyridine, is an ultra-short-acting agent. In perioperative patients, it produces a 4% to 5% reduction in SBP within 2 to 4 minutes of initiating the infusion. After initiation, each 1- to 2-mg/h increase typically decreases systolic BP by an additional 2 to 4 mm Hg. Full recovery of BP is achieved in 5 to 15 minutes after discontinuation of the infusion. Clevidipine is lipophilic and rapidly metabolized by red blood cell and extravascular tissue esterases; as a result, drug clearance is independent of the liver or kidney.

The cerebrovascular effects of clevidipine have not been studied. It has been shown to be safe and effective in the treatment of perioperative hypertension neurosurgical patients[38] as well as for rapid BP reduction in critically ill ICH patients.[39] A 7-patient subgroup of the this trial demonstrated that there was no clinically meaningful change in CPP or ICP while the SBP was reduced.[40] The place in therapy of clevidipine compared with nicardipine has yet to be determined.

Angiotensin-Converting Enzyme Inhibitor

The renin-angiotensin system (RAS) may contribute to many hypertensive states, including hypertensive emergencies. Angiotensin-converting enzyme inhibitors (ACEIs) are thought to effective in 3 ways: (1) by decreasing systemic concentrations of angiotensin II, (2) by inhibiting local vascular effects of angiotensin II, and (3) by increasing concentrations of the vasodilator, bradykinin. Several agents are available for oral administration. However, only oral captopril and intravenous enalaprilat are used for hypertensive crises.

Captopril

Unlike the direct vasodilators, which increase CBF and inhibit cerebral autoregulation, ACEIs appear to increase CBF and shift the autoregulatory curve. When captopril was administered intravenously to normotensive or spontaneously hypertensive rats, both the upper and lower limits of autoregulation were shifted and the plateau curve was shortened.[41] Captopril appears to influence autoregulation by inhibiting angiotensin II–mediated vascular tone in large cerebral arteries while small resistant vessels vasoconstrict.[42,43] As BP decreases, these vessels have an increased capacity to dilate. Effects on ICP have not been widely studied. In patients with normal-pressure hydrocephalus, captopril reduces MAP without altering ICP or CBF. In addition, literature suggests that ACEIs and angiotensin receptor blocking agents (ARBs) may have neuroprotective effects beyond their BP-lowering properties due to additional effects on RAS and other substances.

Enalaprilat

Enalaprilat lowers BP largely by decreasing SVR. Cardiac output and heart rate are not significantly altered. Unlike direct vasodilators, these agents do not result in reflex sympathetic activation, allowing them to be safely used in patients with ischemic heart disease. The onset of action of enalaprilat is 15 minutes, with a duration of action of 12 to 24 hours. Enalaprilat is administered via slow intravenous push at doses of 0.625 to 2.5 mg.

Enalaprilat is the only intravenous ACEI available in the United States. An unpredictable dose response and long duration of action limit its widespread use. Enalaprilat should not be used in patients with acute renal dysfunction. However, some compelling literature suggests that ACEIs and ARBs may be neuroprotective. Additional research may advance the use of these agents, particularly in neurologically impaired patients.

α-2 Adrenergic Receptor Agonists

The α-2 receptors are a subgroup of noradrenergic receptors distributed broadly within and outside the central nervous system. Stimulation of presynaptic α-2 receptors inhibits norepinephrine release from the presynaptic neuron. The antihypertensive agent clonidine has an affinity for α-2 receptors vs α-1 receptors of 200:1. In comparison, dexmedetomidine, which is used for primarily for sedation and anxiety, has an affinity ratio of 1620:1.

Clonidine

Clonidine is a centrally acting α-2 agonist. Arterial BP reduction results from reduction of cardiac output due to a decrease in heart rate, relaxation of capacitance vessels, and reduction in peripheral vascular resistance. Oral clonidine is the only formulation available in the United States, limiting its use to hypertensive urgencies. The half-life of oral clonidine is 8 to 12 hours. After ingestion, BP reduction starts within 30 minutes, with significant reduction at 1 hour. The maximum effect is seen between 2 and 4 hours. While several aggressive dosing regimens have been described, doses should generally be limited to 0.1 to 0.2 mg every 6 to 8 hours.

There is a lack of data on the cerebrovascular effects of clonidine in patients with neurological injuries. In animal studies, α-2 agonists decrease cerebral blood flow, but they do not alter the cerebral metabolic rate, suggesting a direct vasoconstrictor effect. Human studies have been consistent, with animal studies showing a reduction in CBF of up to 28% from baseline.[44] Animal studies have raised concerns that clonidine may reduce CBF without decreasing cerebral metabolic rate, potentially limiting adequate cerebral oxygenation of brain tissue at risk for ischemic injury. However, no evidence of global cerebral ischemia in animal studies with dogs was observed.[45,46]

Drawbacks to clonidine include an inconveniently long dosing interval for acute reduction of BP and the risk of an excessive reduction in BP, which may be difficult to reverse. Many of the side effects of clonidine are disadvantageous in neurologically impaired patients, including sedation, orthostatic hypotension, and dizziness. Secondary to the unknown effects on the cerebrovasculature as well as its side effect profile, clonidine should be limited to second or third line in patients with neurological impairments.

SHOCK OVERVIEW

Shock can be defined as poor perfusion resulting in widespread cellular hypoxia, an inability to meet increased oxygen demand, or inadequate oxygen utilization. Stated simply, shock is an imbalance between oxygen supply and demand. Shock is typically characterized by arterial hypotension, evidence of tissue hypoperfusion, and elevated serum lactate levels resulting in metabolic acidosis. A lack of perfusion compromises oxygen and nutrient delivery and can result in accumulation of toxins. Timely restoration of adequate oxygen can reverse the effects of shock and prevent irreversible complications, which include multiorgan failure and death. Thus, the primary goal of the treatment of shock is to restore adequate perfusion to tissues. This is broadly achieved through correction of the underlying cause, administration of oxygen, restoring blood volume with fluids and/or blood products, and, when necessary, vasopressors and inotropes.[47]

Invasive monitoring is often needed for patients in shock. An arterial catheter can monitor arterial BP while a central venous catheter can be used to assess fluid status and central venous oxyhemoglobin saturation, as well as enable administration of fluids, blood products, and vasoactive medications. Both can be used to facilitate frequent blood draws. Pulmonary arterial catheterization is not associated with improved patient outcomes and is limited by significant complications. While it can be used to measure the pulmonary artery occlusion pressure and mixed venous oxyhemoglobin saturation, this monitoring strategy should be used with caution in the management of patients with shock.[48] Noninvasive continuous electronic monitoring of hemodynamic parameters (eg, BP, heart rate, rhythm) should be used for all patients with shock on vasopressors and/or inotropes to facilitate dose titration, direct interventions, and ensure achievement of BP goals.

The following section describes different types of shock and their management. It is important to note that multiple types of shock may coexist, and treatment should be tailored to the individual patient.

Hypovolemic Shock

Hypovolemic shock is characterized by a reduced blood volume, which is commonly seen in patients with trauma and significant blood loss. This results in widespread vasoconstriction, increased heart rate, and ventricular contractility. Typical symptoms include cool clammy skin, tachycardia, increased respiratory rate, orthostasis, altered mental status, and oliguria. A lack of oxygen causes a shift to anaerobic glycolysis, which is unable to meet metabolic demand. Lactate, a by-product of anaerobic metabolism, accumulates and can cause a metabolic acidosis. Serum lactate can be serially measured to aid in the assessment of therapeutic response. As inadequate intravascular volume due to blood loss is often the cause of hypovolemic shock, interventions generally target restoration of blood volume by limiting further blood loss and replacement of blood volume with fluids and/or blood products.[49,50]

Cardiogenic Shock

Cardiogenic shock is characterized by persistent hypotension, reduced cardiac index (<2.2 L/min/m^2 with support or <1.8 L/min/m^2 in the absence of support), decreased mixed venous oxygen saturation, and normal or elevated filling pressures in one or both ventricles.[51] Cardiogenic shock most commonly occurs in the setting of an acute myocardial infarction (AMI), but it can also be seen in cardiac surgery, cardiomyopathy, cardiac arrhythmias, and in patients with valvular disease. In addition to other symptoms of shock, pulmonary congestion and jugular venous distention are usually present.

Severe heart failure reduces cardiac output and causes a release of adrenaline and aldosterone. This results in systemic vasoconstriction, increased afterload, and cardiac metabolic demand. The primary target of interventions in cardiogenic shock is early reperfusion if appropriate. In patients with shock due to arrhythmias, clinicians should evaluate for shockable rhythm/antiarrhythmic therapy in accordance with the advanced cardiac life support guidelines. In shock due to AMI, clinicians should consider administration of antiplatelets, anticoagulants, coronary revascularization therapy, and/or use of an intra-aortic balloon pump to restore flow.[52]

Distributive Shock

Distributive shock can occur with systemic infection, anaphylaxis, or systemic inflammatory response syndrome. Distributive shock is characterized by widespread peripheral vasodilation, resulting in impaired oxygen exchange and delivery as well as a fluid shift to the interstitium and increased intravascular space. The net effect is a relative hypovolemia as blood remains in the venous system. Septic shock is the most common type of shock in patients admitted to the intensive care unit.[47] In 2016, septic shock was redefined as life-threatening organ dysfunction caused by an abnormality in the regulation of the patient's response to an infection in combination with a vasopressor requirement to maintain goal MAP (at least 65 mm Hg) and serum lactate (>2 mmol/L) despite adequate volume resuscitation.[53] Therapeutic targets in distributive shock include fluid resuscitation, increased vascular tone (vasopressors), and, if present, treatment of infection.[50]

Neurogenic Shock

Neurogenic shock is a type of distributive shock that can occur after traumatic spinal cord injury or severe traumatic brain injury. As a result of the central nervous system injury, there is a loss of control of vascular tone, systemic vasodilation, and subsequent relative hypovolemia often accompanied by bradycardia.

Secondary ischemic injury and worse outcomes are associated with hypotension and low cerebral perfusion pressure.[54] Traumatic spinal cord injury guidelines recommend to maintain MAP at least 85 to 90 mm Hg for the first 7 days following acute spinal cord injury to prevent secondary ischemic injury, but this recommendation is based on low-quality evidence, and the use of vasopressors in this population has been associated with an increased rate of complications.[55–58] In contrast, severe traumatic brain injury (TBI) guidelines recommend a less aggressive goal SBP greater than 90 mm Hg with a CPP of 50 to 70 mm Hg.[59] Interventions to treat neurogenic shock include vasopressors to increase SVR as well as blood products and fluids to increase preload.

Cerebrovascular Pathophysiology in Shock

Global ischemia causes cellular injury and end-organ damage. Specific to the brain, global hypoxic-ischemic encephalopathy can occur. In the injured brain, inadequate cerebral perfusion can lead to secondary injury. In addition, the blood-brain barrier may be compromised in septic shock, resulting in exposure to potentially toxic inflammatory mediators and cytokines.[60] Immediate restoration of adequate blood flow and delivery of oxygen and nutrients is essential to preserve cerebral tissue.

Fluid Resuscitation

Fluid resuscitation should be initiated immediately while the cause of shock is evaluated. Isotonic crystalloids are generally preferred for patients who are neurocritically ill and in severe sepsis, and septic shock crystalloids are the initial fluid of choice.[50] There is little evidence suggesting a reduction in mortality or enhanced efficacy with a specific resuscitation fluid, although hydroxyethyl starches should be avoided as described below.[50,61–63] Intravenous fluids are administered to optimize cardiac filling pressures to increase intravascular volume, cardiac output, and peripheral blood flow. Treatment goals may target BP, a normalized heart rate, or adequate urine output. When available, pulmonary-capillary wedge pressure (PCWP) in combination with arterial oxygen saturation can help assess efficacy of fluid resuscitation. While imperfect, central venous pressure (CVP) is often used in combination with the physical examination to assess fluid status.[50]

In practice, crystalloids are used as first-line therapy due to their favorable side effect profile and low cost. In TBI, normal saline is preferred as albumin administration is associated with increased mortality. Albumin is not associated with harm in other critically ill populations, but its use is limited by cost and the lack of a clear advantage over crystalloids.[64] Albumin may have a role in the treatment of patients with severe sepsis and septic shock who require large volumes of crystalloids.[50] Hydroxyethyl starch solutions carry a black box warning due to the risk of increased mortality and severe renal injury when administered to critically ill patients and should not be used in the treatment of shock. Similarly, while hypertonic saline is an effective intervention for elevated intracranial pressure, it has not been shown to be beneficial for fluid resuscitation in patients with TBI.[65]

General limitations of intravenous fluids include interstitial edema, pulmonary edema, and exacerbation of congestive heart failure. Other adverse effects vary among resuscitation fluids. Administration of large volumes of normal saline can result in a non–anion gap hyperchloremic metabolic acidosis. Restriction of chloride by preferentially administering balanced salt solutions such as lactated Ringer's solution may reduce the risk of acute kidney injury and need for renal replacement therapy in critically ill patients.[66] Conversely, administration of large volumes of lactated Ringer's solution can cause a metabolic alkalosis due to generation of bicarbonate from lactate metabolism. Lactated Ringer's solution is incompatible with blood due to clotting, necessitating use of a separate line.

Another important consideration, particularly in patients with neurologic injury, is fluid tonicity. In patients with acute spinal cord injury, excess fluids can cause further cord swelling and damage. Similarly, administration of hypotonic fluids in susceptible patients can exacerbate cerebral edema and intracranial pressure. Therefore, isotonic solutions are preferred in patients with acute neurologic injury, and both hypovolemia and hypervolemia should be avoided.

When immediately available, some centers prefer to provide blood products in place of fluids to restore blood volume in trauma patients with severe blood loss, but this remains controversial. Advanced Trauma Life Support guidelines discuss the use of a delayed fluid resuscitation strategy.[67] For patients with neurologic injury in particular, this strategy should be used with caution as the lower BP goals that are used as part of this therapy may compromise cerebral perfusion and contribute to the risk of mortality.[68]

Vasopressor Therapy

Vasopressor therapy is indicated for the treatment of shock that persists after adequate fluid resuscitation. Vasopressors can also be used to induce hypertension to maintain adequate cerebral perfusion in the setting of symptomatic vasospasm. These agents support BP through peripheral vasoconstriction and may also increase cardiac output. Due to their rapid onset and short half-life, the vasopressors presented below are readily titratable with trained personnel and appropriate monitoring. All vasopressors can compromise perfusion of the extremities and are vessel irritants. While it may be necessary to emergently initiate vasopressor therapy at a low dose while only peripheral access is present, central access should be established as soon as possible to prevent local tissue injury. If extravasation occurs, the infusion should be stopped immediately, the line should not be flushed, and administration of an antidote may be required.

Early use of vasopressors in hemorrhagic shock is associated with an increased risk of mortality.[69] Of note, patients with severe TBI and spinal cord injury were excluded from this trial. Vasopressors should generally be avoided in the treatment of hypovolemic shock unless there is persistent hypotension despite administration of adequate fluids. Vasopressors are limited in the treatment of cardiogenic shock as they generally are not targeting the underlying issue and may further stress compromised cardiac tissue. Vasopressors exert their effect primarily by increasing SVR, but these patients often already have an elevated SVR, and this effect increases cardiac work and PCWP. In the treatment of shock, vasopressin is usually added on as a second or third agent. In the absence of severe hypotension, dobutamine can be a useful alternative to vasopressors in the setting of cardiogenic shock.

Vasopressors should be initiated at a low dose and then can be rapidly titrated to the desired hemodynamic effect. Typical dose ranges are presented below, but higher doses have been described in the setting of refractory shock, and the concurrent use of multiple vasopressors may be required. Tachyphylaxis can develop over time with continued use of vasopressors requiring higher doses to maintain the same effect. Sudden interruptions in vasopressor therapy may precipitate hypotension; therefore, incremental weaning of vasopressors is recommended.

Vasopressors differ with regard to receptor selectivity and in some cases exhibit a dose-dependent effect. Agonism of the α_1 or vasopressin$_1$ receptor results in an increase in systemic vascular resistance while β-1 or phosphodiesterase agonism primarily increases cardiac output. Commonly used vasopressors (norepinephrine, dopamine, epinephrine, phenylephrine, and vasopressin) and their properties are described below.

Norepinephrine

Norepinephrine is an α-1 and β-1 agonist with both vasopressor and inotropic properties. It causes vasoconstriction except in the coronary and cerebral vessels, which dilate, resulting in increased preload (PCWP), afterload (SVR), venous return, and myocardial metabolic demand. Norepinephrine is the drug of choice in hypovolemic shock, septic shock, and cardiogenic shock over dopamine due to reduced mortality.[50,70] The typical dose is 2 to 12 mcg/min (0.025–0.15 mcg/kg/min). In contrast to dopamine and epinephrine, the heart rate is usually minimally affected by norepinephrine.

Dopamine

The usual dose of dopamine is 2 to 20 mcg/kg/min. Dopamine exerts its pharmacologic effect through stimulation of dopamine and adrenergic receptors (α and β, dose dependent). Norepinephrine is preferred over dopamine unless the patient is at low risk of tachyarrhythmias and bradycardia is present since dopamine is associated with a higher mortality rate in patients with cardiogenic or septic shock.[50,70,71] At the lower end of the dose range used for shock, increased inotropic and chronotropic effects are observed due to β-1 agonism, while vasoconstriction related to α-1 agonism is observed at the high end of the dose range. Dopamine can cause significant tachycardia, increased myocardial oxygen consumptions, and immunosuppression. In critically ill patients, dopamine administration has been associated with sick euthyroid syndrome.[72] In addition, it should be avoided in patients with pheochromocytoma, ventricular fibrillation, or a severe sulfite allergy.

Epinephrine

Epinephrine is primarily a β-1 agonist at low doses with α-1 agonist effects and moderate β-2 agonist effects at high doses. As a result, it has both vasopressor and chronotropic properties. The usual dose is 1 to 10 mcg/min (0.014–0.14 mcg/kg/min). At low doses, epinephrine increases cardiac output, decreases SVR, and has a variable effect on MAP, while at higher doses, epinephrine increases cardiac output, SVR, and MAP. Epinephrine is used first-line for anaphylactic shock and is a second-line agent after norepinephrine for the treatment of septic shock.[50] Adverse effects of epinephrine include dysrhythmias, increased serum lactate levels, and reduced mesenteric perfusion.

Phenylephrine

Phenylephrine is an α agonist that increases vascular tone and BP. The typical dose is 20 to 180 mcg/min (0.25–2 mcg/kg/min). Phenylephrine is used to treat symptomatic cerebral vasospasm, as an adjunctive therapy in shock refractory to other vasopressors and vasopressin, in patients who are unable to tolerate other vasopressors due to tachyarrhythmias or persistent hypotension in the setting of high cardiac output.[50] Significant adverse effects of phenylephrine include decreased cardiac output in patients with cardiac dysfunction and reflex bradycardia; therefore, it should be used with caution in patients with acute spinal cord injury.

Vasopressin

Vasopressin is usually given at a constant dose of 0.03 to 0.04 U/min as doses above 0.04 U/min can cause cardiac ischemia. It should not be used as a first-line vasopressor, but it can be useful as an adjunctive therapy for patients with inadequate response to 1 or more vasopressors. Vasopressin 0.03 U/min can be helpful in septic shock when added to norepinephrine to further augment MAP or reduce the dose of norepinephrine. The higher 0.04-U/min dose can also be used but is recommended only in refractory cases.[50] As vasopressin may decrease stroke volume and cardiac output in the setting of cardiac dysfunction, it should be reserved for patients with adequate cardiac output. Finally, vasopressin administration can cause hyponatremia, which may be particularly problematic in patients with neurologic injury.

Inotropes

Rather than directly increasing BP, inotropes improve cardiac contractility, which increases cardiac output. In fact, inotropes should be used with caution in shock due to the risk of hypotension. They are commonly used alone or in combination with vasopressors in the treatment of cardiogenic shock in patients without severe hypotension. Dobutamine and milrinone are 2 commonly used inotropes.

Dobutamine

Dobutamine is a β-1 agonist that increases cardiac contractility, cardiac output, and heart rate. At high doses (0.5–20 mcg/kg/min), dobutamine also exhibits β-2 agonism, which results in increased sympathetic tone and cardiac output. Dobutamine is a first-line option for patients in cardiogenic shock with low cardiac output with adequate BP. While hypotension is a concern, BP may actually improve slightly in patients with shock due to myocardial dysfunction. Therefore, dobutamine may be useful for patients with sepsis who have evidence of myocardial dysfunction or persistent hypoperfusion in the setting of sufficient intravascular volume and MAP.[50] Contraindications to dobutamine include idiopathic hypertrophic and subaortic stenosis.

Milrinone

Milrinone has a unique mechanism of action. It is a phosphodiesterase type III inhibitor with vasodilatory and inotropic properties that increase cardiac contractility and at high doses can increase heart rate and cause peripheral vasodilation and hypotension, as well as ventricular arrhythmias. Milrinone may be advantageous when used in addition to β agonists or in patients with diminished response to β agonists. The usual dose is 0.125 to 0.75 mcg/kg/min, which must be reduced in patients with renal impairment. Due to its prolonged half-life and propensity to cause hypotension, milrinone cannot be rapidly titrated unlike the other vasopressors and inotropes presented in this chapter.

CONCLUSION

Uncontrolled hypertension or hypotension can harm the patient with acute neurologic injury. Careful hemodynamic management to rapidly attain and maintain hemodynamic goals is critical to support positive patient outcomes. Antihypertensives, vasopressors, and inotropes should be employed as appropriate, often in combination with invasive monitoring, to achieve these goals.

References

1. Chobanian AV, Bakris GL, Black HR, et al. The seventh report of the Joint National Committee on Prevention, Detection, Evaluation, and Treatment of High Blood Pressure. *JAMA*. 2003;289(19):2560–2572.
2. Mozaffarian D, Benjamin EJ, Go AS, et al, on behalf of the American Heart Association Statistics Committee and Stroke Statistics Subcommittee. Heart disease and stroke statistics—2015 update: a report from the American Heart Association. *Circulation*. 2015;131: e29–e322.
3. Deshmukh A, Kumar G, Kumar N, et al. Effect of Joint National Committee VII report on hospitalizations for hypertensive emergencies in the United States. *Am J Cardiol*. 2011;108(9):1277–1282.
4. Baumann BM, Cline DM, Pimenta E. Treatment of hypertension in the emergency department. *J Am Soc Hypertens*. 2011;5(5):366–377.
5. Palmer AJ, Bulpitt CJ, Fletcher AE. Relation between blood pressure and stroke mortality. *Hypertension*. 1992;20(5):601–605.
6. Leonardi-Bee J, Bath PMW, Phillips SJ, Sandercock PAG, for the IST Collaborative Group. Blood pressure and clinical outcomes in the International Stroke Trial. *Stroke*. 2002;33(5):1315–1320.
7. Alqadri SL, Sreenivasan V, Qureshi AI. Acute hypertensive response management in patients with acute stroke. *Curr Cardiol Rep*. 2013;15(12):426–433.
8. Wallace JD, Levy LL. Blood pressure after stroke. *JAMA*. 1981;246(19):2177–2180.
9. Lang EW, Lagopoulos J, Griffith J, et al. Cerebral vasomotor reactivity testing in head injury: the link between pressure and flow. *J Neurol Neurosurg Psychiatry*. 2003;74(8): 1053–1059.
10. Vemmos KN, Tsivgoulis G, Spengos K, et al. U-shaped relationship between mortality and admission blood pressure in patients with acute stroke. *J Intern Med*. 2004;255(2): 257–265.
11. Astrup J, Siesjo BK, Symon L. Thresholds in cerebral ischemia-the ischemic penumbra. *Stroke*. 1981;12(6):726–730.
12. Jauch EC, Saver JL, Adams HP Jr, et al. Guidelines for the early management of patients with acute ischemic stroke: a guideline for healthcare professionals from the American Heart Association/American Stroke Association. *Stroke*. 2013;44(3):870–947.
13. Fofelholm R, Avikainen S, Murros K. Prognostic value and determinants of first-day mean arterial pressure in spontaneous supratentorial intracerebral hemorrhage. *Stroke*. 1997;28(7):1396–1400.
14. Zhang Y, Reilly KH, Tong W, et al. Blood pressure and clinical outcome among patients with acute stroke in inner Mongolia, China. *J Hypertens*. 2008;26(7):1446–1452.

15. Davis SM, Broderick J, Hennerici M, et al. Hematoma growth is a determinant of mortality and poor outcome after intracerebral hemorrhage. *Neurology*. 2006;66(8): 1175–1181.

16. Anderson CS, Huang Y, Wang JG, et al. Intensive blood pressure reduction in acute cerebral haemorrhage trial (INTERACT): a randomized pilot trial. *Lancet Neurol*. 2008;7(5):391–399.

17. Anderson CS, Heeley E, Huang Y, et al. Rapid blood-pressure lowering in patients with acute intracerebral hemorrhage. *N Engl J Med*. 2013;368(25):2355–2365.

18. Hemphill JC, Greenberg SM, Anderson CS, et al. Guidelines for the management of spontaneous intracerebral hemorrhage: a guideline for healthcare professionals from the American Heart Association/American Stroke Association. *Stroke*. 2015;46:2032–2060.

19. Connolly ES Jr, Rabinstein AA, Carhuapoma JR, et al. Guidelines for the management of aneurysmal subarachnoid hemorrhage: a guideline for healthcare professionals from the American Heart Association/American Stroke Association. *Stroke*. 2012;43:1711–1737.

20. Teunissen LL, Rinkel GJE, Algra A, et al. Risk factors for subarachnoid hemorrhage: a systematic review. *Stroke*. 1996;27(3):544–549.

21. Kruszyna H, Kruszyna R, Smith RP, et al. Red blood cells generate nitric oxide from directly acting, nitrogenous vasodilators. *Toxicol Appl Pharmacol*. 1987;91(3):429–438.

22. Murphy C. Hypertensive emergencies. *Emerg Med Clin North Am*. 1995;13(4):973–1007.

23. O'Malley K, Segal JL, Israeli ZH, et al. Duration of hydralazine action in hypertension. *Clin Pharmacol Ther*. 1975;18(5, pt 1):581–586.

24. Skinhoj E, Overgaard J. Effect of dihydralazine on intracranial pressure in patients with severe brain damage. *Acta Med Scand Suppl*. 1983;678:83–87.

25. Overgaard J, Skinhoj E. A paradoxical cerebral hemodynamic effect of hydralazine. *Stroke*. 1975;6(4):402–410.

26. Alaniz C, Watts B. Monitoring cyanide toxicity in patients receiving nitroprusside therapy. *Ann Pharmacother*. 2005;39(2):388–389.

27. Cottrell JE, Casthely P, Brodie JD, et al. Mechanism and prevention of tachyphylaxis and cyanide toxicosis after nitroprusside-induced hypotension. *Surg Forum*. 1978;29: 308–310.

28. Marsh ML, Aidinis SJ, Naughton KVH, et al. The technique of nitroprusside administration modifies the intracranial pressure response. *Anesthesiology*. 1979;51(6):538–541.

29. Turner JM, Powell D, Gibson RM, et al. Intracranial pressure changes in neurosurgical patients during hypotension induced with sodium nitroprusside or trimethaphan. *Br J Anesth*. 1977;49(5):419–425.

30. Gagnon RL, Marsh ML, Smith RW, et al. Intracranial hypertension caused by nitroglycerin. *Anesthesiology*. 1979;51(1):86–87.

31. Morris PJ, Todd M, Philbin D. Changes in canine intracranial pressure in response to infusions of sodium nitroprusside and trinitroglycerin. *Br J Anaesth*. 1982;54(9): 991–995.

32. Rogers MC, Hamburger C, Owen K, et al. Intracranial pressure in the cat during nitroglycerin-induced hypotension. *Anesthesiology*. 1979;51(3):227–229.

33. Griffith DNW, James IM, Newbury PA, et al. The effect of β-adrenergic receptor blocking drugs on cerebral blood flow. *Br J Clin Pharmacol*. 1979;7(5):491–494.

34. Orlowski JP, Shiesley D, Vidt DG, et al. Labetalol to control blood pressure after cerebrovascular surgery. *Crit Care Med*. 1988;16(8):765–768.

35. Flamm ES. The potential use of nicardipine in cerebrovascular disease. *Am Heart J*. 1989;117(1):236–242.

36. Sabbatini M, Strocchi P, Amenta F. Nicardipine and treatment of cerebrovascular diseases with particular reference to hypertension-related disorders. *Clin Exp Hypertens.* 1995;17(5):719–750.

37. Huang BR, Chang PC, Yeh WL, et al. Anti-neuroinflammatory effects of the calcium channel blocker nicardipine on microglial cells: implications for neuroprotection. *PLoS ONE.* 2014;9(3):e91167.

38. Bekker A, Didehvar S, Kim S, et al. Efficacy of clevidipine in controlling perioperative hypertension in neurosurgical patients: initial single-center experience. *J Neurosurg Anesthesiol.* 2010;22(4):330–335.

39. Graffagnino C, Bergese S, Love J, et al. Clevidipine rapidly and safely reduces blood pressure in acute intracerebral hemorrhage: the ACCELERATE trial. *Cerebrovasc Dis.* 2013;36(3):173–180.

40. Graffagnino C, Riker RR, Bergese S, et al. Assessment of cerebral perfusion pressure (CPP) and intracranial pressure (ICP) in patients with acute intracerebral hemorrhage (ICH) receiving aggressive blood pressure management with clevidipine: an ACCELERATE analysis. Poster presented at 5th Annual NECC; 2010. http://www.thenecc.org/images/Williams.pdf. Accessed December 20, 2016.

41. Barry DI, Paulson OB, Jarden JO, et al. Effects of captopril on cerebral blood flow in normotensive and hypertensive rats. *Am J Med.* 1984;76(5B):79–85.

42. Waldemar G, Paulson OB. Angiotensin converting enzyme inhibition and cerebral circulation-a review. *Br J Clin Pharmacol.* 1989;28(suppl 2):177S–182S.

43. Paulson OB, Waldemar G, Andersen AR, et al. Role of angiotensin in autoregulation of cerebral blood flow. *Circulation.* 1988;77(6, pt 2):I55–I58.

44. Bertel O, Conen D, Radü EW, et al. Nifedipine in hypertensive emergencies. *BMJ.* 1983;286:19–21.

45. Fale A, Kirsch JR, McPherson RW. α2-adrenergic agonist effects on normocapnic and hypercapnic cerebral blood flow in the dog are anesthetic dependent. *Anesth Analg.* 1994;79(5):892–898.

46. McPherson RW, Koehler RC, Traystman RJ. Hypoxia, alpha-2-adrenergic, and nitric oxide–dependent interactions on canine cerebral blood flow. *Am J Physiol.* 1994;266: H476–H482.

47. Vincent JL, De Backer D. Circulatory shock. *N Engl J Med.* 2013;369(18):1726–1734.

48. Richard C, Warszawski J, Anguel N, et al. Early use of the pulmonary artery catheter and outcomes in patients with shock and acute respiratory distress syndrome: a randomized controlled trial. *JAMA.* 2003;290(20):2713–2720.

49. Seymour CW, Rosengart MR. Septic shock: Advances in diagnosis and treatment. *JAMA.* 2015;314(7):708–717.

50. Dellinger RP, Levy MM, Rhodes A, et al. Surviving sepsis campaign: international guidelines for management of severe sepsis and septic shock. *Crit Care Med.* 2013;41(2): 580–637.

51. Reynolds HR, Hochman JS. Cardiogenic shock: current concepts and improving outcomes. *Circulation.* 2008;117(5):686–697.

52. Thiele H, Ohman EM, Desch S, et al. Management of cardiogenic shock. *Eur Heart J.* 2015;36(20):1223–1230.

53. Singer M, Deutschland CS, Seymour CW, et al. The third international consensus definitions for sepsis and septic shock (Sepsis-3). *JAMA.* 2016;315(8):801–810.

54. Andrews PJ, Sleeman DH, Statham PF, et al. Predicting recovery in patients suffering from traumatic brain injury by using admission variables and physiological data: a

comparison between decision tree analysis and logistic regression. *J Neurosurg.* 2002;97(2): 326–336.

55. Arabi B, Hadley MN, Dhall SS, et al. Management of acute traumatic central cord syncope (ATCCS). *Neurosurgery.* 2013;72(suppl 2):195–204.

56. Inoue T, Manley GT, Patel N, Whetstone WD. Medical and surgical management after spinal cord injury: vasopressor usage, early surgeries, and complications. *J Neurotrauma.* 2014;31(3):284–291.

57. Readdy WJ, Whetstone WD, Ferguson AR, et al. Complications and outcomes of vasopressor usage in acute traumatic central cord syndrome. *J Neurosurg Spine.* 2015;23(5): 1–7.

58. Readdy WJ, Saigal R, Whetstone WD, et al. Failure of mean arterial pressure goals to improve outcomes fallowing penetrating spinal cord injury. Neurosurgery. 2016;79(5): 708–714.

59. Brain Trauma Foundation. Guidelines for the management of severe traumatic brain injury. 2016. braintrauma.org/uploads/03/12/Guidelines_for_Management_of_Severe _TBI_4th_Edition.pdf. Accessed December 20, 2016.

60. Iacobone E, Bailly-Salin J, Polito A, et al. Sepsis-associated encephalopathy and its differential diagnosis. *Crit Care Med.* 2009;37(10)(suppl):S331–S336.

61. Perel P, Roberts I. Colloids versus crystalloids for fluid resuscitation in critically ill patients. *Cochrane Database Syst Rev.* 2013;(2):CD000567.

62. Bunn F, Trivedi D. Colloid solutions for fluid resuscitation. *Cochrane Database Syst Rev.* 2012;(7):CD001319.

63. Cotton BA, Jerome R, Collier BR, et al. Guidelines for prehospital fluid resuscitation in the injured patient. *J Trauma.* 2009;67(2):389–402.

64. SAFE Study Investigators. Saline or albumin for fluid resuscitation in patients with traumatic brain injury. *N Engl J Med.* 2007;357(9):874–884.

65. Cooper DJ, Myles PS, McDermott FT, et al. Prehospital hypertonic saline resuscitation of patients with hypotension and severe traumatic brain injury: a randomized controlled trial. *JAMA.* 2004;291(11):1350–1357.

66. Yunos NM, Bellomo R, Hegarty C, et al. Association between a chloride-liberal vs chloride-restrictive intravenous fluid administration strategy and kidney injury in critically ill adults. *JAMA.* 2012;308(15):1566–1572.

67. ATLS Subcommittee, American College of Surgeons' Committee on Trauma, International ATLS Working Group. Advanced trauma life support (ATLS®), 9e. *J Trauma Acute Care Surg.* 2013;74(5):1363–136.

68. Winchell RJ, Simons RK, Hoyt DB. Transient systolic hypotension: a serious problem in the management of head injury. *Arch Surg.* 1996;131(5):533–539.

69. Plurad DS, Talving P, Lam L, et al. Early vasopressor use in critical injury is associated with mortality independent from volume status. *J Trauma.* 2011;71(3):565–570.

70. De Backer D, Biston P, Devriendt J, et al. Comparison of dopamine and norepinephrine in the treatment of shock. *N Engl J Med.* 2010;362(9):779–789.

71. De Backer D, Aldecoa C, Njimi H, and Vincent JL. Dopamine versus norepinephrine in the treatment of septic shock: a meta-analysis. *Crit Care Med.* 2012;40(3):725–730.

72. Van den Berghe G, de Zegher F, Lauwers P. Dopamine and the sick euthyroid syndrome in critical illness. *Clin Endocrinol (Oxf).* 1994;41(6):731–737.

Antiepileptic Agents for the Prevention and Treatment of Seizures

8

Aaron M. Cook, Norah Liang,
and Viet Nguyen

PATHOPHYSIOLOGY

Seizures are common in the neurologic intensive care unit (ICU) and can be the main reason for admission (eg, status epilepticus) or can occur secondary to other distinct neurologic injuries (eg, traumatic brain injury [TBI], ischemic stroke, and intracerebral and subarachnoid hemorrhage). Specific mechanisms of the pathogenesis of seizures are likely dependent on the primary neurologic pathology as well as the time of seizure occurrence in relation to this injury or insult. Early seizures, usually defined as occurring within 7 days of a primary injury, are acute symptomatic events with a low likelihood of recurrence, while late seizures, which occur weeks or even years after a primary injury, are likely a consequence of persistent brain changes that form an epileptogenic focus and represent epilepsy.

Early seizures occurring after TBI, ischemic stroke, or hemorrhagic stroke share a basic pathophysiologic mechanism: regional neurologic dysfunction produced by the primary neurologic injury causes increased excitation and decreased inhibition in affected brain regions, which then promote synchronous firing of a network of local neurons, resulting in seizures. Numerous specific mechanisms are implicated in the pathogenesis of seizures after neurologic injuries, which are specific to the nature of the injury (Figure 8.1). For instance, during intracerebral hemorrhage (ICH), tissue injury is primarily caused by mechanical damage associated with mass effect from rapid accumulation of blood.[1] In addition, a number of blood plasma components, including

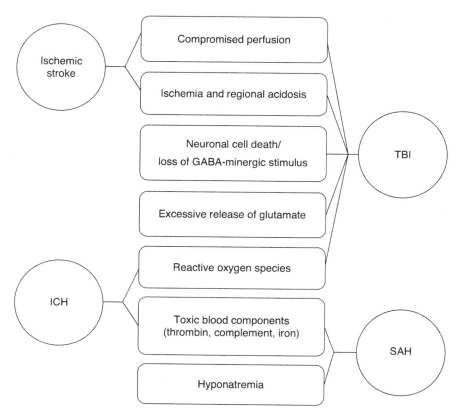

FIGURE 8.1. Pathogenesis of seizures after neurologic injuries. ICH = Intracerebral hemorrhage; TBI = traumatic brain injury; SAH = subarachnoid hemorrhage

coagulation factors, complement components, immunoglobulins, and other molecules, can be cytotoxic and contribute to further tissue damage.[1,2] Excitotoxicity as described above can occur in this setting along with spreading depression that may contribute to generation of seizures. Another major factor that can contribute to seizure generation during hemorrhage is iron deposition after red blood cell lysis. Red blood cell lysis starts to occur at 24 hours and leads to release of hemoglobin and its degradation products, heme and iron.[3] While heme and iron are both directly cytotoxic, iron deposition specifically is known to be seizure-genic, catalyzing a reaction that results in the hyperproduction of hydroxyl radicals and promoting the formation of reactive oxygen species (ROS) that damage the cell wall, leading to cellular depolarization and cell death.[4–6] Another cytotoxic blood plasma component, the coagulation factor thrombin, may contribute specifically to seizure generation. In animal models, thrombin injected into the brain produced immediate focal motor and electrographic seizures, which were eliminated when a thrombin inhibitor was administered.[4]

Neurologic injury is often typified by compromised cerebral perfusion and cell swelling. Altered cerebral blood blow in affected brain regions causes an ischemia-like state that compromises the affected region's ability to maintain cellular ionic membrane potentials, since the high oxygen demands of the brain are largely driven by the increased intracellular energy requirements needed for maintenance of these potentials.[7–9] Ischemia is often present in neurologic injury, either as primary injury (ischemic stroke) or as part of the secondary injury response (TBI, subarachnoid hemorrhage [SAH]). Reduced aerobic metabolism and adenosine triphosphate production leads to generation of ROS, and other proinflammatory mediators lead to a shift of excitatory cations into the intracellular space, which may impair the delicate balance between excitation and inhibition in the brain and can promote seizures.[7–9] Hyponatremia is of particular interest to neurocritical care practitioners, as it leads to increased intracellular edema, further increasing the risk of seizures in susceptible patients.[10]

Most seizures are brief and self-limited. However, when there is a failure of endogenous mechanisms to terminate seizures, status epilepticus can occur.[11] Much of the pathophysiology of status epilepticus is still poorly understood, but similar to the basic mechanisms underlying initial seizure occurrence, the basic mechanisms behind failure to terminate seizures stem from continued excitatory and inhibitory imbalances, which then promote the transformation of a seizure from a single event to a prolonged self-sustaining and self-perpetuating event. The stage for a potentially prolonged seizure may be set in place during the initial seizure onset with the extent of neurotransmitter release and ion channel disturbance that occurs.[12] Protein phosphorylation can then occur, setting the stage for maladaptive processes that affect receptor trafficking and promote self-perpetuation.[13] In animal models, expression of inhibitory $GABA_A$ $\beta2/\beta2$ and $\gamma2$ receptor subunits from the cell surface is effectively reduced through an endocytosis-mediated process while cell surface expression of excitatory N-methyl-D-aspartate (NMDA) receptors is increased within minutes of ongoing seizures and impending status epilepticus.[14–16] Available $GABA_A$ receptors may also undergo modulation, making them less sensitive to $GABA_A$ receptor agonists.[17] This reduction in $GABA_A$ receptor expression and sensitivity contributes to the pharmacoresistance often seen with status epilepticus, especially pharmacoresistance to benzodiazepines. In the subsequent minutes to hours, further maladaptive processes occur, including alterations in excitatory and inhibitory neuropeptide expression, which maintain the hyperexcitable state until spontaneous termination or electrical exhaustion occurs and ending the episode of status epilepticus.[18]

Unlike early seizures, late seizures occurring weeks to months after injury are not a reaction to the acute cellular processes occurring during injury but rather are a consequence of abnormal neuronal rewiring and glial scarring that occur as part of the self-repair process, causing persistent changes in neuronal excitability and connectivity. After injury, degeneration of axonal projections leads to the growth of new axon collaterals via axonal sprouting (also known as mossy fiber sprouting). This process is accepted as a common neuropathological consequence of all brain injury, including TBI, ischemia, and status epilepticus.[19,20] Axonal sprouting then creates new synaptic connections in a process called reactive synaptogenesis. While this mechanism is supposed to aid in the restoration of normal function, it becomes pathologic in certain circumstances and contributes to epileptogenesis by helping to strengthen recurrent excitatory circuitry, creating a focus of hyperexcitable and hyperconnected neurons that can fire in synchrony.[19] A selective and progressive loss of specific vulnerable GABA-ergic interneurons promotes further epileptogenicity.[21] In addition, genetic changes that occur in the days and weeks after status epilepticus promote an extensive molecular plasticity at the transcriptional, translational, and trafficking levels, and epigenetic changes, including genome-wide alterations in hippocampal cell DNA methylation observed in some epilepsy models, may contribute to epileptogenesis.[22,23] Although most epilepsy research has focused on neuronal and synaptic mechanisms, glial scarring and changes in glial functioning can also play a role via altered expression of membrane K^+ and Na^+ channels, resulting in proepileptic changes in the homeostatic control of the extracellular space.[24,25] Last, while early seizures are believed to be a symptomatic reaction to injury and not representative of epileptogenicity, early seizures may promote the development of a permanent seizure focus by reinforcing an abnormal excitatory circuitry and possibly contributing to all of the above changes in a process called kindling.[26,27]

EPIDEMIOLOGY

Traumatic Brain Injury

The reported incidence proportion of seizures after TBI is different based on their classification as early seizures (within 7 days of ictus) or late seizures (greater

TABLE 8.1 Risk Factors for Early Seizures After Traumatic Brain Injury

Severity of injury (GCS <10)

Loss of consciousness

Amnesia lasting >24 hours

Contusion

Subdural hematoma

Skull fracture

Penetrating injury

At least 1 nonreactive pupil

Traumatic intracranial hemorrhage

History of seizure disorder

Note: GCS, Glasgow Coma Scale.

than 7 days from ictus). The incidence of early seizures after TBI varies widely between studies and has been reported to be as high as 25%.[28] Risk factors for posttraumatic seizures have been described in the literature (Table 8.1). A recent case–control study in Stockholm found that the relative risk of seizures was approximately 6 times higher after brain contusion, 4.5 times higher after intracranial hemorrhage, and 42.6 times higher when both brain contusion and intracranial hemorrhage were present compared with a control population.[29] In comparison, the relative risk of seizures after mild TBI was only 2 times that of the control population. The risk for seizures was greatest during the first 6 months after mild and severe TBI but was still elevated more than 10 years afterward. Of note, older studies tended to report clinically evident seizures, often yielding a seizure rate estimated to be approximately 6% to 10%.[30] More recent studies have used continuous electroencephalogram (EEG) monitoring to detect seizures and have consistently reported an increased incidence proportion of seizures. In one of the earliest studies to use continuous EEG monitoring to detect seizure activity in ICU patients specifically after moderate to severe TBI, Vespa et al[31] found that 22% of 94 patients experienced early seizures occurring 7 to 10 days after the initial insult. Of the 22% of patients with seizures, 52% had nonconvulsive or clinically silent seizures, with one-third of the group having status epilepticus. Other subsequent studies have also shown that subclinical seizures, including nonconvulsive status epilepticus, occur more commonly than thought in the ICU. Ronne-Engstrom and Winkler[32] used continuous EEG in 70 patients with TBI and found a 33% incidence of seizures with onset 1 to 5 days after injury.

The incidence proportion of late seizures after TBI has been reported to vary from 9% to 53%.[29,30] Immediate seizures (eg, seizures at the scene of the trauma) have not been linked with any increased risk of developing late seizures, although conflicting evidence exists regarding the impact of early seizures on the rate of developing late seizures.[30] Prevention of early seizures does not appear to decrease the rate of late seizures. The incidence proportion of late seizures after TBI increases with time as many people who did not have early acute symptomatic seizures may still develop an epileptogenic focus after injury and be susceptible to recurrent seizures years after the event. Furthermore, the types of studies that are targeted for long lengths of follow-up skew some of these data. For instance, studies in military populations may follow their cases for decades, such as the Vietnam Head Injury Study, which followed veterans who had penetrating head injuries for 15 years postinjury and reported an incidence proportion of 53%, although the relative risk of developing epilepsy in these patients did drop from 580 times higher than the general age-matched population in the first year after TBI to 25 times higher, after 10 years.[33]

Ischemic and Hemorrhagic Stroke

A multitude of studies looking at seizures after ischemic stroke have been published over the years with definitions of early poststroke seizures that have varied widely from 24 hours poststroke to 4 weeks poststroke. However, for studies that have specifically defined early seizures as occurring within 7 to 15 days of ischemic stroke, the reported incidence proportion of early seizures is reported to be approximately 2.3% to 6% in population- and hospital-based studies.[34-37] Most of these seizures appear to occur within the first 48 to 72 hours after ictus. The impact of early seizures after ischemic stroke on mortality and outcome is unclear. Conflicting evidence exists as to whether early seizures are an independent predictor of early mortality.[34,38] For instance, one study found that early seizures only increased risk of mortality in the first 48 hours after admission. Other studies have also suggested that early seizures may be an independent predictor of the development of late and recurrent seizures.[37]

Primary ICH is typically associated with a higher rate of seizures compared with ischemic stroke. Early seizures (usually defined as occurring within 2 weeks of the primary ICH) can occur after ICH, with a reported incidence proportion ranging from 5.7% to 17%.[39-41] Overall incidence proportions including early and late seizures post-ICH have been reported to range from 5.7% to 25%.[34,37,39-41] Clinically subtle seizures appear commonly in patients with ICH, and the use of continuous EEG (cEEG) monitoring suggests an increased rate of seizures compared with population studies (approximately 28% of patients in one study, despite these patients having been treated with prophylactic phenytoin).[42] Almost 90% of these seizures occurred within the first 72 hours after the insult, and more than three-quarters were nonconvulsive. Similarly, Claassen et al[43] reported a seizure incidence proportion of 31% in all patients with ICH undergoing cEEG monitoring admitted to their center. More than half of the patients in this cohort had subclinical electrographic seizures only detectable by cEEG, with 39% of those having nonconvulsive status epilepticus. Furthermore, almost 95% of these seizures occurred within 48 hours of cEEG initiation. Seizures occurred more frequently in lobar ICH or superficial ICH compared with subcortical locations of hemorrhage.[42,43] Besides location of ICH, seizures may be independently predicted by age, intraventricular extension of blood, initial volume tercile (ie, <30 cc, 30–60 cc, or >60 cc) and by increases in ICH volume of 30% or more between admission and 24-hour follow-up computed tomography scan.[42,43]

The reported incidence proportion of early seizures after aneurysmal SAH (aSAH) is relatively high and dependent on the definition used and the patient sample. Early seizures have been reported in 6.3% to 26% of patients with aSAH, with many studies reporting incidence proportions close to 20%.[44–46] In addition, seizures as an acute symptomatic reaction to the initial acute hemorrhage and acute rebleeding may be more prevalent in this population. One series found that 19% of patients experienced seizures at the onset or within the first 12 hours after SAH, with most occurring during the first few minutes.[45] It is estimated that 90% of all post-SAH seizures are temporally related to acute bleeding. The incidence proportion of seizures occurring postoperatively after aneurysm treatment and the resolution of acute bleeding appears low and has been reported in the 1% to 2% range.[47] Although late seizures and epilepsy occur less frequently than early seizures after aSAH, the incidence proportion of this seems similar to that of ICH and ranges from 4.1% to 14% depending on follow-up period, with many studies reporting incidence proportions in the lower range.[46,48–50] A recent systematic review including 25 studies found the risk of late postoperative seizures to be 5.5%, and the average time to late seizure was over 7 months.[50] Patients who experienced a late seizure were more likely to have middle cerebral artery (MCA) aneurysms, be Hunt/Hess grade III, and have been secured with microsurgical clipping than endovascular coiling. More contemporary study of the development of seizures in the era of endovascular aneurysm management is necessary, as many of the incidence studies were performed when microsurgical clipping was the standard of care and delayed aneurysm obliteration was common.

PROPHYLAXIS OF SEIZURES IN NEUROCRITICAL CARE PATIENTS

Seizure prophylaxis is a commonly implemented intervention in neurocritical care patients. Conceptually, central nervous system (CNS) injury seems likely to be followed by seizure due to physical damage, biochemical response to injury, and ischemia. Seizure prophylaxis has been studied in various neurocritical care populations, including TBI, SAH, ICH, ischemic stroke, brain tumor, and bacterial meningitis. However, little evidence supports the use of anticonvulsant agents (AEDs) for seizure prophylaxis after many acute CNS events except for TBI.

Posttraumatic seizure prophylaxis in patients with moderate to severe TBI can decrease the rate of seizures within 7 days of injury. The current Brain Trauma Foundation guidelines include early seizure prophylaxis with phenytoin as a therapeutic option for clinicians to consider.[28] This recommendation is primarily based on a group of prospective clinical studies with phenytoin.[51–55] Initiation of phenytoin early in the treatment of TBI and continued for 7 days after injury reduces the rate of seizures to approximately 4% in most clinical trials.[51] Despite the fact that individual patients may benefit from prevention of seizures, no data suggest that reducing the seizure rate affects long-term outcome in study populations.[56] Conversely, Dikmen et al[57] suggested that phenytoin exposure early in severe TBI may actually impair performance in neurobehavioral assessments at 1 month after injury. While this impairment of performance was not evident at 1 or 2 years after injury, the impact of early performance after TBI may be a reason to give clinicians pause when initiating prophylaxis in patients with TBI. Phenytoin is not effectively for preventing late seizures (greater than 7 days after the event).[51,58]

Levetiracetam is the emerging alternative to phenytoin for seizure prophylaxis after TBI. Potential advantages compared with phenytoin include predictable pharmacokinetics, the lack of need for therapeutic drug monitoring, less significant drug-drug and drug-nutrient interactions, and potential safety advantages. Limited high-quality clinical data support the use of levetiracetam in TBI. However, several case series and nonrandomized, prospective studies seem to support a potential role for levetiracetam in TBI seizure prophylaxis (although some reports also include non-TBI patients in their analysis).[59–63] The largest study to date was a prospective, nonrandomized trial between 2 major US trauma centers comparing phenytoin and levetiracetam for prevention of early posttraumatic seizures. There was no significant difference in safety or efficacy between the 2 therapies.[60] Other smaller, less-controlled studies have also shown little difference in efficacy when comparing phenytoin and levetiracetam for this indication. The use of levetiracetam for posttraumatic seizure prophylaxis is common and appears to be increasing, although the quality of the evidence supporting levetiracetam use over phenytoin is low.[64]

Agents other than phenytoin have also been evaluated for the prevention of posttraumatic seizures. Phenobarbital was evaluated in a prospective trial in Japan for seizure prevention (when phenobarbital was started 1 month following injury) but showed no impact on the occurrence of late seizures.[54] Phenobarbital is often difficult to use in the acute TBI population due to respiratory and neurologic depression. Carbamazepine was compared with placebo in a prospective, randomized trial in Germany and showed a significant reduction in early but not late seizures.[65] Carbamazepine is currently only available as an oral/enteral formulation, which creates challenges with timely and adequate provision in the context of severe TBI, which limits the utility of carbamazepine in these patients. Valproic acid was compared with phenytoin for early seizure prophylaxis and demonstrated comparable efficacy in preventing early seizures and was similarly safe.[55] However, this trial also reported a trend toward increased mortality in the patients who received valproate compared with phenytoin. The specter of harm suggested by this trial has limited the use of valproate in patients with TBI for prophylaxis.

Routine seizure prophylaxis associated with other major CNS events is not indicated. Several clinical studies and meta-analyses have concluded that seizure prophylaxis should not be given to patients after ICH, ischemic stroke, or diagnosis of brain tumor. One small study investigating seizure prophylaxis after SAH suggests that a brief, 3-day prophylaxis period is associated with a similar seizure rate compared with longer durations of prophylaxis and a lesser incidence of adverse events.[66] It is important to note, however, that longer durations of prophylaxis have not been shown to be beneficial after SAH. On the contrary, some investigators have suggested potential harm.[67] Thus, brief seizure prophylaxis after SAH is unlikely to be effective. Readers are referred to an excellent, recent review of seizure prophylaxis in the neurocritical care patient population for more extensive details.[68]

PHARMACOTHERAPY FOR STATUS EPILEPTICUS

The annual incidence of status epilepticus is approximately 12.5 out of 100,000 individuals in the United States, with adults older than 50 years

TABLE 8.2 Status Epilepticus Dosing Strategies

Name	Dosage Form	Starting Dose	Therapeutic Range
Phenytoin	Injection Capsule Oral solution Chewable tablet	15- to 20-mg/kg load, then 50 mg/kg/d split in 3 doses Use 20 mg/kg in status	Total: 10 to 20 mcg/mL Free: 1 to 2 mcg/mL
Fosphenytoin	Injection	Same as phenytoin (use mg PE)	Same as phenytoin
Valproic acid and derivatives	Valproate: injection, oral liquid Depakote: Capsule, delayed-release capsule, delayed-release sprinkle capsule, delayed-release tablet, extended-release tablet	10 to 15 mg/kg/d Use 20- to 40-mg/kg loading dose in status	50 to 100 mcg/mL
Levetiracetam	Injection, oral solution Tablet, extended-release tablet	1000 mg q12 Use 1000- to 3000-mg loading dose in status	Not available
Lacosamide	Injection, oral solution Tablet	100 mg q12, use 200- to 400-mg loading dose in status	Not available
Midazolam	Injection, oral solution (rarely used in intensive care unit)	0.1- to 0.2-mg/kg bolus, then 0.1 mg/kg/h (suggested maximum dose 0.4 mg/kg/h)	Not applicable, titrate to burst suppression
Pentobarbital	Injection	10-mg/kg slow bolus (over 10 to 20 minutes), then 6 mg/kg/h × 3 hours, then 1-mg/kg/h infusion	15 to 40 mcg/mL, but not typically well associated with antiepileptic effect Titrate to burst suppression
Propofol	Injection	1-mg/kg bolus, then 25 mcg/kg/min	Not applicable, titrate to burst suppression
Ketamine	Injection	1-mg/kg bolus, then 1 mg/kg/h infusion May increase infusion to up to 10 mg/kg/h	Not applicable

Source: Adapted from reference 73.

Note: PE, phenytoin equivalents

having the highest incidence (28.4/100,000).[69] The overall mortality rate from status epilepticus was 8.8% from 2005 to 2010, which represents a relatively static rate since 1979. Status epilepticus, when not treated effectively in a timely manner, is known to become pharmacoresistant in many patients. In addition, nonconvulsive status epilepticus is known to be more treatment refractory and is associated with worse outcomes than convulsive status epilepticus.[57] This may be due to several factors, including receptor changes in the brain that accentuate excitatory transmission, inefficient agent selection, or inadequate timing of effective therapies.[70–72] The most recent status epilepticus guidelines from the Neurocritical Care Society separate therapy into 3 specific groups: emergent therapy, urgent therapy, and refractory therapies (Table 8.2).[73]

Emergent therapy primarily consists of benzodiazepines and should be administered as soon as is feasible. Intravenous lorazepam is the current standard of care and should be given as an intravenous (IV) push injection at a dose of 0.1 mg/kg up to 4 mg, which may be repeated if no clinical response is observed.[74] This therapy leads to resolution of status epilepticus in nearly 3 times the number of patients compared with placebo, with no difference in adverse effects.[74] In fact, respiratory or circulatory complications are more often seen in patients without resolution of seizure than in patients receiving lorazepam.[74] A viable alternative in patients without adequate IV access is intramuscular (IM) midazolam. Emergent IM midazolam appears equally effective to lorazepam early in status epilepticus treatment.[75] Diazepam is also an acceptable option, although rapid redistribution of the drug occurs with single doses, thereby shortening the duration of action.[73,74]

Urgent therapy typically consists of a more traditional antiepileptic agent to keep patients who respond to emergent therapy from going back into status epilepticus or to try another agent in those who do not respond to emergent therapy. There is considerable debate and a paucity of high-quality evidence to guide clinicians in the optimal choice of agents for urgent therapy.[70] Clinical trials aimed at identifying the optimal urgent therapy choice were completed prior to the release of many of the newer antiepileptic agents. The evidence-based guidelines support agents for urgent therapy such as valproate, phenytoin or fosphenytoin, a low-dose midazolam continuous infusion, phenobarbital, or levetiracetam.[73] If a patient is receiving an antiepileptic agent at home prior to admission, consideration for loading of this agent is also reasonable. In all cases, expedient administration of an adequate loading dose of one of the agents listed above is necessary to ensure rapid, adequate serum concentrations.

Optimal therapy for refractory status epilepticus is not well defined. There are numerous options for treatment that have been reported in the literature, although none have rigorous clinical trial evidence to support use. Refractory status epilepticus may be pharmacoresistant due to alterations in the expression of excitatory receptors such as NMDA. An increase in excitatory neurotransmission, coupled with a concomitant decrease in inhibitory transmission via GABA, creates a situation where many of the common antiepileptic agents may not be effective at normal doses.[72] Most commonly, antiepileptic drugs such as lacosamide, topiramate, or any of the urgent therapy options listed above may be considered.[73] Anesthetic infusions such as high-dose midazolam continuous infusion, propofol, or pentobarbital (all typically dosed to burst suppression on EEG) may be used to eliminate electrical activity on EEG, thereby suppressing seizures. These therapies are fraught with complications and are associated with poor outcomes when used, so clinicians should choose patients in whom pharmacologic coma is used very carefully.[76,77] Alternative therapies such as the ketogenic diet, ketamine infusion, inhaled anesthetics, hypothermia, corticosteroids, or surgical management may also be considered, although clinical reports of success are few.[73]

OVERVIEW OF SPECIFIC ANTIEPILEPTIC DRUGS

Levetiracetam

Levetiracetam was first approved in the United States in 2006 as an adjunctive therapy for partial, myoclonic, and generalized seizures. The exact mechanism of levetiracetam is unknown, although binding to synaptic vesicle protein SV2A and modulation of GABA receptors have been proposed to be mechanisms of antiepileptic effect. From a pharmacokinetic perspective, levetiracetam is an ideal agent. Oral absorption of levetiracetam tablets or oral solution is rapid and complete, with Tmax occurring after approximately 1 hour and nearly 100% bioavailability.[78] Oral or enteral nutrition intake has no significant impact on bioavailability.[79] Plasma protein binding is negligible, and a small amount of the drug (24%) is metabolized by hydrolytic enzymes in the liver. Levetiracetam is generally well tolerated, with paradoxical neurologic disturbances being the primary adverse effect. Some patients experience somnolence, while others are "activated" by levetiracetam.[80] The consistent dose-drug concentration relationship and the wide safety index obviate the need for routine therapeutic drug monitoring. Levetiracetam serum monitoring is commercially available and may be helpful to monitor patient adherence. The ideal therapeutic range is not well defined.

Valproic Acid

Valproic acid (VPA) is a short-chain fatty acid that has a wide spectrum of activity in seizure management. It has efficacy in focal and generalized seizures, cortical myoclonus, and absence seizures. Although the exact mechanism of action is not clear, valproic acid appears to affect the GABA receptor and may reduce calcium influx into neurons. Valproic acid is available as the sodium salt or the valproate-complex, divalproex, which is converted to valproate in vivo. The bioavailability of oral formulations is near 100% and is minimally affected by oral or enteral intake. VPA binds to albumin in a concentration-dependent fashion. The free fraction is approximately 10% at serum concentrations of 40 µg/mL but increases to 18.5% at 130 µg/mL. VPA is almost completely metabolized by the liver, with up to 50% of the dose undergoing glucuronide conjugation and over 40% via mitochondrial β-oxidation. Hepatic metabolism of valproate is susceptible to effects by common CYP450 enzyme inhibitors and inducers. Valproate is also known to reduce plasma protein binding of concomitant agents, most notably phenytoin.

VPA is well tolerated in most individuals, with gastrointestinal intolerance or somnolence being the most common adverse effects. However, in select individuals, more severe adverse effects may occur and often lead to discontinuation of valproate and the need for other treatment. Valproate is associated with hepatic toxicity, thrombocytopenia, and pancreatitis, all of which may be related to the serum concentration. While thrombocytopenia (within a week of initiation) and hepatic toxicity (within 6 months of initiation) typically occur early in therapy, pancreatitis may occur at any point after initiation. Hyperammonemia may also occur, particularly in patients with preexisting hepatic dysfunction, those receiving high doses of valproate, those who are critically ill, and, perhaps, those who are malnourished. Supplementation of levocarnitine and discontinuation of valproate is typically sufficient to reduce ammonia concentrations to desirable concentrations and aid in resolution of encephalopathy associated with the hyperammonemia.

The recommended therapeutic range for total valproate serum concentrations is 50 to 100 mcg/mL.[1,15] Routine serum concentration monitoring is necessary in nearly all patients receiving valproate for seizures because of the relatively narrow therapeutic window. Consideration for obtaining free concentrations in patients who may exhibit a higher than expected valproate free fraction may be necessary (those with liver or renal disease, who have hypoalbuminemia, who are elderly, or who are malnourished).

Phenytoin

Phenytoin is perhaps the most studied antiepileptic drug in the neurocritical care population and can be used for focal and generalized seizures. Phenytoin is a reversible inhibitor of fast-inactivation sodium channels in neurons. Phenytoin is available as an IV solution and capsule (phenytoin sodium), chewable tablet and suspension (phenytoin acid), and solution for IV or intramuscular injection (fosphenytoin, a phosphorylated phenytoin prodrug). The bioavailability of oral phenytoin is approximately 80% to 100%, although time to maximal absorption is prolonged and proportional to the dose administered. Phenytoin exhibits a 10% fraction unbound from albumin under normal physiologic conditions, although this often increases in the context of hypoalbuminemia or use of other protein-binding displacers such as valproate. Hepatic clearance is primarily through CYP450 2C9 and 2C19 and is susceptible to effects by common CYP450 inhibitors and inducers. Uniquely, phenytoin metabolism is saturable, often at concentrations within the normal therapeutic window. This begets a situation where nonlinear, dramatic increases in phenytoin concentration may occur with subtle dose changes.

Phenytoin IV and oral liquid dosage forms are associated with unique pharmaceutical considerations. Intravenous phenytoin is buffered to a pH of 12 and contains several diluents such as propylene glycol (40%) and ethanol (10%), which contribute to infusion-related reactions such as phlebitis, hypotension, and cardiac arrhythmias. A slow infusion rate (5–10 mg/min) should be considered upon initiation to mitigate these potential adverse effects. Infusion via a central venous catheter also minimizes the risk of phlebitis and extravasation. The phenytoin infusion rate can be titrated to higher infusion rates (not to exceed 50 mg/min) as the patient tolerates. Fosphenytoin is more water soluble and does not require these diluents or central venous administration. Thus, it is associated with less infusion-related reactions and can be given at a faster infusion rate (not to exceed 150 mg/min). Oral or enteral phenytoin can be problematic depending on the dose and formulation. Oral or enteral doses of more than 400 mg may have delayed time to absorption and a slightly lower bioavailability.[81] Clinicians should consider dividing the daily doses such that an individual dose administered does not exceed 400 mg in most patients. In addition, the precise bioavailability of phenytoin suspension is not well defined and appears to be susceptible to drug-nutrient interactions with certain enteral nutrition products.

Clinicians may often be faced with unique dosing issues with phenytoin, including dosing in obese patients and boosting subtherapeutic concentrations. Phenytoin is a lipophilic agent that distributes well into adipose tissue. This requires the prescriber to consider the actual body weight of the patient when prescribing a loading dose. In fact, due to the predilection of phenytoin to distribute preferentially into adipose tissue, adjusted body weights that often exceed actual body weights have been proposed.[82] The variability of phenytoin pharmacokinetics also often leads to subtherapeutic concentrations, particularly in critically ill patients.[51] Clinicians may need to provide smaller loading doses to quickly boost phenytoin concentrations back into the desired range in certain patients. Generally, empiric use of the volume of distribution and desired increase in concentration can be considered when providing such a "mini-load" (X mg/kg to raise the concentration by X mcg/mL), although clinicians should be aware of factors such as altered protein binding and likelihood of saturation of hepatic metabolism, which may confound this strategy. Likewise, increases in the maintenance dose of phenytoin in light of subtherapeutic concentrations should be done cautiously to avoid abrupt increases in concentration due to saturable metabolism. Use of pharmacokinetic equations such as the Ludden method or empiric changes in dose of 0.25 to 1 mg/kg/d are typically reasonable approaches for most patients.[83]

Phenytoin is also associated with various other classic, severe adverse effects such as rash and purple glove syndrome. Rash associated with phenytoin may be idiosyncratic, although in many patients, it may be a result of a genetic polymorphism in metabolism. In these patients, accumulation of a toxic epoxide metabolite leads to an immune response that can lead to hepatitis, conjunctival damage, and erythema multiforme. The rash can progress to Stevens-Johnson syndrome with continued phenytoin exposure. Clinicians should rapidly transition patients exhibiting signs and symptoms of this adverse effect to an alternative antiepileptic drug. Specific agents that are not likely to cross-react with this adverse effect include levetiracetam, lacosamide, and valproic acid. Purple glove syndrome is an infusion-related reaction, primarily associated with phenytoin. The precise cause is not well defined but may have something to do with the lack of water solubility of IV phenytoin sodium. Microemboli in the extremities cause a purple, cyanotic appearance and lead to digital ischemia. Supportive care and cessation of phenytoin (whenever possible) appear to be the best course of action for patients experiencing this unique adverse effect.

Therapeutic drug monitoring of phenytoin is necessary in all patients due to the various factors that affect drug exposure such as saturable hepatic metabolism and perturbations in protein binding. Total phenytoin concentrations are widely available and useful in most patients, particularly those who do not have critical illness or hypoalbuminemia or are not receiving medications that are protein-binding displacers. In patients at risk of having an elevated free fraction (those listed above), a free concentration should also be obtained to evaluate the actual concentration of phenytoin responsible for pharmacologic action. Equations may be used to estimate the impact of hypoalbuminemia, although correlation with actual free concentrations may not be precise in all patients.

Lacosamide

Lacosamide was first approved in the United States in 2008 with indication for partial seizures. It can be used as monotherapy or as an adjunct to other seizure medications. Lacosamide has a unique mechanism of action in that it enhances slow inactivation of sodium channels in neurons. This results in selective inhibition of activity in neurons that are repetitively firing and provides a more sustained blockade than other antiepileptic agents that work on internal membrane fast inactivation of sodium channels. Lacosamide exhibits nearly 100% bioavailability after oral administration. Plasma protein binding of lacosamide is negligible and nearly 40% of the dose is excreted unchanged in the urine. However, lacosamide is partially metabolized in the liver by CYP 3A4, 2C9, and 2C19. Lacosamide is relatively well tolerated and exhibits few adverse effects that cause discontinuation of therapy. The most common side effects for lacosamide are double vision, headaches, dizziness, and nausea. It can also increase the PR interval on electrocardiography (ECG) readings, especially when it is given together with other medications that have the same effect. Bradycardia may be evident in patients with PR prolongation, so close monitoring of patients at risk of this adverse effect may be necessary.

Benzodiazepines

Benzodiazepines stimulate $GABA_A$ receptor activity, which leads to increased chloride influx into neurons, thereby causing an inhibition of neurotransmission.[84] The onset of this mechanism of action appears to be optimal early in the treatment of seizures, and the commonly used agents in this class all exhibit pharmacokinetic characteristics, which make them ideal for emergent use. Lorazepam (IV) and midazolam (IM) are currently the agents of choice for emergent therapy in status epilepticus and are commonly used as abortive therapy in patients with isolated seizure.[73] Diazepam may also be used in the emergent setting (IV or rectal), whereas other orally available agents such as clonazepam are typically used as maintenance therapies only.

Lorazepam is long-acting benzodiazepine that can be effectively administered intravenously (or less commonly intranasally) for seizures. Oral, sublingual, and deep intramuscular routes may also be used, although these routes may not be advantageous in patients with active seizures. The half-life of lorazepam is approximately 12 hours, and unlike many other benzodiazepines, lorazepam is not subject to cytochrome P450 metabolism. Lorazepam undergoes hepatic glucuronidation to an inactive metabolite.[55] Lorazepam is less fat soluble than midazolam and diazepam, which may cause a slower, less complete distribution through the blood-brain barrier penetration compared with more lipid-soluble agents. However, the time difference is of minimal importance clinically as rapidly administered IV doses of lorazepam appear to abate seizures as quickly as other benzodiazepines.[74,75] In addition, the long terminal half-life of lorazepam ensures that sufficient concentrations are present for several hours after the dose.[85] In patients with seizures, this lingering effect may reduce the likelihood of acute seizure recurrence.

Diazepam is a long-acting benzodiazepine that can be effectively administered intravenously or rectally for seizures. Diazepam has a fast onset of action for seizures due to high lipophilicity. With single doses, diazepam quickly distributes into and out of the central compartment, causing the initial (α) half-life to be quite short.[86] This may lead to seizure recurrence if additional doses of diazepam or other AEDs are not given after the redistribution period.[87] However, with repeated doses, redistribution is less obvious, and the much longer β half-life leads to accumulation of diazepam. Diazepam is hepatically oxidized by CYP3A4 and 2C19 into active metabolites nordiazepam and temazepam (and ultimately oxazepam).[84] The rectal formulation of diazepam (Diastat) is well absorbed, exhibiting 90% bioavailability. However, the peak concentration occurs approximately 1.5 hours after rectal administration.[88] While rectal diazepam remains a valuable abortive therapy for primarily parents and caregivers of patients with epilepsy, the delayed onset of action can be a limitation.

Midazolam is a short-acting benzodiazepine that can be effectively administered intravenously, intramuscularly, buccally, or intranasally for seizures. The formulation for midazolam is unique in that the solution for injection has a low pH (3), resulting in midazolam existing in an open-ring, salt form, increasing the water solubility. When administered in vivo, the physiologic pH (7.40) causes the midazolam ring to close, creating a much more lipid-soluble molecule, capable of rapid distribution through the blood-brain barrier and into adipose tissue. Whereas intramuscular injection often is associated with a slow absorption profile, this unique physiochemical property is also the reason that intramuscular administration of midazolam is an effective option in status epilepticus.[75] Midazolam is hydroxylated via cytochrome P450 3A4 to a less potent but active metabolite. Single doses of midazolam typically exhibit a short half-life of approximately 60 minutes. Another potential advantage of the intramuscular route is that the full distribution of the drug is delayed, thereby prolonging the serum half-life and potentially reducing the likelihood of acute seizure recurrence. Intranasal midazolam administration appears to be comparable to other systemic methods of administration and appears to have a faster onset than rectal diazepam, which may lead more practitioners to use intranasal midazolam as a home abortive therapy.

Barbiturates and Intravenous Anesthetics

Phenobarbital is a long-acting barbiturate that has long been used for seizures. Barbiturates are lipophilic agents that act at the $GABA_A$ receptor to potentiate chloride influx in neurons. These agents also appear to potentiate the binding of endogenous GABA to its receptor and promote benzodiazepine binding to $GABA_A$ receptors.[84] Phenobarbital exhibits a large volume of distribution and a very long half-life; therefore, an adequate loading dose is required to rapidly attain therapeutic effect. Those effects (or any potential adverse effects such as sedation) may linger for hours to days depending on the level of phenobarbital accumulation. Phenobarbital is cleared primarily by hepatic metabolism (glycosylation and oxidation), although approximately 25% is cleared unchanged in the urine.[84] The therapeutic window for phenobarbital is relatively small, and supratherapeutic concentrations are well associated with adverse effects. Therefore, therapeutic drug monitoring is often necessary for patients receiving phenobarbital. Common adverse effects can range from mild to severe and include sedation, hypotension, and respiratory depression. As more AEDs with different mechanisms of action and a better safety profile are developed, the use of phenobarbital has waned. The role of phenobarbital in status epilepticus is virtually nugatory in contemporary practice, despite having been studied relatively extensively in early status epilepticus trials.[70]

Intravenous anesthetic infusions may be used in patients with super-refractory status epilepticus. Sedative agents used in this setting include high-dose midazolam infusion, pentobarbital, and propofol. The goal of these therapies is to achieve an isoelectric pattern (ie, burst suppression) on EEG. To achieve this goal, large doses of these agents are required. Pentobarbital differs from phenobarbital in that pentobarbital exhibits a higher level of lipophilicity, and it also appears to prevent calcium influx in neurons as well as its actions on $GABA_A$.[84] This broader mechanism is likely the reason that pentobarbital has more utility in inducing pharmacologic coma than phenobarbital. The initial pharmacologic half-life of pentobarbital is brief due to rapid distribution in and out of the CNS. However, once the volume of distribution in vivo (ie, the adipose tissue) has been saturated, the half-life of pentobarbital is prolonged (approximately 18–24 hours in most individuals), resulting in accumulation and, in some patients, prolonged time to emergence from the pharmacologic coma. Propofol is much shorter acting than pentobarbital, although accumulation with long-term, high-dose use is common in the setting of status epilepticus. The mechanism of action of propofol is not well defined, but it is able to generate a burst suppression pattern at higher doses (usually >50 mcg/kg/min) than are typically used for routine ICU sedation. Midazolam continuous infusion appears to be comparable to propofol and pentobarbital for burst suppression, particularly when high doses are used (0.4 mg/kg/h).[77] Each of these agents is associated with adverse effects, with hypotension being the most common.[76] Pentobarbital is also associated with numerous other adverse effects, including infection, reduced gastrointestinal motility, and cardiac depression.[89] Use of propofol for prolonged duration and/or high doses may lead to propofol infusion syndrome, which is characterized by cardiovascular collapse, profound metabolic acidosis, and increased mortality.[90] Outcomes associated with these therapies are poor.[73,76] Clinicians should consider this therapeutic strategy as a last-line therapy whenever possible.

Ketamine is a unique sedative agent with an ideal pharmacokinetic profile for use in patients with acute seizures. Ketamine is a racemic mixture of 2 enantiomers, S(+) and R(–) ketamine. Although quite water soluble, at physiologic pH, ketamine is capable of exhibiting extensive lipid solubility, which leads to a high volume of distribution and excellent tissue penetration into the brain, heart, and other tissues. CNS effects are evident within 1 to 5 minutes of IV infusion.[91] The α half-life of ketamine is approximately 11 minutes, while the β half-life is approximately 2.5 hours.[92] Ketamine is demethylated by hepatic cytochrome P450 enzymes to nor-ketamine, a less potent active metabolite. Nor-ketamine is renally eliminated or may be further metabolized to inactive metabolites, which are also renally eliminated.

Ketamine has several mechanisms of action, which lead to a multitude of physiologic effects. The cardiovascular effects of ketamine distinguish it from most other IV anesthetic agents. Inhibition of neuronal uptake of catecholamines and other neurotransmitters leads to increases in heart rate, cardiac output, and blood pressure. Respiratory depression is unlikely in most cases, and airway protection reflexes remain intact. The CNS effects of ketamine are primarily due to the noncompetitive binding to the NMDA receptor. Ketamine binds to the intramembrane phencyclidine receptor, causing a conformational change to the calcium channel.[93] Antagonism of this receptor appears to be greater if the NMDA channel has previously been opened by glutamate. The S-isomer of ketamine has greater potency at this binding site (approximately 4 times more potent than the R-isomer). The potent binding of the S(+) enantiomer to mu and kappa receptors also allows the drug to produce analgesic properties at subanesthetic doses. NMDA antagonism likely represents the mechanism of action of ketamine in refractory status epilepticus, given the role of glutamate and NMDA in this clinical context.

CONCLUSION

Numerous antiepileptic drugs are now available for acute use in hospitalized patients for prevention and treatment of seizures. The use of agents other than phenytoin for seizure prophylaxis after TBI is emerging, but rigorous clinical trials have not defined a specific preferential agent. Emergent treatment of status epilepticus with a benzodiazepine and urgent treatment with an antiepileptic drug are essential for prompt seizure cessation. Numerous options for refractory status epilepticus exist, including agents that may induce a pharmacologic coma such as midazolam or pentobarbital. Overall, the pharmacologic armamentarium of antiepileptic drugs is growing, but the use of many of these agents carries with them a level of complexity that requires consistent attention and expert monitoring to ensure safe and effective use.

References

1. Aronowski J, Zhao X. Molecular pathophysiology of cerebral hemorrhage: secondary brain injury. *Stroke.* 2011;42(6):1781–1786.
2. Xi G, Keep RF, Hoff JT. Mechanisms of brain injury after intracerebral haemorrhage. *Lancet Neurol.* 2006;5(1):53–63.
3. Willmore LJ, Sypert GW, Munson JB. Recurrent seizures induced by cortical iron injection: a model of posttraumatic epilepsy. *Ann Neurol.* 1978;4(4):329–336.
4. Lee KR, Drury I, Vitarbo E, Hoff JT. Seizures induced by intracerebral injection of thrombin: a model of intracerebral hemorrhage. *J Neurosurg.* 1997;87(1):73–78.
5. Kabuto H, Yokoi I, Habu H, et al. Reduction in nitric oxide synthase activity with development of an epileptogenic focus induced by ferric chloride in the rat brain. *Epilepsy Res.* 1996;25(2):65–68.
6. Rubin JJ, Willmore LJ. Prevention of iron-induced epileptiform discharges in rats by treatment with antiperoxidants. *Exp Neurol.* 1980;67(3):472–480.
7. Algattas H, Huang JH. Traumatic brain injury pathophysiology and treatments: early, intermediate, and late phases post-injury. *Int J Mol Sci.* 2014;15(1):309–341.
8. Prins M, Greco T, Alexander D, Giza CC. The pathophysiology of traumatic brain injury at a glance. *Dis Model Mech.* 2013;6(6):1307–1315.

9. Werner C, Engelhard K. Pathophysiology of traumatic brain injury. *Br J Anaesth.* 2007;99(1):4–9.

10. Sherlock M, O'Sullivan E, Agha A, et al. The incidence and pathophysiology of hyponatraemia after subarachnoid haemorrhage. *Clin Endocrinol (Oxf).* 2006;64(3):250–254.

11. Lado FA, Moshe SL. How do seizures stop? *Epilepsia.* 2008;49(10):1651–1664.

12. Betjemann JP, Lowenstein DH. Status epilepticus in adults. *Lancet Neurol.* 2015; 14(6):615–624.

13. Chen JW, Naylor DE, Wasterlain CG. Advances in the pathophysiology of status epilepticus. *Acta Neurol Scand.* 2007;115:7–15.

14. Naylor DE, Liu H, Niquet J, Wasterlain CG. Rapid surface accumulation of NMDA receptors increases glutamatergic excitation during status epilepticus. *Neurobiol Dis.* 2013;54:225–238.

15. Goodkin HP, Sun C, Yeh JL, et al. GABA(A) receptor internalization during seizures. *Epilepsia.* 2007;48(suppl 5):109–113.

16. Naylor DE, Liu H, Wasterlain CG. Trafficking of GABA(A) receptors, loss of inhibition, and a mechanism for pharmacoresistance in status epilepticus. *J Neurosci.* 2005;25(34):7724–7733.

17. Kapur J, Macdonald RL. Rapid seizure-induced reduction of benzodiazepine and Zn2+sensitivity of hippocampal dentate granule cell GABAA receptors. *J Neurosci.* 1997;17(19):7532–40.

18. Liu H, Mazarati AM, Katsumori H, et al. Substance P is expressed in hippocampal principal neurons during status epilepticus and plays a critical role in the maintenance of status epilepticus. *Proc Natl Acad Sci USA.* 1999;96(9):5286–5291.

19. Buckmaster PS. Mossy fiber sprouting in the dentate gyrus. In: Noebels JL, Avoli M, Rogawski MA, et al, eds. *Jasper's Basic Mechanisms of the Epilepsies.* 4th ed. Bethesda, MD: Oxford University Press; 2012.

20. Dudek FE, Shao LR. Mossy fiber sprouting and recurrent excitation: direct electrophysiologic evidence and potential implications. *Epilepsy Curr.* 2004;4(5):184–187.

21. Dudek FE, Shao LR. Loss of GABAergic interneurons in seizure-induced epileptogenesis. *Epilepsy Curr.* 2003;3(5):159–161.

22. Roopra A, Dingledine R, Hsieh J. Epigenetics and epilepsy. *Epilepsia.* 2012;53(suppl 9):2–10.

23. Elliott RC, Miles MF, Lowenstein DH. Overlapping microarray profiles of dentate gyrus gene expression during development- and epilepsy-associated neurogenesis and axon outgrowth. *J Neurosci.* 2003;23(6):2218–2227.

24. D'Ambrosio R. The role of glial membrane ion channels in seizures and epileptogenesis. *Pharmacol Ther.* 2004;103(2):95–108.

25. Rusan ZM, Kingsford OA, Tanouye MA. Modeling glial contributions to seizures and epileptogenesis: cation-chloride cotransporters in *Drosophila melanogaster. PLoS ONE.* 2014;9:e101117.

26. Bertram E. The relevance of kindling for human epilepsy. *Epilepsia.* 2007;48(suppl 2):65–74.

27. McNamara JO. Kindling model of epilepsy. *Adv Neurol.* 1986;44:303–318.

28. Carney N, Totten AM, O'Reilly C, et al, on behalf of The Brain Trauma Foundation. Guidelines for the Management of Severe Traumatic Brain Injury, Fourth Edition. *Neurosurgery.* 2016. [ePub ahead of print]

29. Mahler B, Carlsson S, Andersson T, et al. Unprovoked seizures after traumatic brain injury: a population-based case-control study. *Epilepsia.* 2015;56(9):1438–1444.

30. Annegers JF, Hauser WA, Coan SP, Rocca WA. A population-based study of seizures after traumatic brain injuries. *N Engl J Med*. 1998;338(1):20–24.
31. Vespa PM, Nuwer MR, Nenov V, et al. Increased incidence and impact of nonconvulsive and convulsive seizures after traumatic brain injury as detected by continuous electroencephalographic monitoring. *J Neurosurg*. 1999;91(5):750–760.
32. Ronne-Engstrom E, Winkler T. Continuous EEG monitoring in patients with traumatic brain injury reveals a high incidence of epileptiform activity. *Acta Neurol Scand*. 2006;114(1):47–53.
33. Salazar AM, Jabbari B, Vance SC, et al. Epilepsy after penetrating head injury. I. Clinical correlates: a report of the Vietnam Head Injury Study. *Neurology*. 1985;35(10):1406–1414.
34. Reith J, Jorgensen HS, Nakayama H, et al. Seizures in acute stroke: predictors and prognostic significance. The Copenhagen Stroke Study. *Stroke*. 1997;28(8):1585–1589.
35. Bladin CF, Alexandrov AV, Bellavance A, et al. Seizures after stroke: a prospective multi center study. *Arch Neurol*. 2000;57(11):1617–1622.
36. Labovitz DL, Hauser WA, Sacco RL. Prevalence and predictors of early seizure and status epilepticus after first stroke. *Neurology*. 2001;57(2):200–206.
37. So EL, Annegers JF, Hauser WA, et al. Population-based study of seizure disorders after cerebral infarction. *Neurology*. 1996;46(2):350–355.
38. Arboix A, Comes E, Massons J, et al. Relevance of early seizures for in-hospital mortality in acute cerebrovascular disease. *Neurology*. 1996;47(6):1429–1435.
39. Qian C, Lopponen P, Tetri S, et al. Immediate, early and late seizures after primary intracerebral hemorrhage. *Epilepsy Res*. 2014;108(4):732–739.
40. Passero S, Rocchi R, Rossi S, et al. Seizures after spontaneous supratentorial intracerebral hemorrhage. *Epilepsia*. 2002;43(10):1175–1180.
41. Tatu L, Moulin T, El Mohamad R, et al. Primary intracerebral hemorrhages in the Besancon stroke registry: initial clinical and CT findings, early course and 30-day outcome in 350 patients. *Eur Neurol*. 2000;43(4):209–214.
42. Vespa PM, O'Phelan K, Shah M, et al. Acute seizures after intracerebral hemorrhage: a factor in progressive midline shift and outcome. *Neurology*. 2003;60(9):1441–1446.
43. Claassen J, Jette N, Chum F, et al. Electrographic seizures and periodic discharges after intracerebral hemorrhage. *Neurology*. 2007;69(13):1356–1365.
44. Fung C, Balmer M, Murek M, et al. Impact of early-onset seizures on grading and outcome in patients with subarachnoid hemorrhage. *J Neurosurg*. 2015;122(2):408–413.
45. Hart RG, Byer JA, Slaughter JR, et al. Occurrence and implications of seizures in subarachnoid hemorrhage due to ruptured intracranial aneurysms. *Neurosurgery*. 1981;8(4):417–421.
46. Rhoney DH, Tipps LB, Murry KR, et al. Anticonvulsant prophylaxis and timing of seizures after aneurysmal subarachnoid hemorrhage. *Neurology*. 2000;55(2):258–265.
47. Lin CL, Dumont AS, Lieu AS, et al. Characterization of perioperative seizures and epilepsy following aneurysmal subarachnoid hemorrhage. *J Neurosurg*. 2003;99(6):978–985.
48. Claassen J, Peery S, Kreiter KT, et al. Predictors and clinical impact of epilepsy after subarachnoid hemorrhage. *Neurology*. 2003;60(2):208–214.
49. Huttunen J, Kurki MI, von Und Zu Fraunberg M, et al. Epilepsy after aneurysmal subarachnoid hemorrhage: A population-based, long-term follow-up study. *Neurology*. 2015;84(22):2229–2237.
50. Raper DM, Starke RM, Komotar RJ, et al. Seizures after aneurysmal subarachnoid hemorrhage: a systematic review of outcomes. *World Neurosurg*. 2013;79(5–6):682–690.
51. Temkin NR, Dikmen SS, Wilensky AJ, et al. A randomized, double-blind study of phenytoin for the prevention of post-traumatic seizures. *N Engl J Med*. 1990;323(8):497–502.

52. Young B, Rapp RP, Norton JA, et al. Failure of prophylactically administered phenytoin to prevent post-traumatic seizures in children. *Childs Brain*. 1983;10(3):185–192.

53. Young B, Rapp R, Brooks WH, et al. Posttraumatic epilepsy prophylaxis. *Epilepsia*. 1979;20(6):671–681.

54. Manaka S. Cooperative prospective study on posttraumatic epilepsy: risk factors and the effect of prophylactic anticonvulsant. *Jpn J Psychiatry Neurol*. 1992;46(2):311–315.

55. Temkin NR, Dikmen SS, Anderson GD, et al. Valproate therapy for prevention of post-traumatic seizures: a randomized trial. *J Neurosurg*. 1999;91(4):593–600.

56. Haltiner AM, Newell DW, Temkin NR, et al. Side effects and mortality associated with use of phenytoin for early posttraumatic seizure prophylaxis. *J Neurosurg*. 1999;91(4):588–592.

57. Dikmen SS, Temkin NR, Miller B, et al. Neurobehavioral effects of phenytoin prophylaxis of posttraumatic seizures. *JAMA*. 1991;265(10):1271–1277.

58. Young B, Rapp RP, Norton JA, et al. Failure of prophylactically administered phenytoin to prevent late posttraumatic seizures. *J Neurosurg*. 1983;58(2):236–241.

59. Jones KE, Puccio AM, Harshman KJ, et al. Levetiracetam versus phenytoin for seizure prophylaxis in severe traumatic brain injury. *Neurosurg Focus*. 2008;25(4):E3.

60. Inaba K, Menaker J, Branco BC, et al. A prospective multicenter comparison of levetiracetam versus phenytoin for early posttraumatic seizure prophylaxis. *J Trauma Acute Care Surg*. 2013;74(3):766–773.

61. Caballero GC, Hughes DW, Maxwell PR, et al. Retrospective analysis of levetiracetam compared to phenytoin for seizure prophylaxis in adults with traumatic brain injury. *Hosp Pharm*. 2013;48(3):757–761.

62. Kruer RM, Harris LH, Goodwin H, et al. Changing trends in the use of seizure prophylaxis after traumatic brain injury: a shift from phenytoin to levetiracetam. *J Crit Care*. 2013;28(5):883.e9–13.

63. Szaflarski JP, Sangha KS, Lindsell CJ, Shutter LA. Prospective, randomized, single-blinded comparative trial of intravenous levetiracetam versus phenytoin for seizure prophylaxis. *Neurocrit Care*. 2010;12(2):165–172.

64. Szaflarski JP. Is there equipoise between phenytoin and levetiracetam for seizure prevention in traumatic brain injury? *Epilepsy Curr*. 2015;15(2):94–97.

65. Glötzner FL, Haubitz I, Miltner F, et al. Seizure prevention using carbamazepine following severe brain injuries [in German]. *Neurochirurgia (Stuttg)*. 1983;26(3):66–79.

66. Chumnanvej S, Dunn IF, Kim DH. Three-day phenytoin prophylaxis is adequate after subarachnoid hemorrhage. *Neurosurgery*. 2007;60(1):99–103.

67. Rosengart AJ, Huo JD, Tolentino J, et al. Outcome in patients with subarachnoid hemorrhage treated with antiepileptic drugs. *J Neurosurg*. 2007;107(2):253–260.

68. Rowe AS, Goodwin H, Brophy GM, et al. Seizure prophylaxis in neurocritical care: a review of evidence-based support. *Pharmacotherapy*. 2014;34(4):396–409.

69. Dham BS, Hunter K, Rincon F. The epidemiology of status epilepticus in the United States. *Neurocrit Care*. 2014;20(3):476–483.

70. Treiman DM, Meyers PD, Walton NY, et al. A comparison of four treatments for generalized convulsive status epilepticus. Veterans Affairs Status Epilepticus Cooperative Study Group. *N Engl J Med*. 1998;339(12):792–798.

71. Cascino GD, Hesdorffer D, Logroscino G, Hauser WA. Treatment of nonfebrile status epilepticus in Rochester, Minn, from 1965 through 1984. *Mayo Clin Proc*. 2001;76(1):39–41.

72. Chen JW, Wasterlain CG. Status epilepticus: pathophysiology and management in adults. *Lancet Neurol*. 2006;5(3):246–256.

73. Brophy GM, Bell R, Claassen J, et al. Guidelines for the evaluation and management of status epilepticus. *Neurocrit Care.* 2012;17(1):3–23.

74. Alldredge BK, Gelb AM, Isaacs SM, et al. A comparison of lorazepam, diazepam, and placebo for the treatment of out-of-hospital status epilepticus. *N Engl J Med.* 2001; 345(9):631–637.

75. Silbergleit R, Durkalski V, Lowenstein D, et al. Intramuscular versus intravenous therapy for prehospital status epilepticus. *N Engl J Med.* 2012;366(7):591–600.

76. Claassen J, Hirsch LJ, Emerson RG, Mayer SA. Treatment of refractory status epilepticus with pentobarbital, propofol, or midazolam: a systematic review. *Epilepsia.* 2002;43(2):146–153.

77. Fernandez A, Lantigua H, Lesch C, et al. High-dose midazolam infusion for refractory status epilepticus. *Neurology.* 2014;82:359–365.

78. Strolin Benedetti M, Whomsley R, Nicolas JM, et al. Pharmacokinetics and metabolism of 14C-levetiracetam, a new antiepileptic agent, in healthy volunteers. *Eur J Clin Pharm.* 2003;59(8–9):621–630.

79. Fay MA, Sheth RD, Gidal BE. Oral absorption kinetics of levetiracetam: the effect of mixing with food or enteral nutrition formulas. *Clin Ther.* 2005;27(5):594–598.

80. UCB Inc. Levetiracetam (Keppra) [package insert]. 2013.

81. Record KE, Rapp RP, Young AB, Kostenbauder HB. Oral phenytoin loading in adults: rapid achievement of therapeutic plasma levels. *Ann Neurol.* 1979;5(3):268–270.

82. Abernethy DR, Greenblatt DJ. Phenytoin disposition in obesity: determination of loading dose. *Arch Neurol.* 1985;42(5):468–471.

83. Ludden TM, Hawkins DW, Allen JP, Hoffman SF. Letter: Optimum phenytoin-dosage regimens. *Lancet.* 1976;1(7954):307–308.

84. Charney DS, Mihic SJ, Harris RA. Hypnotics and sedatives. In: Hardman JG, Limbird LE, eds. *Goodman and Gilman's The Pharmacological Basis of Therapeutics.* 10th ed. New York, NY: McGraw-Hill, 2001:399–428.

85. Wermeling DP, Miller JL, Archer SM, et al. Bioavailability and pharmacokinetics of lorazepam after intranasal, intravenous, and intramuscular administration. *J Clin Pharmacol.* 2001;41(11):1225–1231.

86. Mandelli M, Tognoni G, Garattini S. Clinical pharmacokinetics of diazepam. *Clin Pharmacokinet.* 1978;3(1):72–91.

87. Cock HR, Schapira AH. A comparison of lorazepam and diazepam as initial therapy in convulsive status epilepticus. *QJM.* 2002;95(4):225–231.

88. Cloyd JC, Lalonde RL, Beniak TE, Novack GD. A single-blind, crossover comparison of the pharmacokinetics and cognitive effects of a new diazepam rectal gel with intravenous diazepam. *Epilepsia.* 1998;39(5):520–526.

89. Cook AM, Weant KA. Pharmacologic strategies for the treatment of elevated intracranial pressure: focus on metabolic suppression. *Adv Emerg Nurs J.* 2007;29(4):309–318.

90. Vasile B, Rasulo F, Candiani A, Latronico N. The pathophysiology of propofol infusion syndrome: a simple name for a complex syndrome. *Intensive Care Med.* 2003; 29(9):1417–1425.

91. White PF, Way WL, Trevor AJ. Ketamine—its pharmacology and therapeutic uses. *Anesthesiology.* 1982;56(5):119–136.

92. Wieber J, Gugler R, Hengstmann JH, Dengler HJ. Pharmacokinetics of ketamine in man. *Der Anaesthesist.* 1975;24(6):260–263.

93. Mion G, Villevieille T. Ketamine pharmacology: an update (pharmacodynamics and molecular aspects, recent findings). *CNS Neurosci Ther.* 2013;19(6):370–380.

Neuropharmacologic Therapies for Recovery Following Traumatic Brain Injury and Ischemic Stroke

9

A. Shaun Rowe
and Lisa Kurczewski

INTRODUCTION

The use of medications for the treatment of cognitive disorders following acute neurologic disease states has been evaluated in several small clinical trials. In addition to the excitatory effects of these medications, it is theorized that they may have some effect on neuroplasticity,[1] thus improving the recovery of devastating disease states such as traumatic brain injury and ischemic stroke. The medications that have been studied in these disease states include amphetamines and structurally similar medications such as methylphenidate, modafinil, and armodafinil. In addition, amantadine has been evaluated for its effect on cognitive recovery following traumatic brain injury. The purpose of this chapter is to focus on the use of these medications and their effect on the recovery of patients who have experienced either a traumatic brain injury or ischemic stroke.

PHARMACOLOGY OF MEDICATIONS FOR RECOVERY FOLLOWING TRAUMATIC BRAIN INJURY AND ISCHEMIC STROKE

Amphetamines

In the central nervous system, amphetamines increase the release of norepinephrine, dopamine, histamine, adenosine, and serotonin. In addition, amphetamines inhibit the reuptake of monoamines.[2,3] It is hypothesized that amphetamines' effect on norepinephrine, dopamine, and serotonin in the central nervous system is at least partially responsible for the observed effect on stroke recovery.[2,3] Dexamphetamine has US Food and Drug Administration (FDA) labeling for the treatment of narcolepsy and attention-deficit disorder with hyperactivity.

The most common adverse events associated with amphetamines are dose related and include anxiety, agitation, mood swings, insomnia, and loss of appetite. In addition, more serious adverse events, such as myocardial infarction and stroke, have been associated with amphetamines. Amphetamines should not be used in combination with other medications that may increase the release of or prevent the breakdown of catecholamines such as serotonin, norepinephrine, or dopamine.

Methylphenidate

Methylphenidate is structurally similar to amphetamine and has a similar yet distinct mechanism of action. In the central nervous system, methylphenidate blocks the reuptake of norepinephrine and dopamine into presynaptic neurons, appearing to stimulant the cerebral cortex and subcortical structures. Methylphenidate is indicated for the treatment of narcolepsy and attention-deficit disorders.

Due to its structural similarity to amphetamine, methylphenidate shares many of the same adverse events; however, it is comparatively a milder stimulant medication. Adverse events are dose related and include anxiety, agitation, mood swings, insomnia, and loss of appetite. In addition, more serious adverse events, such as myocardial infarction and stroke, have been associated with large doses. As with amphetamines, methylphenidate should be used with caution in patients who are also taking medications that prevent the breakdown of or increase the release of catecholamines.

Modafinil/Armodafinil

While its mechanism of action remains unclear, modafinil is postulated to inhibit the posterior hypothalamus and increase levels of glutamate in these regions. Unlike methylphenidate and amphetamine, modafinil has little effect on catecholamine, serotonin, histamine, adenosine, and monoamine oxidase B systems.[4-7] Modafinil carries FDA-approved indications for narcolepsy, obstructive sleep apnea, or sleep-wake disturbances (SWD) due to shift work.[8]

Armodafinil is a longer acting enantiomer of racemic modafinil and has been shown to improve wakefulness in patients with narcolepsy, obstructive sleep apnea, and shift-work disorder.[9]

Both modafinil and armodafinil are associated with anxiety, insomnia, and nausea. In addition, more serious adverse reactions such as hypertension and

Stevens-Johnson syndrome have been associated with both medications. An increased risk of adverse events can occur when modafinil and armodafinil are used in conjunction with monoamine oxidase inhibitors, selective serotonin reuptake inhibitors, and serotonin and norepinephrine reuptake inhibitors. In addition, modafinil is an inducer of CYP3A4; therefore, methylphenidate should be used with caution in patients taking medications that are substrates of that enzyme.

Amantadine

Amantadine is a nonstimulant medication unrelated to amphetamine. The mechanism of action related to its effect on cognitive recovery remains unclear but is possibly related to its effect on N-methyl-D-aspartate and dopamine.[10,11] Amantadine carries FDA indications for the treatment of influenza A, Parkinson disease, and extrapyramidal disease.

The use of amantadine is associated with adverse events such as ataxia, confusion, dizziness, and insomnia. More serious adverse events such as agranulocytosis and neuroleptic malignant syndrome are rare but have been documented with the use of amantadine. To decrease the risk of adverse events, amantadine should be used with caution in patients concurrently taking memantine and bupropion.

TRAUMATIC BRAIN INJURY

Traumatic brain injury (TBI) is defined as a blow or jolt to the head resulting in disruption of normal brain function. The severity of injury ranges from mild to severe depending on the patient's Glasgow Coma Scale score, duration of unconsciousness, and presence of posttraumatic amnesia.[12–14] TBI is a significant contributor to overall death and disability in the United States. The Centers for Disease Control and Prevention (CDC) estimated that 2.5 million emergency department visits, hospitalizations, and deaths were attributed to TBI in 2010. The indirect costs due to lack of productivity and chronic disability due to TBI totaled more than $60 billion in the United States in 2000.[15,16] Because untreated TBIs and those treated in outpatient or military settings were excluded from the CDC report, the true incidence and economic burden of this disease are underestimated.[17,18]

It is reported that 3.2 to 5.3 million persons in the United States are living with a TBI-related disability.[19–21] These disabilities include cognitive disturbances such as difficulties with memory, attention, learning, and processing. Commonly, patients appreciate symptoms from several of those domains.[22,23]

Nearly all patients experience some type of neuropsychiatric sequelae during the acute phase of the brain injury. While most patients with mild TBI will fully recover, it is estimated that somewhere between 30% and 80% of all patients with mild to moderate TBI continue to experience these symptoms 3 months after injury. Of those patients, approximately 15% will retain symptoms beyond 3 months.[22,24] Psychiatric complications can impede the process of rehabilitation and affect a TBI survivor's ability to live autonomously. The most recent edition of the *DSM-5* (American Psychiatric Association DSM-5 Task Force), released in 2013, attributes significant consideration to the diagnosis of TBI with neuropsychiatric sequelae. Despite this, there remains a challenge in diagnosing functional consequences of TBI.[25,26] Several stimulant medications have been evaluated for the treatment of these cognitive and functional complications of TBI. These include methylphenidate, modafinil, and armodafinil. In addition, the dopaminergic agent, amantadine, has been studied it this population for a similar indication. The purpose of this portion of the chapter is to review the use of these medications for the treatment of cognitive disorders and SWD secondary to TBI. Common dosages, indications, and adverse events associated with the medications in this section can be found in Table 9.1.

Cognitive Disorders

Oftentimes, patients with TBI with a secondary generalized cognitive disorder will have difficulty following conversations, will perseverate, or have trouble completing a thought. The severity of the disorder depends on the size and location of the damage, as well as the degree of diffuse axonal injury. A possible mechanism for these cognitive complications is related to the disruption of ascending catecholaminergic and serotonergic pathways resulting in inattention and impairment in information processing. These impairments have been associated with poorer overall outcomes in TBI survivors.[27–30]

In the acute phase of TBI, cognitive disturbance may occur as part of postconcussive syndrome. Symptoms may resolve in certain patients within a few weeks of injury with full recovery obtained by 3 to 6 months. A study involving 200 patients aged 11 to 22 years demonstrated that most symptoms resolved within 14 days of injury. Symptoms that lasted the longest included irritability, sleep disturbance, frustration, and poor concentration. At day 90, 15% of patients reported continued symptoms.[31,32] Symptoms lasting longer than 3 months should be worked up more thoroughly for cognitive impairment. It has been proposed that the restoration of functional anatomy is dependent on improving these cognitive deficits.[14,33]

TABLE 9.1 Medications Used to Treat Complications Associated With Traumatic Brain Injury

Medication	Dose	Duration	Indication	Adverse Drug Reactions
Methylphenidate	0.25 to 0.3 mg/kg twice daily	1 to 6 weeks	Attention and speed of information processing Mental fatigue Depression	Increases in blood pressure and heart rate, headache, insomnia, and irritability. Gastrointestinal intolerances (decreased appetite, dry mouth, nausea and vomiting)
Modafinil	100 to 200 mg daily	6 weeks	Sleep-wake disturbances	Headache, anxiety, nausea, and dizziness
Armodafinil	50 to 250 mg daily	Up to 12 months	Sleep-wake disturbances	Headache, anxiety, nausea, and dizziness
Amantadine	200 to 400 mg/d divided twice daily	4 weeks	Cognitive deficits Irritability and aggression (all off-label)	Neuroleptic malignant syndrome, orthostatic hypotension, increased irritability

Despite the lack of well-designed trials supporting the use of methylphenidate, the Neurobehavioral Guidelines Working Group in 2006 recommended the use of methylphenidate at doses of 0.25 to 0.3 mg/kg twice a day for the treatment of deficits in attention and speed of information processing.[34] This recommendation for treating general cognitive dysfunctions (consciousness, attention, and memory) was primarily based off one small, double-blind, placebo-controlled randomized trial of 23 patients with TBI with ages ranging from 16 to 64 years. The severity of injury ranged from mild to severe. Methylphenidate was administered at 0.3 mg/kg twice daily. Thirty-day follow-up could be performed on 12 patients, and 90-day follow-up was performed on 9 patients. The Disability Rating Scale (DRS) was significantly improved at day 30 in terms of attention and motor performance. However, no significant differences between the groups were seen at 90 days. The DRS is an outcome scale designed to measure the functional changes and progress of patients with TBI during their recovery and rehabilitation. The authors of the study concluded that methylphenidate appeared to enhance the rate of cognitive recovery but not the ultimate level of recovery as measured by the DRS.[35] With regard to the use of methylphenidate for deficits in attention and speed of recovery, some studies have found benefits in sustained attention, while others with similar methodology found no improvements.[35–39] Similarly, these same studies produced conflicting results with regard to the speed of processing. One study showed potential positive outcomes for methylphenidate in the treatment of post-TBI anger.[40]

There were several limitations with these trials. While most of the studies used placebo controls and randomization, the outcomes measured and study methodologies were different in nearly every study. The types of symptoms patients were experiencing, the amount of time that passed after their initial injury, and means of measuring improvements all varied. In addition, limited details were presented regarding the mechanism of injury and anatomical locations of the injuries. Methylphenidate was most commonly studied at 0.3 mg/kg twice daily; however, doses ranging from 0.15 mg/kg up to 30 mg daily were studied. The duration of methylphenidate exposure ranged from 1 to 6 weeks, and follow-up ranged from 1 week to 1 year after study drug discontinuation. This variation in duration of treatment and follow-up periods questions the ideal medication dosage and the plausibility for sustained effect after discontinuation. All studies were single-centered with small sample sizes ranging from 10 to a few dozen. Most patients were enrolled during their rehabilitation, of which a minimum amount of time ranging for 3 to 12 months after injury was required to pass before therapy initiation. However, a maximum amount of time since the initial injury was not provided in the exclusion criteria of most trials, thus allowing for the enrollment of patients decades after their initial injury. Last, little is mentioned regarding controlling for the confounding effects of other medications and therapies.[35–42]

A more recent study published in 2015 demonstrated that escalating doses of methylphenidate were well tolerated and improved mental fatigue and processing speed. This trial examined 51 adult patients with mild TBI who had symptoms of mental fatigue for at least 6 months. Methylphenidate dosing was titrated weekly to a maximum daily dosage of either 15 mg or 60 mg. The outcome measures were performed at the end of the study, a total of 12 weeks of follow-up for the patients. Treatment with methylphenidate was shown to reduce ratings on the Mental Fatigue Scale (MFS), and these results were dose dependent. The MFS is a self-assessment scale used to rate common symptoms occurring after TBI in 15 categories (including mental fatigue, concentration, memory, and irritability). No long-term effects were reported. Of note, 6 patients withdrew from the study due to adverse effects or minimal benefit.[43]

One of the few studies to examine the use of methylphenidate in the inpatient setting was performed by Willmott et al[42] in 2009 This randomized, crossover, placebo-controlled, double-blinded study included 40 adult inpatients, a mean of 68 days postinjury, with moderate to severe TBIs. Methylphenidate dosed 0.3 mg/kg twice daily was used and treatment periods lasted 2 weeks.

Methylphenidate was shown to significantly enhance processing speed, especially in patients with greater severity of injury. Unfortunately, methylphenidate did not improve speed of processing for tasks that are more complex. This signified minimal effect on working memory or strategic control of attention. Another inpatient trial by Moein et al[44] examined the effect of methylphenidate on intensive care unit (ICU) and hospital length of stays. Forty patients with moderate to severe TBI were randomized on day 2 of admission to receive methylphenidate 0.3 mg/kg twice daily or placebo until day of discharge. Patients receiving the stimulant had reductions in ICU length of stay by 23% to 26%, while only patients with severe TBI demonstrated an additional reduction in hospital length of stay.

There is substantial evidence supporting that depression is a commonly seen complication post-TBI. While the reported incidence varies greatly, patients with TBI appear to have several risk factors for depression, including the aforementioned neurotransmitter imbalances and frustration with previously described cognitive impairments.[45] Based on the similar neurotransmitter disruption seen in depression and cognitive impairments following TBI, Lee et al[46] investigated the effects of methylphenidate (20 mg/d) or sertraline (100 mg/d) compared with placebo in 30 patients with mild to moderate TBI. The 4-week double-blind, parallel-group trial allocated 10 patients per group and assessed outcomes 4 weeks later. The authors found similar improvements in depressive symptoms with both methylphenidate and sertraline compared with placebo. In addition, methylphenidate provided cognitive and alertness improvements, whereas the sertraline and placebo groups did not.

Based on current trials, methylphenidate appears safe in patients with brain injury and seizure disorders.[47] However, some studies have demonstrated small effects on blood pressure and increased heart rate,[36,41,48,49] as well as infrequent reports of reduced appetite.[50] The side effects reported with methylphenidate tended to be infrequent and typically had the same frequencies as placebo; however, this could be due to the inability of small sample sizes to detect a difference in the groups. Patients initiated on this therapy should be monitored closely for cardiovascular effects (increases in blood pressure and heart rate), central nervous system effects (headache, insomnia, and irritability), and gastrointestinal intolerances (decreased appetite, dry mouth, nausea, and vomiting).

Another cognitive-enhancing medication with promising outcomes in the TBI population is amantadine. Although not classified as a neurostimulant medication, amantadine is one of the most commonly prescribed medications for patients undergoing neurorehabilitation after cognition disorders. Specifically in patients with TBI, an international, multicenter, placebo-controlled trial by Giacino and colleagues[51] has found that amantadine accelerates functional recovery when administered to patients with nonpenetrating head injury presenting in a minimally conscious or vegetative state 4 to 16 weeks prior to treatment initiation. In total, 184 eligible patients with ages ranging from 16 to 65 years were randomized to receive placebo or amantadine 100 mg twice daily for a total of 4 weeks. Doses could be increased during treatment weeks 3 and 4 if no improvements were seen on the DRS. While both study groups had significantly improved DRS scores from baseline at week 4, the amantadine group demonstrated a significantly increased rate of recovery and decreased number of dose titrations. After a 2-week wash-out period, DRS scores were largely indistinguishable between treatment groups, suggesting a dose-dependent effect. Adverse effects were similar between the groups, with 1 amantadine patient dying of a cardiac arrest. Whether or not amantadine improves long-term outcomes was not addressed by this study and remains unknown. This study has limitations, including not using the Glasgow Coma Scale to describe TBI severity or the Coma Recovery Scale–Revised (CRS-R), which evaluates clinically relevant neurobehavioral markers, as a prespecified outcome. However, it remains the highest level of evidence available regarding the use of amantadine in this patient population. The remaining evidence is limited to smaller studies and highly variable meta-analyses with conflicting results on the potential benefits of amantadine on agitation, aggression, mood, and attentional deficits in the acute and rehabilitation settings.[11,52–54]

While the long-term efficacy of amantadine use in this patient population remains largely unknown, the treatment appears safe and well tolerated when started as early as 4 weeks after insult or as late as 6 months. If initiating amantadine, it is important to monitor renal function and blood pressure. As with all dopaminergic agents, the risk of neuroleptic malignant syndrome increases with higher doses and abrupt discontinuation. This is should be monitored for during titrations.

Sleep-Wake Disturbances

Another complication of TBI is posttraumatic SWD. These can be further classified into insomnia, increased sleep need, or excessive daytime sleepiness (EDS). SWD have significant effects on patients' outcomes and recovery. These disturbances can also exacerbate the negative effects of other neurobehavioral sequelae, including the cognitive impairment and psychological disorders as previously described.[55] While the reported incidence varies, a meta-analysis determined around 50% of all TBI survivors have some form of SWD, as defined by increased sleep need over 24 hours and excessive daytime sleepiness.[56] Quantifying the presence of SWD is variable because most reporting is based on subjective questionnaires and not objective gold standards of sleep disorder diagnoses, such as polysomnography. In patients with mild TBI, it has been reported that 56% of patients self-report postconcussive symptoms affecting their ability to return to work 2 weeks after initial injury. Poor concentration, poor memory, and sleep disorders were among the commonly reported complications.[57] A recent prospective, controlled trial attempted to quantify the presence of SWD and EDS. Similar to previously published literature, these authors found an increase in EDS by 38% for objective measures in the patients with TBI compared with controls. They also found subjective measures of sleep to be underreported in the TBI group compared with objective measures.[58]

While the pathophysiology of SWD and EDS is largely unknown, damage to hypothalamic neurons and other wake-promoting neurons (such as hypocretin 1 and histamine) is postulated to be affected in TBI.[59–61] In addition, environmental and social factors may contribute.[62,63] Research regarding the pharmacologic treatment of these SWD is very limited.[64,65] Most clinicians rely on the treatment data for non–TBI patients with primary sleep disorders to help guide therapy. The data are lacking even more so in the acute setting. Medications used to treat insomnia (eg, benzodiazepines, antihistamines, and hypnotics) are often avoided in the acute setting as they may interfere with the assessment of cognitive function and precipitate delirium. Although the management of insomnia may be a more difficult situation based on medication side effects profiles, there is still the option of treating daytime sleepiness with neurostimulant medications.

Methylphenidate has been extensively reviewed in the previous section of this chapter; however, minimal, controversial data exist on the medication's utility for EDS.[46,66] Overall, the use of methylphenidate does not appear to have any adverse effects on sleep-wake cycles, but it has not demonstrated any effectiveness on the regulation of EDS. Another pharmacologic agent that has data that are more promising for SWD and EDS in TBI is the mild central nervous system (CNS) stimulant, modafinil.

Conflicting results exist regarding this particular therapy for SWD secondary to TBI. In an open-label trial, modafinil demonstrated positive results in 2 of 5 patients with regard to the resolution of posttraumatic hypersomnia or narcolepsy.[67] These patients received modafinil 200 mg/d with no titrations and were only seen outside of the 3-month follow-up period if they experienced an adverse event. Modafinil 100 to 200 mg/d was evaluated in a prospective, double-blind, randomized, placebo-controlled pilot study of 20 patients experiencing EDS, fatigue, or both following TBI. Modafinil demonstrated significant effects on the improvement of EDS with no effect on fatigue after 6 weeks of treatment.[68] While these studies demonstrated positive results, the study populations are heterogenic and sample sizes are very small. In contrast, a double-blind, placebo-controlled, crossover trial demonstrated no benefit in self-reported wakefulness from 400 mg/d modafinil in 46 patients with TBI within 1 year of injury. Modafinil was titrated up over 14 days, and the maintenance dose of 400 mg was provided for 8 weeks with a 4-week washout period between groups. Similar to the previously mentioned studies, this trial further supports that modafinil is well tolerated; however, efficacy is questioned in this patient population.[69] Sheng and colleagues' meta-analysis[70] published in 2013 examined the use of modafinil for the treatment of EDS and fatigue associated with several neurological disorders. Of the 10 randomized controlled trials included, only 2 were from the TBI population. Beneficial effects of modafinil use were not seen in the TBI subgroup. After examining a total of 534 participants with neurological disorders, the authors concluded that existing trial data for modafinil provide inconsistent results among small patient populations and therefore cannot be recommended in these medical conditions. Of note, modafinil was reported to be well tolerated, with only insomnia and nausea reported more often with this agent compared with placebo.

Despite the limited objective data available, modafinil at a dose of 200 mg/d could be considered for the treatment of TBI-related insomnia and EDS in patients who do not respond to other treatments. If used, patients should be monitored for adverse effects, including hypertension, headache, insomnia, gastrointestinal disturbances, and severe dermatologic reactions.

One phase III study evaluated the usefulness of armodafinil for EDS associated with mild to moderate TBI.[71] This randomized, placebo-controlled, double-blind trial examined armodafinil doses at 50 mg, 150 mg, or 250 mg per day (titrated over 8 days) for 12 weeks with an optional 12-month open-label extension. Adult patients were included if they were diagnosed with a TBI in the preceding 1 to 10 years. Due to low enrollment, the study was terminated early after approximately 74% of the 117 enrolled patients completed the 12-week treatment period. Only the 250-mg daily dose was shown to reduce objective EDS. Among armodafinil recipients, the most commonly cited adverse effects causing withdrawal were headache, anxiety, nausea, and dizziness.

Overall, the evidence supporting or refuting the use of CNS stimulants, most notably modafinil and armodafinil, is lacking. Very small, often flawed, trials exist for each agent with conflicting outcomes. Furthermore, patients with underlying psychiatric disorders or previously diagnosed sleep disturbances prior to TBI were excluded from all trials. This makes the treatment of SWD with neurostimulants less generalizable to the TBI population as a whole. In addition, these agents have little to no evidence for utility in the acute setting as most studies enrolled patients 1 year postinjury. Considerations must be made for the potential of these agents to exacerbate cognitive and somatic complications already experienced by TBI survivors. Last, it is important to keep in mind the addictive and abuse potentials of these medications as they are federally designated scheduled IV controlled substances.

ISCHEMIC STROKE

Globally, ischemic stroke is one of the leading causes of death and disability. In the United States, death due to ischemic stroke is declining. However, since 2003, the prevalence rate for ischemic stroke has continued to rise. In 2010, the prevalence rate of ischemic stroke in adults aged between 20 and 64 years was estimated to be 176 per 100,000 people.[72] The reduced mortality rate with a continued increase in prevalence can increase stroke's societal burden. In 2012, the total cost attributed to stroke was estimated to be $33 billion. This number is estimated to triple by 2030.[73]

Depending on the location of vessel occlusion, tissue in the motor, sensory, and deep brain areas can be affected by a stroke. Oftentimes, this damage leads to significant disability in patients who have experienced an ischemic stroke. The hope is that the use of stimulant medications may increase the plasticity of the brain, thus improving the recovery of deficits caused by the stroke. Because of the potential for improved recovery, there is much interest in the use of stimulant medications to alleviate morbidities associated with ischemic stroke. This portion of the chapter will focus on the use of neurostimulants for cognitive and physical rehabilitation. The neurostimulants discussed include amphetamine, methylphenidate, and modafinil. Common dosages, indications, and adverse events associated with the medications in this section can be found in Table 9.2.

Functional Recovery

Following an ischemic stroke, lesions in the motor and sensory areas of the cerebral cortex can be debilitating. Therefore, there has been great interest in exploring therapies to improve the extent and time of recovery. A laboratory study by Feeney and colleagues[74] described a lab model to evaluate the use of amphetamines in rats after motor cortex injury. Due to the significant

TABLE 9.2 Medications Used to Treat Complications Associated With Ischemic Stroke

Medication	Dose	Duration	Indication	Adverse Drug Reactions
Amphetamine	2.5 mg to 10 mg PO once or twice daily Administered prior to physical and occupational therapy	One day to 5 weeks	Functional recovery of motor and speech deficits	Increases in blood pressure and heart rate, headache, insomnia, and irritability. Gastrointestinal intolerances (decreased appetite, dry mouth, nausea and vomiting).
Methylphenidate with levodopa	Methylphenidate 20 mg/levodopa 125 mg PO prior to physiotherapy	5 days a week for 15 sessions	Functional recovery of motor function	Increases in blood pressure and heart rate, headache, insomnia, and irritability. Gastrointestinal intolerances (decreased appetite, dry mouth, nausea and vomiting).
Methylphenidate	5 to 30 mg PO twice daily	3 weeks	Apathy, depression, and fatigue	Increases in blood pressure and heart rate, headache, insomnia, and irritability. Gastrointestinal intolerances (decreased appetite, dry mouth, nausea and vomiting).
Modafinil	400 mg PO daily	90 days	Fatigue	Headache, anxiety, nausea, and dizziness

Note: PO, per os.

improvements in recovery after a single dose of amphetamine, interest sparked in the use of amphetamines to help speed the recovery of patients who have experienced a stroke. Since that time, several small studies and case reports have evaluated the use of amphetamines in the setting of ischemic stroke recovery. The most commonly used amphetamine in these trials was dexamphetamine.[75] This was followed by d,l-amphetamine and methamphetamine.

In 2007, a meta-analysis published by The Cochrane Collaboration described 10 trials related to the use of amphetamine in stroke recovery.[75] These 10 trials comprised a total of 287 patients. The dosing regimens, duration of treatment, and medication used in the described trials varied greatly. Amphetamine doses ranged from 2.5 to 10 mg once or twice daily, and the duration of therapy was anywhere from 1 day to 5 weeks. The time from medication administration to when specific stroke recovery training began varied from 30 to 60 minutes. Due to these variabilities, it is difficult to estimate the true effect amphetamine may have on stroke recovery. Despite these limitations, there was a statistically significant improvement in motor and language function when patients were treated with amphetamines and underwent targeted therapy for these problems. However, the use of amphetamines did not affect the activities of daily living, depression, or combined outcome of death and disability. Treatment with amphetamines was also associated with a statistically significant increase in heart rate and blood pressure, as well as a slower decrease in blood pressure during the first week after stroke onset. Due to the variabilities in the trials and the potential for adverse events, the beneficial effects observed in this meta-analysis should be interpreted with caution.

In 2008, Sprigg et al[76] published a meta-analysis on the use of amphetamines in stroke recovery. The authors found similar results to the previously published meta-analysis; however, they did not observe a significant improvement in motor recovery or language function. As with the previous meta-analysis, they observed a significant increase in hemodynamics in those patients taking amphetamines.[76]

Few trials have been published on the use of amphetamines for stroke recovery since 2008. However, in 2011, Schuster et al[77] published a study of 16 patients in which they evaluated the use of dexamphetamine for upper extremity rehabilitation after stroke. Patients in the study were 14 to 60 days poststroke and received twice-weekly doses of dexamphetamine (10 mg) up to 3 hours prior to a 1-hour physiotherapy session. The authors observed a statistically significant increase in both activities of daily living and motor function in the upper extremity. In addition, there were no reported adverse events. Although the results of this trial are promising, the small size of the trial and conflicting results from previous trials leave many unanswered questions.

Another medication, methylphenidate, has been evaluated for its utility in improving motor recovery after stroke. When used in combination with levodopa, methylphenidate's effect on motor recovery in patients with stroke was evaluated in a small double-blind trial.[78] Compared with placebo, the combination did show a modest improvement in motor recovery and activities of daily. However, the study was very small, and there was no clear distinction as to the best time window for administration of therapy.

The utility of amphetamines and methylphenidate to improve functional recovery after an ischemic stroke is still not fully elucidated. Although the meta-analyses published on this topic did not find any significant heterogeneity, differences in the way the studies were designed could affect the outcome. Laboratory evidence suggests that the dose response of amphetamines for recovery is U-shaped. Thus, we do not know the most appropriate dose, duration of therapy, or timing prior to physiotherapy. These questions need to be answered before amphetamines can be recommended for routine use in patients with ischemic stroke to improve functional recovery.

Psychological Recovery

Although not as physically visible, depression and fatigue can cause significant disability in patients who have experienced an ischemic stroke. Younger patients, female patients, those with multiple comorbidities, and those who have functional disabilities are at the highest risk of depression. Up to 50% of patients who survive an ischemic stroke may experience some symptoms of depression. Stimulants have a long history as adjuncts to other antidepressant medications for the treatment of depression.

When administered to patients in the rehabilitation period, methylphenidate has been associated with acute improvements in mood and depression as measured by the Hamilton Depression Rating Scale.[79] However, as the authors of that article point out, it was a relatively small sample, and some of the statistically significant results may not have been clinically significant. The successful use of methylphenidate for the treatment of depression and apathy after a stroke has been described in other small case series and case reports as well.[80–82]

As far as safety is concerned, methylphenidate can be associated with many side effects. Some of these include tachycardia, hypertension, headache, and decreased appetite. However, none of the studies reported a significant increase in adverse events.

Although small studies have shown efficacy with methylphenidate, many questions remain unanswered about the use of this medication for poststroke recovery. As with amphetamines, the best dose and time widow to start treatment are not fully elucidated. The observed success of methylphenidate needs to be confirmed with larger, more robust trials.

Researchers have also evaluated the use of modafinil for poststroke fatigue.[83–85] In a randomized, placebo-controlled trial by Poulsen et al,[86] 41 patients were evaluated for poststroke fatigue; 21 of these patients received modafinil. Patients received either modafinil 400 mg/d or placebo for 90 days. Although the investigators did not observe a significant change in the primary end point, those patients who received modafinil had better Fatigue Severity Scale scores (36 [24–41] vs 49.5 [37–55]; $P = .019$). The Fatigue Severity Scale is a 9-item questionnaire used to evaluate fatigue. A lower score is associated with less fatigue. In addition, the investigators did not see a statistical difference in adverse events.

Due to the possibility of medication-related side effects and paucity of data on the use of modafinil in patients who have experienced an ischemic stroke, modafinil cannot be recommended for routine use in poststroke patients. However, the results of current trials are promising, and this medication warrants further investigation.

CONCLUSION

It remains a challenge to ascertain which neurologically injured patients would benefit from neurostimulant therapy. Although results are promising with regard to motor, cognitive, and psychologic recovery, differences in clinical trial design provoke many unanswered questions. The ideal timing, dose, and duration of therapy remain unknown. Due to this, the applicability of clinical trials to current practice is limited. When considering these limitations, the current evidence does not suggest stimulant medications have a routine place in the recovery of patients who have experienced a TBI or an ischemic stroke. However, the use of stimulant medications to speed the recovery in select patients cannot be ruled out.

References

1. Butefisch CM, Davis BC, Sawaki L, et al. Modulation of use-dependent plasticity by d-amphetamine. *Ann Neurol.* 2002;51:59–68.
2. Rosser N, Floel A. Pharmacological enhancement of motor recovery in subacute and chronic stroke. *NeuroRehabilitation.* 2008;23:95–103.
3. Walker-Batson D. Amphetamine and post-stroke rehabilitation: indications and controversies. *Eur J Phys Rehabil Med.* 2013;49:251–260.
4. Lin JS, Hou Y, Jouvet M. Potential brain neuronal targets for amphetamine-, methylphenidate-, and modafinil-induced wakefulness, evidenced by c-fos immunocytochemistry in the cat. *Proc Natl Acad Sci USA.* 1996;93:14128–14133.
5. Ferraro L, Tanganelli S, O'Connor WT, et al. The vigilance promoting drug modafinil decreases GABA release in the medial preoptic area and in the posterior hypothalamus of the awake rat: possible involvement of the serotonergic 5-HT3 receptor. *Neurosci Lett.* 1996;220:5–8.
6. Chew E, Zafonte RD. Pharmacological management of neurobehavioral disorders following traumatic brain injury—a state-of-the-art review. *J Rehab Res Dev.* 2009;46:851–879.
7. Ishizuka T, Murotani T, Yamatodani A. Modafinil activates the histaminergic system through the orexinergic neurons. *Neurosci Lett.* 2010;483:193–196.

8. Provigil [package insert]. North Wales, PA: Teva Pharmaceuticals; 2015. http://www.provigil.com/pdfs/prescribing_info.pdf. Accessed December 21, 2016.

9. Nuvigil [package insert]. North Wales, PA: Teva Pharmaceuticals; 2015. http://www.nuvigil.com/PDF/Full_Prescribing_Information.pdf. Accessed December 21, 2016.

10. Brown F, Redfern PH. Studies on the mechanism of action of amantadine. *Br J Pharmacol.* 1976;58:561–567.

11. Sami MB, Faruqui R. The effectiveness of dopamine agonists for treatment of neuropsychiatric symptoms post brain injury and stroke. *Acta Neuropsychiatr.* 2015;27:317–326.

12. Centers for Disease Control and Prevention (CDC). Basic information about traumatic brain injury and concussion. http://www.cdc.gov/traumaticbraininjury/basics.html. Accessed December 21, 2016.

13. Powell JM, Ferraro JV, Dikmen SS, et al. Accuracy of mild traumatic brain injury diagnosis. *Arch Phys Med Rehab.* 2008;89:1550–1555.

14. Writer BW, Schillerstrom JE. Psychopharmacological treatment for cognitive impairment in survivors of traumatic brain injury: a critical review. *J Neurospych Clin Neurosci.* 2009;21:362–370.

15. Faul M, Xu L, Wald MM, Coronado VG. Traumatic brain injury in the United States: emergency department visits, hospitalizations and deaths 2002–2006. https://www.cdc.gov/traumaticbraininjury/pdf/blue_book.pdf. Accessed December 21, 2016.

16. Finkelstein E, Corso PS, Miller TR. *The Incidence and Economic Burden of Injuries in the United States.* New York, NY: Oxford University Press; 2006:68, 105–106.

17. Schootman M, Fuortes LJ. Ambulatory care for traumatic brain injuries in the US, 1995–1997. *Brain Injury.* 2000;14:373–381.

18. Sosin DM, Sniezek JE, Thurman DJ. Incidence of mild and moderate brain injury in the United States, 1991. *Brain Injury.* 1996;10:47–54.

19. Selassie AW, Zaloshnja E, Langlois JA, et al. Incidence of long-term disability following traumatic brain injury hospitalization, United States, 2003. *J Head Trauma Rehab.* 2008;23:123–131.

20. Thurman DJ, Alverson C, Dunn KA, et al. Traumatic brain injury in the United States: a public health perspective. *J Head Trauma Rehab.* 1999;14:602–615.

21. Zaloshnja E, Miller T, Langlois JA, Selassie AW. Prevalence of long-term disability from traumatic brain injury in the civilian population of the United States, 2005. *J Head Trauma Rehab.* 2008;23:394–400.

22. Riggio S, Wong M. Neurobehavioral sequelae of traumatic brain injury. *Mt Sinai J Med.* 2009;76:163–172.

23. Langlois JA, Rutland-Brown W, Wald MM. The epidemiology and impact of traumatic brain injury: a brief overview. *J Head Trauma Rehab.* 2006;21:375–378.

24. Lundin A, de Boussard C, Edman G, Borg J. Symptoms and disability until 3 months after mild TBI. *Brain Injury.* 2006;20:799–806.

25. American Psychiatric Association, DSM-5 Task Force. *Diagnostic and Statistical Manual of Mental Disorders.* 5th ed. Arlington, VA: APA; 2013:624–627.

26. Wortzel HS, Arciniegas DB. The DSM-5 approach to the evaluation of traumatic brain injury and its neuropsychiatric sequelae. *NeuroRehabilitation.* 2014;34:613–623.

27. Nicholl J, LaFrance WC Jr. Neuropsychiatric sequelae of traumatic brain injury. *Semin Neurol.* 2009;29:247–255.

28. Scheid R, Walther K, Guthke T, et al. Cognitive sequelae of diffuse axonal injury. *Arch Neurol.* 2006;63:418–424.

29. Povlishock JT, Katz DI. Update of neuropathology and neurological recovery after traumatic brain injury. *J Head Trauma Rehab.* 2005;20:76–94.

30. Hamill RW, Woolf PD, McDonald JV, et al. Catecholamines predict outcome in traumatic brain injury. *Ann Neurol.* 1987;21:438–443.

31. Eisenberg MA, Meehan WP III, Mannix R. Duration and course of post-concussive symptoms. *Pediatrics.* 2014;133:999–1006.

32. Rao V, Koliatsos V, Ahmed F, et al. Neuropsychiatric disturbances associated with traumatic brain injury: a practical approach to evaluation and management. *Semin Neurol.* 2015;35:64–82.

33. Rassovsky Y, Satz P, Alfano MS, et al. Functional outcome in TBI II: verbal memory and information processing speed mediators. *J Clin Exp Neuropsychol.* 2006;28: 581–591.

34. Neurobehavioral Guidelines Working Group, Warden DL, Gordon B, et al. Guidelines for the pharmacologic treatment of neurobehavioral sequelae of traumatic brain injury. *J Neurotrauma.* 2006;23:1468–1501.

35. Plenger PM, Dixon CE, Castillo RM, et al. Subacute methylphenidate treatment for moderate to moderately severe traumatic brain injury: a preliminary double-blind placebo-controlled study. *Arch Phys Med Rehab.* 1996;77:536–540.

36. Whyte J, Hart T, Schuster K, et al. Effects of methylphenidate on attentional function after traumatic brain injury: a randomized, placebo-controlled trial. *Am J Phys Med Rehab.* 1997;76:440–450.

37. Whyte J, Hart T, Vaccaro M, et al. Effects of methylphenidate on attention deficits after traumatic brain injury: a multidimensional, randomized, controlled trial. *Am J Phys Med Rehab.* 2004;83:401–420.

38. Speech TJ, Rao SM, Osmon DC, Sperry LT. A double-blind controlled study of methylphenidate treatment in closed head injury. *Brain Injury.* 1993;7:333–338.

39. Gualtieri CT, Evans RW. Stimulant treatment for the neurobehavioural sequelae of traumatic brain injury. *Brain Injury.* 1988;2:273–290.

40. Mooney GF, Haas LJ. Effect of methylphenidate on brain injury-related anger. *Arch Phys Med Rehab.* 1993;74:153–160.

41. Kaelin DL, Cifu DX, Matthies B. Methylphenidate effect on attention deficit in the acutely brain-injured adult. *Arch Phys Med Rehab.* 1996;77:6–9.

42. Willmott C, Ponsford J. Efficacy of methylphenidate in the rehabilitation of attention following traumatic brain injury: a randomised, crossover, double blind, placebo controlled inpatient trial. *J Neurol Neurosurg Psychiatry.* 2009;80:552–557.

43. Johansson B, Wentzel AP, Andrell P, et al. Methylphenidate reduces mental fatigue and improves processing speed in persons suffered a traumatic brain injury. *Brain Injury.* 2015;29:758–765.

44. Moein H, Khalili HA, Keramatian K. Effect of methylphenidate on ICU and hospital length of stay in patients with severe and moderate traumatic brain injury. *Clin Neurol Neurosurg.* 2006;108:539–542.

45. Kim E, Lauterbach EC, Reeve A, et al. Neuropsychiatric complications of traumatic brain injury: a critical review of the literature (a report by the ANPA Committee on Research). *J Neurospych Clin Neurosci.* 2007;19:106–127.

46. Lee H, Kim SW, Kim JM, et al. Comparing effects of methylphenidate, sertraline and placebo on neuropsychiatric sequelae in patients with traumatic brain injury. *Hum Psychopharm.* 2005;20:97–104.

47. Wroblewski BA, Leary JM, Phelan AM, et al. Methylphenidate and seizure frequency in brain injured patients with seizure disorders. *J Clin Psychiatry*. 1992;53:86–89.

48. Johansson B, Wentzel AP, Andrell P, et al. Evaluation of dosage, safety and effects of methylphenidate on post-traumatic brain injury symptoms with a focus on mental fatigue and pain. *Brain Injury*. 2014;28:304–310.

49. Burke DT, Glenn MB, Vesali F, et al. Effects of methylphenidate on heart rate and blood pressure among inpatients with acquired brain injury. *Am J Phys Med Rehab*. 2003;82:493–497.

50. Alban JP, Hopson MM, Ly V, Whyte J. Effect of methylphenidate on vital signs and adverse effects in adults with traumatic brain injury. *Am J Phys Med Rehab*. 2004;83:131–141.

51. Giacino JT, Whyte J, Bagiella E, et al. Placebo-controlled trial of amantadine for severe traumatic brain injury. *N Engl J Med*. 2012;366:819–826.

52. Frenette AJ, Kanji S, Rees L, et al. Efficacy and safety of dopamine agonists in traumatic brain injury: a systematic review of randomized controlled trials. *J Neurotrauma*. 2012;29:1–18.

53. Hammond FM, Bickett AK, Norton JH, Pershad R. Effectiveness of amantadine hydrochloride in the reduction of chronic traumatic brain injury irritability and aggression. *J Head Trauma Rehab*. 2014;29:391–399.

54. Schneider WN, Drew-Cates J, Wong TM, Dombovy ML. Cognitive and behavioural efficacy of amantadine in acute traumatic brain injury: an initial double-blind placebo-controlled study. *Brain Injury*. 1999;13:863–872.

55. Aloia MS, Arnedt JT, Davis JD, et al. Neuropsychological sequelae of obstructive sleep apnea-hypopnea syndrome: a critical review. *JINS*. 2004;10:772–785.

56. Mathias JL, Alvaro PK. Prevalence of sleep disturbances, disorders, and problems following traumatic brain injury: a meta-analysis. *Sleep Med*. 2012;13:898–905.

57. Haboubi NH, Long J, Koshy M, Ward AB. Short-term sequelae of minor head injury (6 years experience of minor head injury clinic). *Disabil Rehab*. 2001;23:635–638.

58. Imbach LL, Valko PO, Li T, et al. Increased sleep need and daytime sleepiness 6 months after traumatic brain injury: a prospective controlled clinical trial. *Brain*. 2015;138:726–735.

59. Parcell DL, Ponsford JL, Redman JR, Rajaratnam SM. Poor sleep quality and changes in objectively recorded sleep after traumatic brain injury: a preliminary study. *Arch Phys Med Rehab*. 2008;89:843–850.

60. Baumann CR, Bassetti CL, Valko PO, et al. Loss of hypocretin (orexin) neurons with traumatic brain injury. *Ann Neurol*. 2009;66:555–559.

61. Baumann CR, Stocker R, Imhof HG, et al. Hypocretin-1 (orexin A) deficiency in acute traumatic brain injury. *Neurology*. 2005;65:147–149.

62. Ouellet MC, Beaulieu-Bonneau S, Morin CM. Sleep-wake disturbances after traumatic brain injury. *Lancet Neurol*. 2015;14:746–757.

63. Duclos C, Dumont M, Blais H, et al. Rest-activity cycle disturbances in the acute phase of moderate to severe traumatic brain injury. *Neurorehabil Neural Repair*. 2013;28:472–482.

64. Wiseman-Hakes C, Murray B, Moineddin R, et al. Evaluating the impact of treatment for sleep/wake disorders on recovery of cognition and communication in adults with chronic TBI. *Brain Injury*. 2013;27:1364–1376.

65. Wiseman-Hakes C, Victor JC, Brandys C, Murray BJ. Impact of post-traumatic hypersomnia on functional recovery of cognition and communication. *Brain Injury*. 2011;25:1256–1265.

66. Al-Adawi S, Burke DT, Dorvlo AS. The effect of methylphenidate on the sleep-wake cycle of brain-injured patients undergoing rehabilitation. *Sleep Med*. 2006;7:287–291.

67. Castriotta RJ, Atanasov S, Wilde MC, et al. Treatment of sleep disorders after traumatic brain injury. *J Clin Sleep Med.* 2009;5:137–144.

68. Kaiser PR, Valko PO, Werth E, et al. Modafinil ameliorates excessive daytime sleepiness after traumatic brain injury. *Neurology.* 2010;75:1780–1785.

69. Jha A, Weintraub A, Allshouse A, et al. A randomized trial of modafinil for the treatment of fatigue and excessive daytime sleepiness in individuals with chronic traumatic brain injury. *J Head Trauma Rehab.* 2008;23:52–63.

70. Sheng P, Hou L, Wang X, et al. Efficacy of modafinil on fatigue and excessive daytime sleepiness associated with neurological disorders: a systematic review and meta-analysis. *PLoS ONE.* 2013;8:e81802.

71. Menn SJ, Yang R, Lankford A. Armodafinil for the treatment of excessive sleepiness associated with mild or moderate closed traumatic brain injury: a 12-week, randomized, double-blind study followed by a 12-month open-label extension. *J Clin Sleep Med.* 2014;10:1181–1191.

72. Krishnamurthi RV, Moran AE, Feigin VL, et al. Stroke prevalence, mortality and disability-adjusted life years in adults aged 20–64 years in 1990–2013: data from the Global Burden of Disease 2013 Study. *Neuroepidemiology.* 2015;45:190–202.

73. Mozaffarian D, Benjamin EJ, Go AS, et al. Heart disease and stroke statistics—2016 update: a report from the American Heart Association. *Circulation.* 2015;33(4):e38–e360.

74. Feeney DM, Gonzalez A, Law WA. Amphetamine, haloperidol, and experience interact to affect rate of recovery after motor cortex injury. *Science.* 1982;217:855–857.

75. Martinsson L, Hardemark H, Eksborg S. Amphetamines for improving recovery after stroke. *Cochrane Database Sys Rev.* 2007;(1):CD002090.

76. Sprigg N, Gray LJ, England T, et al. A randomised controlled trial of triple antiplatelet therapy (aspirin, clopidogrel and dipyridamole) in the secondary prevention of stroke: safety, tolerability and feasibility. *PLoS ONE.* 2008;3:e2852.

77. Schuster C, Maunz G, Lutz K, et al. Dexamphetamine improves upper extremity outcome during rehabilitation after stroke: a pilot randomized controlled trial. *Neurorehabil Neural Repair.* 2011;25:749–755.

78. Lokk J, Salman Roghani R, Delbari A. Effect of methylphenidate and/or levodopa coupled with physiotherapy on functional and motor recovery after stroke—a randomized, double-blind, placebo-controlled trial. *Acta Neurol Scand.* 2011;123:266–273.

79. Grade C, Redford B, Chrostowski J, et al. Methylphenidate in early poststroke recovery: a double-blind, placebo-controlled study. *Arch Phys Med Rehabil.* 1998;79:1047–1050.

80. Johnson ML, Roberts MD, Ross AR, Witten CM. Methylphenidate in stroke patients with depression. *Am J Phys Med Rehab.* 1992;71:239–241.

81. Spiegel DR, Kim J, Greene K, et al. Apathy due to cerebrovascular accidents successfully treated with methylphenidate: a case series. *J Neuropsych Clin Neurosci.* 2009;21:216–219.

82. Watanabe MD, Martin EM, DeLeon OA, et al. Successful methylphenidate treatment of apathy after subcortical infarcts. *J Neurospych Clin Neurosci.* 1995;7:502–504.

83. Berkowitz HL. Modafinil in poststroke depression. *Psychosomatics.* 2005;46:93–94.

84. Geffen S, Shum K, Tan HM. Novel use of modafinal to treat severe physical and cognitive impairment post-stroke. *Intern Med J.* 2013;43:338.

85. Goyal MK, Kumar G, Sahota PK. Isolated hypersomnia due to bilateral thalamic infarcts. *J Stroke Cerebrovasc Dis.* 2012;21:146–147.

86. Poulsen MB, Damgaard B, Zerahn B, et al. Modafinil may alleviate poststroke fatigue: a randomized, placebo-controlled, double-blinded trial. *Stroke.* 2015;46:3470–3477.

Intracerebroventricular and Intrathecal Drug Therapies

10

Theresa Human, Jennifer Bushwitz,
and Olabisi Falana

INTRODUCTION

Medication access to the central nervous system (CNS) is limited. Two physiologic barriers, the blood-brain barrier (BBB) and the blood–cerebrospinal fluid barrier (BCSFB), impair the entry of all large and 98% of small drug molecules into therapy targets in the CNS.[1] Rapid metabolism and active efflux pumps further limit the availability of molecules that are able to cross the BBB. To adequately address the drug therapy needs of critically ill patients with neurologic injury, utilization of systemic medications and dosing strategies that gain access to the CNS must sometimes be combined with direct, local administration. Direct administration of medications into the CNS remains a complex, incompletely understood intervention. Critical care pharmacists play a unique role in assisting with drug product selection and assessment of the appropriateness of intracerebroventricular (IVT) or intrathecal (IT) drug administration based on a medication's physiochemical properties. This chapter will further discuss the specific therapeutic approaches considered within the neurological critically ill population.

CEREBROSPINAL FLUID PHYSIOLOGY OVERVIEW

Cerebrospinal Fluid Production and Flow

The majority of cerebrospinal fluid (CSF) is produced by the cells of the choroid plexus located in the lateral, third, and fourth ventricles of the brain and by the dura of nerve root sleeves in the spine. Through a combination of passive plasma filtration and active transport of select substances, roughly 400 to 600 mL/d of CSF is produced in adults at a rate of approximately 0.3 mL/min.[2,3] The total volume of CSF in adults is approximately 150 mL and is split nearly evenly between the ventricles and spinal space. In children, the volume of CSF is much smaller and begins at ~50 mL total volume and increases with age.[3]

CSF circulates between the meningeal layers of the pia and arachnoid mater in the subarachnoid space where the flow of CSF is continuous and multidirectional. From the choroid plexus to arachnoid villi, located throughout the CNS where absorption takes place, the flow of CSF is unidirectional and pulsatile. While the precise flow pattern of CSF has not been fully elucidated, broad flow patterns have been identified. Beginning in the choroid plexus of the lateral ventricles, CSF travels through the third and fourth ventricle and then rostrally or caudally through the cranial or spinal subarachnoid space, respectively.[3]

CSF is absorbed primarily through the arachnoid villi, which drain into the venous sinuses and ultimately the systemic venous vasculature. The arachnoid villi, or arachnoid granulations, are endothelium-lined meningeal protrusions that extend through the dura mater to the venous sinuses. The rate of CSF resorption varies with fluctuations in pressure. Under normal physiologic conditions, as pressure builds, the surface area of the arachnoid villi increases, accelerating the rate of CSF absorption.[3]

Physiologic Barriers to Medication Entry

Medication entry into the CNS is limited by the BBB and the BCSFB. The BBB is a complex cell layer predominantly formed by brain capillary endothelial cells (BCECs) joined by tight junctions lining the microvasculature of the CNS. It limits systemic medications from freely entering the brain parenchyma.[4] The BCSFB is established predominantly by the epithelia cells of the choroid plexus and acts as a barrier between blood and CSF.[5,6] These barriers are important structures in maintaining brain homeostasis, allowing selective uptake of nutrients, and limiting passage of potentially noxious substances. Disruption of these barriers occurs due to lack of uniformity within the BBB itself as well as under certain pathologic conditions.[7] Medications can overcome these barriers through passive diffusion or by using the active transport systems of BCECs.

The physiochemical properties of systemic medications, specifically their ionization, lipophilicity, molecular weight, and protein binding, determine the extent to which they can enter the brain. It is thought that passage of these molecules is accomplished by passive diffusion through small, transiently available pores. Lipophilic, uncharged, small molecules (<500 Daltons) are able to pass through the BBB more easily than their counterparts.[5,6] Alteration of any of these properties significantly diminishes drug permeability.[6] Plasma protein binding also strongly influences drug penetration into the CSF, as bound drug is unable to freely cross the BBB secondary to sheer size.[5]

A number of systemically administered medications gain entry into the CNS by taking advantage of absorptive-, carrier-, and receptor-mediated active transport systems present in BCECs. These transport systems are the subject of extensive research with only a few currently used in clinical practice. Absorptive-mediated transcytosis occurs as a result of an electrostatic interaction between cationic molecules and the negatively charged BCEC plasma membrane surface. Once initiated, endosome formation and transport occur. This process is downregulated in the BBB but is the method by which a number of medications, including heparin and aspirin, gain access to the brain parenchyma.[4,6,7] Carrier-mediated transport uses substrate-specific transporters present on the luminal cell surface to enter the CNS. It is the principal mechanism by which essential amino acids, vitamins, and some neuropeptides enter the brain.[4] A number of medications with structural similarities to endogenous substances use these transporters, including levodopa, gabapentin, and melphalan.[6] Receptor-mediated endocytosis is the method a number of large molecules, notably insulin and transferrin, enter the brain parenchyma.[4,7]

Only a small proportion of commercially available medications are able to take advantage of these entry mechanisms to gain access to the CNS. One method of bypassing the BBB is to administer medications directly into the CNS through IT or IVT injection. These methods of drug delivery present a unique set of challenges and considerations.

PHYSIOCHEMICAL CONSIDERATIONS FOR INTRACEREBROVENTRICULAR/INTRATHECAL DRUG ADMINISTRATION

When selecting a medication for IT/IVT administration, the physiochemical properties of the drug must be carefully considered in conjunction with its therapeutic indication. Drug volume, pH, osmolarity, drug preservatives, and intrinsic neurotoxicity significantly affect the safety and efficacy of IT/IVT administration.

Drug Volume/Concentration

The average adult cranial and spinal space holds approximately 140 to 160 mL of CSF, with 50% located within the ventricles.[4,6,8] Increases in CSF volume may lead to an intolerable rise in intracranial pressure (ICP) and associated adverse effects. To date, definitive recommendations are lacking regarding maximum rate and volume of administration into the IT or IVT space. However, instilling small volumes (less than 3 mL) into the lateral ventricles over 1 to 2 minutes appears to be safe.[8] In cases where there may be concern for increased ICP, one may consider removing the same volume of CSF prior to instillation of the medication. In addition, in some situations, removed autologous CSF may be used to reconstitute and dilute particular medications for IT/IVT instillation.

pH

The physiologic pH range of CSF is 7.27 to 7.37 and does not have the buffering capacity of the blood and is thus more susceptible to alterations in pH resulting from drug administration. Alterations in CSF pH, especially acidification of CSF, may cause neuronal injury. Adverse effects from pH changes have been noted more commonly with medications administered through the IT route compared with IVT. The larger volume of CSF within the lateral ventricles allows greater opportunity for medication diffusion and dilution, which may partially explain this disparity.

Osmolarity

Administration of hyper- or hypotonic solutions may cause adverse effects, including dipsogenesis, syndrome of inappropriate antidiuretic hormone, and cerebral edema. The osmolarity of CSF is approximately 281 mOsm/L, with solutions ranging from 230 to 330 mOsm/L generally considered isotonic.[5,8] Adverse effects may be minimized by selecting and administering only isotonic medications or by limiting the volume of hyper- or hypotonic solutions administered.

Hydrophilicity and Lipophilicity

Lipophilic medications are generally able to diffuse into and out of the CSF more freely than their hydrophilic counterparts. Many hydrophilic medications become trapped within the CNS at high concentrations immediately following IT/IVT administration. For these hydrophilic medications, because the rate of CSF elimination exceeds the rate of medication dissolution, drug elimination is mostly dependent on CSF flow.[1,8] Patients requiring CSF diversion or

TABLE 10.1 Common Diluents/Preservatives

Additive	Products That May Contain Additive	Adverse Effects
Sodium metabisulfite	Gentamicin, tobramycin, amikacin	Seizures
EDTA	Gentamicin, tobramycin	Seizures
Benzyl alcohol	Bacteriostatic NS	Metabolic acidosis, cerebral palsy
Chlorobutanol	Ketamine	Neurotoxicity
Propylene glycol	Lorazepam	None reported

Source: Reference 8.

Note: NS, normal saline.

those with other pathologies that interfere with the normal outflow of CSF may be at higher risk of experiencing sub- or supratherapeutic local drug concentrations across a dosing interval. In addition, because hydrophilic medications diffuse poorly into the brain parenchyma, they may be less effective at treating disorders outside of the immediate IT/IVT space.

Preservatives and Intrinsic Toxicity

Although not all preservatives carry the same risk of neurotoxicity, the presence of preservatives and their risk for adverse effects should be investigated prior to IT/IVT drug administration.[9,10] A number of commonly used medication preservatives, including benzyl alcohol and chlorobutanol, have demonstrated varying degrees of neurotoxicity in both animal models and human case reports.[8,9] Ideally, both parent medication and any drug diluents should be preservative free.

Aside from preservative-containing formulations, the epileptogenicity of drug compounds themselves must also be considered. Administration of agents known to be directly irritating to the brain parenchyma, such as beta-lactams, is ultimately futile as the epileptogenic risk outweighs any possible benefit (Table 10.1).[8]

CSF Clearance

The rate of clearance of medications from the CSF space appears to be dependent on the patients' CSF production, volume, and elimination. Higher CSF volumes secondary to increased production or external drug administration may result in increased CSF clearance to maintain ICP homeostasis. This increase in CSF clearance can ultimately result in faster drug elimination from the central compartment. CSF elimination can be further complicated by CSF diversion catheters, CSF albumin concentrations, and concomitant systemic medication administration.[11] In situations where CSF flow is obstructed and hydrocephalus occurs, the volume of distribution of IVT-administered medications may be increased with resulting lower peak concentration as a result of the dilution. To further complicate matters, CSF diversion catheters placed for treatment of hydrocephalus may hasten drug elimination and lead to subtherapeutic drug concentrations within the CSF. In cases where IT/IVT-administered medications are able to diffuse readily out of the central compartment due to their physiochemical properties, concomitant systemic medications may slow drug elimination from the CSF compartment by diminishing the concentration gradient across the BBB, ultimately potentiating the drug effects.

COMMON METHODS OF INTRACEREBROVENTRICULAR/ INTRATHECAL DRUG ADMINISTRATION

Antibiotics, chemotherapy agents, medications for chronic pain and spasticity, and fibrinolytics have all been administered directly into the CNS via the IT or IVT route. This can be achieved through direct injection, placement of a temporary external catheter, or implantation of an indwelling device for long-term use. Many medications administered via the IT/IVT route require repeated administrations. For this reason, temporary or indwelling catheters are frequently used to minimize the risk of complications related to serial CSF lumbar punctures such as infection, hemorrhage, direct neuronal injury, and CSF fistulae formation.

Intrathecal

IT administration consists of drug delivery into the lumbar cistern, a large pocket of CSF located in the lower lumbar spine. Direct injection into this space may be accomplished via lumbar puncture. Indwelling pump devices are also available for long-term medication administration. These pumps are typically implanted into subcutaneous abdominal tissue and deliver a continuous infusion or bolus doses of medication into the IT space. The pump's medication reservoir is typically refilled every 1 to 3 months. IT pumps are used most commonly to administer medications for pain and spasticity.

Intraventricular

IVT administration is accomplished by directly instilling drug into the lateral ventricles. Short-term access to the lateral ventricles may be achieved through placement of a ventriculostomy, or external ventricular device (EVD). These catheters have a number of other therapeutic uses and are not placed solely for medication administration under usual circumstances. IVT administration of drug is usually followed by clamping the catheter for at least 15 minutes to allow adequate drug exposure.[8] Disease states in which ventriculostomy clamping would lead to significantly increased intracranial pressures could pose a challenge to drug delivery as cessation of CSF drainage may be detrimental to the patient. In cases where there may be concern for increased ICP, one may consider removing the same volume of CSF prior to instillation of the medication. Long-term access to the lateral ventricles is achieved most commonly through the implantation of an Ommaya reservoir. This device contains a refillable reservoir that sits under the scalp with a catheter that runs to the ventricles.

ANTIBIOTICS

Direct administration of antibiotics into the cerebral compartment may be considered after failure to eradicate the bacteria from the CSF with adequate systemic therapy or in situations where systemic administration cannot produce high enough concentrations in the CSF without producing serious adverse effects. When treating meningitis related to indwelling hardware, IVT treatment has been shown be most successful when administered with concomitant systemic antibiotics and the hardware is removed.

Glycopeptides (Vancomycin/Teicoplanin)

Numerous reports have described the relative efficacy and safety of IT/IVT administration of vancomycin for the treatment of infections caused by gram-positive organisms with reported efficacy between 66% and 95%.[12,13] Dose strategies reported in the literature range from 10 to 20 mg administered IVT daily. For a more tailored regimen, therapeutic drug monitoring has been described to adjust subsequent doses and frequency to achieve a goal CSF trough that is adequate above the MIC.[14–16] Desired CSF vancomycin concentration goals are unclear, however, and the relationship between CSF concentrations and efficacy or toxicity has not yet been elucidated.[17] Overall, in studies where CSF concentrations were measured following IT/IVT administration, results were generally much higher than predicted and extremely variable using customary pharmacokinetic models.[14,15] Goal peak levels obtained approximately 60 minutes after drug administration range from 15 to 40 mg/mL. Higher peak concentrations have been reported with successful outcomes and no increase in side effects, indicating that a peak target concentration is likely unnecessary.

Assuming time-dependent effects in the serum also apply to the CSF, trough CSF concentrations of 10 to 20 mcg/mL would ensure adequate concentrations above the minimum inhibitory concentration (MIC).[18] Higher trough concentrations may be targeted in cases where there is lack of clinical response; in patients with hydrocephalus due to increased volume of distribution; in cases of recurrent infections, abscesses, or fulminant ependymitis; in cases with persistent positive cultures; or when in vitro sensitivity data indicate higher concentrations are desirable. There seems to be a saturable clearance mechanism for the elimination of vancomycin from the CSF as clearance appears to be reduced when higher CSF concentrations are documented.[17] Furthermore, when concomitant systemic vancomycin is given, CSF diffusion out of the central compartment is slowed, resulting in increased CSF concentrations.[19] This suggests that it might be beneficial to administer systemic vancomycin when employing IT/IVT vancomycin therapy.

The possible toxicities associated with administering vancomycin directly into the CSF are controversial. It is difficult to determine if neurologic sequelae reported are secondary to the underlying disease process or adverse effects from the route of administration. Rarely, CSF eosinophilia, headache, and CSF leukocytosis have been reported and do not appear to correlate with CSF drug concentrations. Reports in the literature demonstrate vancomycin CSF levels of more than 500 mcg/mL without adverse effects.[19] No cases of ototoxicity or nephrotoxicity have been described in the literature with IT/IVT therapy. Due to the pH of vancomycin and the lack of buffering capabilities within the CSF, arachnoiditis is possible and may be more common when drug concentrations are elevated.

Duration of treatment requires clinical judgment and can range from 7 to 21 days and is dependent on clinical response, normalization of CSF parameters, and evidence of bacteriologic eradication. Source control is generally necessary, requiring the removal of indwelling devices in some cases.

Another glycopeptide, teicoplanin, has also been successfully administered via the IT/IVT route in doses that range from 5 to 40 mg/d.[20] Although fewer reports have been published with teicoplanin than vancomycin, the medication appears to be well tolerated and carries similar success rates.

Aminoglycosides

Aminoglycosides are bactericidal agents that are active against many strains of gram-negative bacteria, but penetration across the BBB is limited and variable.[21–23] In patients receiving conventional systemic dosing strategies of aminoglycosides, little or no correlation between serum and CSF concentrations has been observed.[24,25] Furthermore, there is a paucity in data evaluating the impact of extended-interval dosing strategies on corresponding CSF concentrations. Meningeal inflammation may enhance CSF penetration slightly but is generally not considered significant enough to produce necessary concentrations to treat CSF infections.

The dose of IV/IVT gentamicin ranges from 1 to 10 mg/d, with the most commonly recommended dose being 4 mg/d. Tobramycin and amikacin doses reported in the literature range from 5 to 20 mg/d and 10 to 50 mg/d, respectively, with the most commonly recommended doses being tobramycin 5 mg/d and amikacin 20 mg/d. Therapeutic drug monitoring has been investigated for the aminoglycosides. Studies evaluating ventricular and lumbar concentrations in relationship to the administration site (IT vs IVT) have given insight into CSF flow and the importance of choosing the correct IT or IVT route for drug delivery. Gentamicin doses of 5 to 10 mg/d administered into the lateral ventricles resulted in peak ventricular concentrations of 12 to 40 mcg/mL and peak lumbar concentrations of 11 to 28 mcg/mL. In comparison, doses of 5 to 10 mg/d administered into the lumbar space resulted in peak ventricular concentrations less than 2.1 mcg/mL and lumbar concentrations of 27 to 81 mcg/mL. Both ventricular and lumber trough concentrations at 24 hours were similar between routes of administration at 3 to 5 mcg/mL. Other studies have evaluated CSF concentrations after IVT administration of 4 to 8 mg/d of gentamicin. Ventricular peak concentrations were reported between 20 and 50 mcg/mL and trough values between 5 and 20 mcg/mL. The half-life in the CSF appears to be prolonged compared with the half-life of systemically administered aminoglycosides, supporting a once-daily dosing interval.

When administered directly into the cerebral compartment, aminoglycosides appear to have the second highest risk of seizures, after beta-lactams, especially when concentrations are greater than 20 mg/L. Tobramycin may be less eleptogenic than gentamicin and may carry a lower risk for seizures than other aminoglycosides.[26] Nephrotoxicity and ototoxcity, common adverse effects seen with systemic aminoglycoside administration, do not appear to be a concern. Amikacin is currently not available in a preservative-free formulation; therefore, careful consideration must be taken when IT or IVT therapy is warranted. The lack of a preservative-free formulation may be the cause for a higher incidence of adverse effects compared with other aminoglycosides. Of note, relapse in infection appears to less common when administered with concomitant systemic antibiotics.[23,27]

Beta-lactams

Penicillin G is a well-known epileptic agent, with seizures reported during both high-dose systemic therapy or after IVT administration.[8] Caution should be used when considering IT/IVT administration of beta-lactam, carbapenem, or cephalosporin antibiotics secondary to reported toxicities, including seizures, tremulousness, supraventricular tachyarrhythmia, incontinence, headache, nausea, and vomiting.[28] Many of the cephalosporins and carbapenems readily cross the BBB when given systemically and therefore eliminate the need to administer directly into the central compartment.

Colistin

With the rise in multiresistant gram-negative CNS infections, IT/IVT administration of colistin, administered as colistin methanesulfonate, has become more frequently reported. Intravenous colistin has poor distribution into the CSF. Studies report CSF concentrations of 11% to 25% of serum concentrations after systemic administration in patients with inflamed meninges.[29–31] IVT doses reported in the literature range from 2 to 10 mg/d, with success rates as high as 89%. Pharmacokinetic studies describe doses greater than 5.22 mg/d result in CSF concentrations continuously above the MIC of 2 mcg/mL and trough concentrations between 2 and 9.7 mcg/mL. The conversion of the pro-drug to the active form in the CSF is not fully understood and appears to have a large patient variability. The elimination of colistin from the CSF appears to be dose independent and monoexponential, with 10% eliminated every hour. Elimination, however, may be higher in cases where there is large CSF diversion via a ventriculostomy drain, and doses of 10 mg/d should be considered in such cases. Toxicities, although rare, include reversible chemical ventriculitis and meningitis, seizures, hypotonia, diaphragmatic paralysis, and cauda equine syndrome.

Daptomycin

CNS infections associated with a neurosurgical procedures are frequently caused by gram-positive organisms, including staphylococci, streptococci, and entero-cocci, including vancomycin-resistant strains. Multidrug resistance is occurring more frequently in both nosocomial and community-acquired infections. Daptomycin, a cyclic lipopeptide, has been shown to be rapidly bactericidal against enterococci, including vancomycin-resistant strains. Daptomycin penetrates poorly into the CSF compartment when given via the systemic route, and therefore IVT administration may be considered for the treatment of CNS infections caused by resistant strains that do not respond to conventional therapy.

IVT doses of daptomycin reported range between 5 and 10 mg/d. Small pharmacokinetic studies have evaluated the ventricular CSF peak and trough concentrations after 5- and 10-mg/d doses. Peak concentrations of 112 and 483 mcg/mL and trough concentrations of 1.34 and 23 mcg/mL, respectively, for each dose were reported.[32,33] After 3 days of daily administration, daptomycin appears to accumulate in the CSF and may increase the risk of toxicities with continued administration. Due to this accumulation, daily administration for 3 consecutive days followed by a reduction in the frequency to every 72 hours has been recommended. CSF peak and trough concentrations reported with every 3-day administration are 139 mcg/mL and 9.9 mcg/mL, respectively. Toxicities with IVT daptomycin appear rare, and the authors are not aware of any reports of toxicities in the literature, although its use in this capacity is relatively new.

Chloramphenicol

In contrast to previously described antibiotics, chloramphenicol has relatively good CSF penetration when administered systemically with a CSF/serum concentration ratio of 0.67. Chloramphenicol may be considered bacteriocidal against *Streptococcus pneumoniae*, *Haemophilus influenzae*, and *Neisseria meningitidis*, but in other bacterial infections, its bacteriostatic nature may be cause to directly instill into the central compartment. Direct IT or IVT instillation may be also required in refractory infections or in rare cases where in vitro sensitivity data indicate a higher MIC.[34] Doses reported in the literature range from 25 to 100 mg/d and should be combined with systemic therapy to improve CSF concentrations by minimizing rapid redistribution out of the CNS compartment. Combined IVT with systemic administration revealed significantly higher CSF concentrations between 18 and 134 mcg/mL compared with systemic administration alone with CNS concentrations from 0.4 to 23 mcg/mL. Few toxicities have been reported in the literature with direct cerebral instillation (Table 10.2).

THROMBOLYTIC THERAPY

The first use of intracerebroventricular thrombolytic therapy in humans appeared in the literature in 1991. Neither efficacy nor safety has been firmly established by well-designed studies, but more than 200 published reports have described IT/IVT recombinant tissue plasminogen activator (rt-PA, alteplase) and urokinase for the treatment of primary and secondary intraventricular hemorrhage (IVH). These studies suggest beneficial effects on intraventricular

TABLE 10.2 Antibiotics: Common Dose and Physiochemical Properties

Medication	Most Common Adult IT/IVT Dose	Concentration (Variable Based on Institution and Product Available)	pH	Osmolarity, mOsm/kg
Amikacin	20 mg every 24 hours	1 mg/mL NS	3.5–5.5	349
Amphotericin B	0.5 mg every 24 hours	0.5 mg/3 mL SWFI	5.7	256
Chloramphenicol	25–100 mg every 24 hours	100 mg/1 mL SWFI	4.5–7.5	
Colistin	5–10 mg every 24 hours	10 mg/3 mL NS	7.8	367
Daptomycin	5 mg every 24 hours × 3 doses, then every 72 hours	5 mg/3 mL NS	4–5	304–364
Gentamicin	5 mg every 24 hours	5 mg/1 mL NS	3–5.5	293
Teicoplanin	5–20 mg/d	400 mg/3 mL NS	7.2–7.8	
Tobramycin	5 mg every 24 hours	5 mg/1 mL NS	3–6.5	334
Vancomycin	10–20 mg every 24 hours	10 mg/1 mL NS	2.5–4.5	291

Note: IT, intrathecal; IVT, intracerebroventricular; NS, normal saline; SWFI, sterile water for injection.

clot resolution, ICP, ventricular size, and mortality.[35–40] Urokinase and rt-PA initiate local fibrinolysis by binding to fibrin and convert entrapped plasminogen to plasmin. Administration of these agents directly into the ventricles of the brain requires full consideration of risks and benefits. Urokinanse is no longer available in the United States, and rt-PA is not approved by the US Food and Drug Administration (FDA) for IT/IVT administration.

Several small studies of intraventricular or intracisternal thrombolysis in patients with subarachnoid hemorrhage with IVH have shown promising results. These studies seem to suggest that thrombolytic treatment hastens clearance of blood in the ventricles, normalizes ICP, reduces hydrocephalus, and may prevent vasospasm.[41] In several reported case series, IVT rt-PA was used safely after endovascular aneurysmal coiling.[41] One prospective, randomized trial, published in 2004, evaluated the IVT administration of urokinase, 25,000 IU every 12 hours until clot resolution, in patients with SAH with IVH. Results demonstrated earlier clot resolution in the treatment group compared with placebo, 4.7 days vs 8.5 days, respectively.[42] Shortly after, urokinase was withdrawn from the market due to safety concerns, and rt-PA emerged as the primary thrombolytic for IVT administration.

A systematic review, conducted by Lapointe and Haines,[43] evaluated the safety and efficacy of intracerebrothrombolysis. Ten studies were identified, evaluated, and ultimately excluded for various reasons. The authors concluded that the evidence, albeit weak, may be suggestive that IVT administration of a fibrinolytic agent in patients with IVH or SAH may be safe. They also concluded that IVT fibrinolytic therapy may be a valuable treatment, although the need for a prospective, randomized study is warranted to make a more conclusive recommendation as trials thus far are of insufficient size and quality to allow any determination.

The Clot Lysis Evaluating Accelerated Resolution of Intraventricular Hemorrhage (CLEAR-IVH) trial is a phase II randomized clinical trial using rt-PA to treat IVH in patients with an intracerebral hemorrhage volume less than 30 mL.[44] The end points included time to clot resolution, ICP, cerebral perfusion pressure (CPP), hydrocephalus with need for shunting, vasospasm, and morbidity and mortality. A dose- and interval-finding design was created with doses ranging from 0.3 to 3 mg every 8 or 12 hours. In treated patients, it appears that rt-PA facilitated opening of the ventricular system (18% per day for rt-PA vs 8% per day for placebo; $P < .001$), was associated with a higher rate of successful removal of the EVD (50% rt-PA vs 20% placebo), and improved 30-day outcomes in all prespecified areas. Neither ICP nor CPP differed substantially between the treatment groups on presentation, with EVD closure, or during the active treatment phase. Mortality (19% rtPA vs 23% placebo) and ventriculitis (8% rtPA vs 9% placebo) were substantially lower than expected, and bleeding events remained below the prespecified threshold (23% rtPA vs 5% placebo; $P = .1$).

CLEAR-III is a phase III, randomized, multicenter, double-blind, placebo-controlled study comparing the use of IVT rt-PA to IVT injections of normal saline (placebo) for the treatment of IVH. The primary outcome is a dichotomized modified Rankin Scale of 0 to 3 vs 4 to 6 at 180 days.[37] Clinical secondary outcomes include additional modified Rankin Scale dichotomizations at 180 days (0–4 vs 5–6), ordinal modified Rankin Scale (0–6), mortality and safety events at 30 days, mortality at 180 days, functional status, type and intensity of intensive care unit management, rate and extent of ventricular blood clot removal, and quality-of-life measures. Enrollment was completed in 2015, and results suggest low doses of rt-PA (1.0 mg) given every 8 hours are safe and effective in patients with stable IVH.

Pharmacokinetic data suggest that the half-life of rt-PA in the ventricular cavity is approximately 3 hours, and newer data from the CLEAR-III trial suggest that it may be even longer than originally described. Most investigators have taken the practical approach of closing the ventricular drainage system for 1 hour following fibrinolytic instillation to allow for drug-clot interactions

TABLE 10.3 Recombinant Tissue Plasminogen Activator (Alteplase):
Common Dose and Physiochemical Properties

Medication	Common Adult IT/IVT Dose	Concentration	pH	Osmolarity, mOsm/kg	Preservatives
Alteplase	0.3–3 mg every 8–12 hours	1 mg/mL in SWFI	7.3	215	None

Note: IT, intrathecal; IVT, intracerebroventricular; SWFI, sterile water for injection.

and to optimize clot lysis, but clamping for a longer period of time, if the ICP remains stable, may allow for a longer duration of activity.

IVT thrombolytics have been administered to hundreds of patients worldwide and continues to be widely used despite a paucity of strong evidence demonstrating efficacy or safety. IVT thrombolysis with rt-PA may be considered for patients with a significant amount of IVH that require EVD placement. Precautions and contraindications to consider include unprotected vascular malformation and coagulopathy (Table 10.3).[45]

VASOACTIVE AGENTS

Nitroprusside

Despite the best current medical practices, cerebral vasospasm with delayed cerebral ischemic deficits remains an important cause of permanent neurological injury and death following aneurysmal SAH. Its pathophysiology is poorly understood. One plausible theory to describe the pathophysiology of these delayed ischemic events involves activation of the gene that codes for vasoconstriction while simultaneously removing the influence of the potent vasodilator nitric oxide (NO) via direct binding. This disequilibrium appears to mitigate cerebral vasoconstriction. Sodium nitroprusside (SNP), a direct-acting vasodilator of vascular smooth muscle, works as a NO donor and may be useful to combat NO deficiencies that appear to contribute to this process.[46] Arterial hypotension and the theoretical elevations in ICP that may occur when administering intravenous SNP have deterred clinicians from consistently using this agent. IVT administration of SNP, however, offers a novel therapeutic option for the treatment and/or prophylaxis of refractory cerebral vasospasm following SAH.[47] The direct intracerebroventricular route of administration and the short biological half-life of this medication give the advantage of causing local vasodilation while reducing the risk of systemic complications. For IVT administration, SNP can be reconstituted and diluted in either normal saline or fresh autologous CSF to 0.4% (4 mg/mL) and administered directly into a ventriculostomy or an Ommaya reservoir placed in the ventricular cavity during the clipping of the aneurysm.[47,48]

Several case series have described IVT SNP administration for the treatment of refractory cerebral vasospasm as well as prophylaxis for cerebral vasospasm in high-risk patients.[46–48] Treatment doses were considered when rescue therapy was necessary for severe, symptomatic vasospasm in patients with new neurologic deficits attributable to vasospasm or acute elevations in transcranial Doppler ultrasonography (TCD) velocities were noted. IVT treatment dose strategies described include 1- to 4-mg bolus doses, administered over 1 to 2 minutes, and repeated intermittently, not more frequently than every 5 minutes. Subsequent doses were adjusted according to the patient's clinical response or radiographic response monitored by serial angiography or TCD. Dosing continued until there was resolution of angiographic vasospasm, no resolution of vasoconstriction detected within 30 minutes of the initial dose, or intolerable adverse effects were detected. The majority (83%-100%) of patients treated with at least 30 mg IVT SNP demonstrated reversal or amelioration of vasoconstriction. Total doses administered ranged from 4 to 88 mg. Adverse effects reported included systemic hypotension, nausea, and vomiting, which were successfully treated with vasopressors and antiemetics, respectively. No cases of elevated ICP or cyanide toxicity were observed. Most (70%-76%) of those treated reported good or excellent overall neurological outcome at 3 to 6 months.

Prophylactic dosing strategies are described as either an 8-mg IVT infusion over 60 minutes or more commonly 4- to 8-mg doses administered IVT, over 1 to 2 minutes, 3 times daily continued for 1 to 8 days.[47,48] Although small sample sizes have been reported, no patient receiving prophylaxis with SNP developed clinical vasospasm symptoms. Most of the patients receiving prophylactic therapy experienced nausea (6/10), which could be blunted with pretreatment antiemetic administration. Again, no cases of elevated ICP or cyanide toxicity were observed.

Although safety has been the focus of most studies investigating IVT SNP for the treatment and prophylaxis of refractory cerebral vasospasm, the preliminary data suggest it may be a useful and safe therapy to employ. Careful monitoring of both hemodynamic and ICP remain imperative due to the potential risks of systemic hypotension and intracranial hypertension, although no elevations in ICP have been reported to date in the literature.

Nicardipine

Nicardipine is a dihydropyridine calcium antagonist with potent arterial vasodilator properties. Calcium antagonists have been widely studied for both the treatment and prevention of refractory vasospasm following aneurysmal SAH. The beneficial vasodilating effects are often limited by its hypotensive effects when administered intravenously. IVT administration may offer a more targeted delivery and lessen unwanted systemic effects.

Initial studies evaluated the effects of prophylactic IVT nicardipine on cerebral vasospasm in patients with severe SAH. Doses between 2 and 4 mg, diluted in 10 mL of saline, were administered into cisternal drains placed intraoperatively during aneurysm clipping. Doses were administered every 8 to 12 hours for 10 to 17 days.[49–51] Although not statistically significant, both angiographic and clinical vasospasm were reduced by 20% and 26%, respectively. Outcomes were similar among treated and nontreated groups. Adverse effects, however, may limit the overall utility of this therapy. Adverse events reported with IVT nicardipine include severe headache, nausea, vomiting, increased cerebral infection rate, and increased risk for hypocephalus with increased ventriculoperitoneal shunt requirement. Nicardipine levels in the CSF examined 12 hours after drug administration were 231.44 mcg/mL, which matched the effective concentration revealed in a previous in vitro study and ensured an effective concentration in the CSF at the end of the longest dosing interval.

Nicardipine can also be administered into the CSF via prolonged-release implants; however, the effectiveness of this formulation is limited by the rate of diffusion of the released drug into the CSF.[52–54]

Nimodipine

Nimodipine is a dihydropyridine calcium channel blocker that binds specifically to L-type voltage-gated calcium channels and inhibits calcium ion transfer into vascular smooth muscle cells and thus inhibits contractions of vascular smooth muscle. Nimodipine appears to be more selective for cerebral arteries than systemic arteries due to its high lipophilicity, allowing it to cross the BBB. A plethora of clinical studies have demonstrated the efficacy and safety of systemic nimodipine in reducing the severity of neurological deficits resulting from vasospasm and delayed cerebral ischemia after aneurysmal SAH.[55–57] In addition, the effect of intra-arterial nimodipine on vasospasm is well known and is a common practice during aneurysm surgery at many centers.[58] There are, however, limited human studies on the use of IT/IVT nimodipine.[59–61] IVT

TABLE 10.4 Vasoactive: Common Dose and Physiochemical Properties

Medication	Common Adult IT/IVT Dose	Concentration (Variable Based on Institution and Product Available)	pH	Osmolarity, mOsm/kg
Nitroprusside	Treatment: 1–4 mg IVT every 5 minutes until angiographic resolution of VSP (typical total = 30 mg) Prophylaxis: 1–8 mg IVT 3 times daily or 8 mg IT over 60 minutes	4 mg/mL in NS or autologous CSF	3.5–6	
Nicardipine	2–4 mg IVT every 8–12 hours	1 mg/mL in NS	3.5	300
Nimodipine	0.4-mg/dose IVT bolus followed by 0.4-mg/h IVT infusion	0.02 mg/mL in LR		

Note: CSF, cerebrospinal fluid; IT, intrathecal; IVT, intracerebroventricular; LR, lactated ringer; NS, normal saline; VSP, vasospasm.

nimodipine use has been reported in a small number of patients with refractory cerebral vasospasm. Dose strategies described include an initial 0.4-mg IVT bolus administered via a ventriculostomy drain, followed by an IT infusion at a rate of 0.4 mg/h via an indwelling lumbar catheter for 3 to 9 days.[62] Of the 8 patients described, 3 had improvement in neurological condition during drug therapy, 4 experienced no change, and the neurologic assessment was unable to be attained in 1. CT perfusion and TCD velocities improved slightly in 71% and 67%, respectively. Documented adverse effects included systemic hypotension and bacterial meningitis (Table 10.4).

INTRATHECAL MEDICATIONS ADMINISTERED AS CONTINUOUS INFUSIONS

The first reservoir for IT medication administration was implanted in 1981.[63] Since then, medications administered via implanted IT pumps have been used for the management of a wide variety of conditions associated with pain and spasticity. Recommendations regarding the role of IT therapy in the management of these conditions vary, but in general, the IT route has been reserved for patients who experience an inadequate response to more conservative therapies or who experience intolerable side effects from alternative treatments.

While the IT route of administration has been demonstrated to be safe and effective in select patients, it is associated with a significant initial cost following implantation and is not without risk.[64] The cost-benefit ratio associated with implanted IT devices improves over time, although the "break-even" point is variable. Compared with other implanted systems used for pain management, for example, the IT route becomes more cost-effective when therapy continues beyond 3 months.[64] A variety of economic factors, including individual insurance coverage and background medication regimen prior to IT conversion, influence the economic feasibility of pump implantation for an individual patient.[65] Specific adverse effects vary by medication regimen. Device- and procedure-related complications such as infections, CSF leak, and pump malfunction have been noted with all therapies. Granuloma formation at the catheter tip as a result of stimulation of arachnoid mast cell degranulation has been reported with a number of medications but is predominantly associated with high concentrations of IT opioids. Symptoms of tachyphylaxis or alterations in motor or sensory function should prompt further investigation into the possibility of granuloma formation.[66–69]

Many controversies surrounding the use of IT medications exist. Specifically, variable recommendations exist regarding patient selection, the role of medication trials, initial medication, titration approach, and the role of combination therapy. Heterogeneous patient populations, variability in medication selection, medication combination, and device and administration strategies within the literature complicate resolution of these controversies. Thus, current practice remains largely driven by clinical experience and expert consensus. In this section, medications frequently used as IT continuous infusions via implanted pumps will be discussed and relevant controversies highlighted.

Opioids: Morphine, Hydromorphone, and Fentanyl

Intrathecal opioids have been studied alone and in combination for the management of cancer and noncancer chronic pain. Improved pain scores, quality of life, functional status, and mortality have all been noted with IT opioid therapy to varying degrees in the literature. While improvement in pain has been noted with IT opioid therapy, patients often continue to experience uncontrolled pain. In addition, evidence supporting IT opioid use is overall moderate to low quality.

Respiratory depression, nausea, vomiting, and constipation have been noted with IT opioids.[68,69] Generally, adverse effects from IT opioid administration occur less frequently compared with systemic administration. Respiratory depression remains an important cause of mortality in patients receiving opioids through implanted IT devices.[68,69] The physiochemical characteristics of the various opioids affect the timing of respiratory depression following IT administration. Morphine is more hydrophilic than fentanyl and thus distributes out of the CSF and into tissue more slowly. Thus, respiratory depression following fentanyl administration typically occurs within 30 minutes of administration, while this adverse effect is not typically observed for several hours and may persist for 18 to 24 hours following morphine injection. Strategies to minimize the risk of respiratory depression include frequent monitoring in the 12 to 24 hours following pump implantation, initiation of low doses and slow titration of IT opioids, minimization of concomitant systemic opioid medications following implantation, and appropriate patient selection.[67] While medical comorbidities and conditions that might place patients at an increased risk of respiratory depression should be reviewed and addressed prior to pump implantation, to date there is insufficient evidence to suggest any medical comorbidities to be absolute contraindications to IT therapy.[65] Granuloma formation has also been noted most commonly with high doses of IT opioids, especially morphine. Strategies to minimize IT opioid exposure, including the use of adjuvant therapies, have been suggested to minimize the risk of granuloma formation.[66,70]

A medication trial has been advocated by many to evaluate the safety and efficacy of IT opioid therapy prior to pump implantation.[65] Trialing opioids is a significant point of controversy. Practice varies widely, and there is a lack of support in the literature for any single method that is able to reliably predict success. In addition, the optimal threshold for "passing" or "failing" a trial is unclear. Generally, a reduction in pain scores by 50% or more is considered success. Single- and repeat-bolus IT and/or epidural dosing have been used, as has placement of a temporary external catheter for IT or epidural administration of a continuous infusion. Recommendations regarding equipotent dosing exist, although discrepancies, similar to those described with systemic conversion ratios, also exist. Trialing is usually done in the inpatient setting, and trial duration varies widely.[71]

Morphine, hydromorphone, and fentanyl are opioids that have been successfully administered via the IT route. A preservative-free formulation of morphine for IT use received FDA approval for the treatment of intractable chronic pain in 1990 as an orphan drug. It is currently the only opioid on the market with this designation and is generally considered the first-line opioid for IT use. Hydromorphone and fentanyl have less evidence supporting their use, although their popularity is growing. Evidence suggests patients poorly responsive to morphine or those experiencing intolerable adverse effects may benefit from switching to hydromorphone or fentanyl.

Ziconotide

Ziconotide is a nonopioid analgesic approved by the FDA in 2004 for the treatment of severe, chronic pain. It has been studied alone and in combination with

IT opioids as a part of the management of a variety of cancer and noncancer pain syndromes, including neuropathic pain. Improvements in pain scores and concomitant IT morphine needs have been observed in a variety of settings. In addition, tolerance has rarely been observed in ziconotide trials to date.[72]

Ziconotide is a synthetic derivative of a compound found in the venom of the predatory sea snail, *Conus magnus*. Its precise mechanism of pain inhibition is unclear. It binds N-type calcium channels on the dorsal horn of the spinal column, and this activity is believed to inhibit excitatory neurotransmitter release from afferent nerves, thus interrupting pain signaling. Ziconotide distributes widely through the CSF and diffuses poorly through the BBB. Thus, ziconotide is eliminated from the CSF predominantly through bulk CSF outflow.[72]

Since it has no activity at opioid receptors, ziconotide's adverse effect profile varies significantly from IT opioids commonly used for pain management. In addition, adverse effects of ziconotide generally take several days to appear.[65] Ziconotide has not been observed to have the same risk of respiratory depression or granuloma formation as morphine and consequently has been advocated as an alternative option for patients who experience such complications.[66] Adverse effects that have been frequently observed include nausea, dizziness, and confusion. Some of the most concerning adverse effects noted with ziconotide have been psychiatric in nature and include suicidal ideation, worsening of mood disorders, and new-onset psychosis. These neuropsychiatric effects resulted in a black box warning advocating against use in patients with a history of psychosis.

Most adverse effects have been related to aggressive titration schedules or high doses and are generally reversible. Since coming on the market, slower titration schemes and lower initial doses than those described in the FDA labeling have been advocated to minimize the risk of adverse effects. Specifically, a starting dose of 0.5 mg/d titrated in increments of 0.5 mg/d no more often than once a week has been recommended.[65] Furthermore, complications related to abrupt discontinuation have been infrequently described. Finally, renal failure from rhabdomyolysis has been observed and should be evaluated in patients who experience new muscle pain or weakness.[66]

Baclofen

Baclofen is a $GABA_B$ receptor agonist with a limited ability to pass through the BBB. Oral baclofen entered the US market following FDA approval in 1977. The first report of IT baclofen used for the treatment of severe spasticity was published in 1985 and was later granted FDA approval in 1997 for the treatment of spasticity of cerebral origin.[73] Since then, it has been used in the management of a variety of conditions resulting in pain and spasticity. Compared with other IT agents, baclofen has a large body evidence supporting its use. Favorable spasticity-related outcomes have been demonstrated in most trials regardless of the underlying diagnosis. Data supporting improvement in functional status and quality-of-life measures are less robust.[74] IT baclofen therapy is generally reserved for patients whose spasticity is not well controlled with oral therapy or who experience intolerable side effects with oral therapy such as drowsiness and confusion. Evidence supporting IT baclofen use for the management of chronic pain is less strong but may be effective when pain is muscle spasm related or neuropathic in origin.[75]

Prior to pump implantation, a trial using IT bolus dosing is recommended. An initial bolus dose of 50 mcg should be followed by observation for 4 to 8 hours. This may be done in the inpatient or outpatient setting. Following an initial dose, clinical effects may be observed as early as 30 minutes to 1 hour after administration. A peak effect is usually observed 4 hours after administration and persists for 8 hours. A positive response using the Ashworth Scale or similar objective measure of spasticity within 8 hours is desired. If the patient response is inadequate, additional trials using 75 mcg and 100 mcg may be considered 24 hours later. In severe cases, trials using a continuous infusion via a temporary IT catheter have also been described.[76] After a successful trial dose has been established, the initial maintenance dose is determined by doubling the trial dose and administering it over 24 hours. If the clinical effect of the trial dose extends beyond 8 hours, doubling the dose is not recommended, and administering the trial dose over 24 hours is recommended. Following implantation, the 24-hour dose may be titrated in increments of 5% to 30% every 24 hours.

Adverse effects from IT baclofen are usually minimal but include confusion, drowsiness, and nausea. The greatest risk associated with IT baclofen therapy is acute withdrawal caused by abrupt discontinuation. Acute withdrawal may result in hallucinations, agitation, muscle rigidity, hyperthermia, seizures, multiorgan system failure, and death. A single effective approach to managing acute withdrawal has not been established. Thus, treatment generally consists of supportive care and attempts to minimize CNS complications.[77] Baclofen replacement using oral therapy is generally inadequate given the limited ability of baclofen to diffuse across the BBB and great disparity between CSF concentrations achieved when the IT vs oral route is used.[77,78] Successful management of withdrawal symptoms with the use of a temporary IT catheter and continuous-infusion baclofen has been reported.[79] Benzodiazepines have also

TABLE 10.5 Comparative Properties of Medications Frequently Administered as Continuous Intrathecal Infusions

Medication	pH	Dose	Concentration[a]	Diluents	Preservatives
Morphine	2.5–6.5	1–20 mg/d	0.5 mg/mL 1 mg/mL 10 mg/mL 25 mg/mL	NS	None
Hydromorphone	4–5.5	0.5–10 mg/d	1 mg/mL 2 mg/mL 4 mg/mL 10 mg/mL	NS	None
Fentanyl	4–7.5	0.02–0.3 mg/d	50 mcg/mL	NS	None
Ziconotide	4–5	0.24–19.2 mcg/d	25 mcg/mL 100 mcg/mL	NS	None
Baclofen	5–7	0.05–0.8 mg/d	20 mcg/mL	NS	None

Note: NS, normal saline.

[a]Commercially available products.

been used in the management of acute baclofen withdrawal. Aggressive dosing and rapid titration of benzodiazepines may be required to adequately address withdrawal symptoms that may necessitate airway support. A variety of additional agents have been used in the literature, all with varying degrees of success, including propofol, cyproheptadine, dantrolene, tizanidine, and paralysis (Table 10.5).[77]

INTERFERON-ALPHA

Intraventricular interferon-alpha has been used as an adjunct in the treatment of subacute sclerosing panencephalitis (SSPE), a degenerative and ultimately fatal neurologic complication of measles (rubeola) infection. The pathophysiology of SSPE is incompletely understood. Ongoing immune response caused by incompletely cleared virus is thought to be the primary cause.[80] A variety of antiretroviral and anti-inflammatory therapies have been investigated, but the most effective treatment strategy remains unknown.[80–82]

Interferon-alpha has both antiviral and anti-inflammatory properties, making it an attractive treatment option for SSPE. Intraventricular interferon-alpha has been studied largely in combination with isoprinosine. While data are limited, some reports suggest symptomatic improvement, although without a

Table 10.6 Dosage of Interferon-Alpha-2b for Induction and Maintenance Treatment of Subacute Sclerosing Panencephalitis

Induction	Day 1: 100,000 U/m²
	Day 2: 200,000 U/m²
	Day 3: 400,000 U/m²
	Day 4: 800,000 U/m²
	Day 5: 1,000,000 U/m²
	Day 6: none
	Day 7: none
Maintenance	1,000,000 U/m² two times a week

Source: Reference 84.

survival benefit. Dosages and durations of interferon–alpha used in practice vary. In general, therapy is initiated at a low dose and titrated up over the course of 5 to 10 days to a maintenance dose that is then administered 1 to 3 times per week (Table 10.6).[80–82] Duration varies from months to years and is largely dependent on patient response and complications such as infection. One of the few randomized controlled trials investigating the role of IVT interferon–alpha-2b used the dosing scheme outlined in Table 10.6 and reported a low incidence of adverse effects. Adverse effects associated with IVT interferon include hyperthermia (particularly around the time of administration), headache, and neurologic side effects that are difficult to distinguish between therapy and disease progression.[80–83]

Therapy has shown improvement in modified Rankin Scale over a 12-month period.[84]

Glucocorticosteroids

Glucocorticosteroids are used for the treatment of several inflammatory neurologic diseases, including multiple sclerosis and neuropathic pain syndromes. Systemic glucocorticosteroids have poor CSF bioavailability; intrathecal administration offers an alternative method of delivering these medications into the CSF.[85] For many decades, glucocorticosteroids such as methylprednisolone, dexamethasone, and triamcinolone have been studied for intrathecal administration. Glucocorticosteroids exert their overall anti-inflammatory effect by suppression of inflammatory processes or enhancement of anti-inflammatory mechanisms.[86] Intrathecal glucocorticosteroid is usually administered into the lumbar cistern through a spinal needle during a lumbar puncture. It may also be administered via a temporary indwelling, subcutaneously tunneled catheter. The ideal dosing of these intrathecal glucocorticosteroids is unknown, and the studied doses vary by drug, indication, and severity of the disease state. Methylprednisolone in its acetate form is more commonly used as opposed to the water-soluble succinate formulation. The lack of solubility of the acetate formulation creates a depot that is released over a prolonged period of time when administered into the intrathecal space, with a duration of up to 21 days.[86,87] The use of intrathecal methylprednisolone at doses ranging from 40 to 80 mg weekly for up to 4 weeks resulted in neuropathic pain relief in more than 70% of patients for up to 2 years.[88,89] In contrast, some other studies have shown no benefit in neuropathic pain relief.[85–87] Intrathecal triamcinolone acetonide 40- to 80-mg suspension diluted in 0.9% normal saline every other day up to 5 doses improved spasticity and maximum walking distance in patients with multiple sclerosis.[90] Administration of intrathecal glucocorticosteroid requires full consideration of risks and benefits, including risk for neurotoxicity, paresthesia, CNS infection, intraspinal, cerebral hemorrhage, and arachnoiditis. The commercially available methylprednisolone (Depo-medrol) 40-mg/mL suspension contains polyethylene glycol and myristyl-gamma-picolinium, which have been suggested to be responsible for the neurotoxicity. Of note, there are no preservative-free, commercial formulations of methylprednisolone, but there are several techniques such as centrifugation to decrease the concentrations of these preservatives.[87] Considering its questionable efficacy and current safety concerns, further clinical trials are needed to evaluate the efficacy and safety of intrathecal glucocorticosteroid therapy in inflammatory neurologic diseases. Thus, intrathecal glucocorticosteroids should not be used in place of first-line standard-of-care therapies.

CONCLUSION

Direct administration of medications into the CNS remains a complex intervention that is being considered more frequently in cases where the choice medication does not effectively penetrate the BBB or when intravenous or oral routes have proven to be ineffective. Guidelines are lacking, and therefore instillation of drugs directly into the CSF must be done carefully and with full consideration of factors affecting the efficacy and safety of this route of administration. When selecting a medication for intrathecal or intracerebroventricular administration, the physiochemical properties of the drug must be carefully considered in conjunction with its therapeutic indication. Consultation with a clinical pharmacist is recommended to ensure safe dosing, admixture preparation, and monitoring.

References

1. Pardridge WM. Blood-brain barrier delivery. *Drug Discov Today*. 2007;12:54–61.
2. Lorenzo AV, Page LK, Watters GV. Relationship between cerebrospinal fluid formation, absorption and pressure in human hydrocephalus. *Brain*. 1970;93:679–692.
3. Sakka L, Coll G, Chazal J. Anatomy and physiology of cerebrospinal fluid. *Eur Ann Otorhinolaryngol Head Neck Dis*. 2011;128:309–316.
4. de Boer AG, Gaillard PJ. Strategies to improve drug delivery across the blood-brain barrier. *Clin Pharmacokinet*. 2007;46:553–576.
5. Nau R, Sorgel F, Eiffert H. Penetration of drugs through the blood-cerebrospinal fluid/blood-brain barrier for treatment of central nervous system infections. *Clin Microbiol Rev*. 2010;23:858–883.
6. Patel MM, Goyal BR, Bhadada SV, et al. Getting into the brain: approaches to enhance brain drug delivery. *CNS Drugs*. 2009;23:35–58.
7. de Boer AG, Gaillard PJ. Drug targeting to the brain. *Annu Rev Pharmacol Toxicol*. 2007;47:323–355.
8. Cook AM, Mieure KD, Owen RD, et al. Intracerebroventricular administration of drugs. *Pharmacotherapy*. 2009;29:832–845.
9. Jordan GD, Themelis NJ, Messerly SO, et al. Doxapram and potential benzyl alcohol toxicity: a moratorium on clinical investigation? *Pediatrics*. 1986;78:540–541.
10. Hodgson PS, Neal JM, Pollock JE, Liu SS. The neurotoxicity of drugs given intrathecally (spinal). *Anesth Analg*. 1999;88:797–809.
11. Li X, Wu Y, Sun S, et al. Population pharmacokinetics of vancomycin in postoperative neurosurgical patients. *J Pharm Sci*. 2015;104:3960–3967.
12. Bayston R, Barnicoat M, Cudmore RE, et al. The use of intraventricular vancomycin in the treatment of CSF shunt-associated ventriculitis. *Z Kinderchir*. 1984;39(suppl 2):111–113.
13. Ng K, Mabasa VH, Chow I, Ensom MH. Systematic review of efficacy, pharmacokinetics, and administration of intraventricular vancomycin in adults. *Neurocrit Care*. 2014;20:158–171.
14. Pfausler B, Haring HP, Kampfl A, et al. Cerebrospinal fluid (CSF) pharmacokinetics of intraventricular vancomycin in patients with staphylococcal ventriculitis associated with external CSF drainage. *Clin Infect Dis*. 1997;25:733–735.
15. Chen K, Wu Y, Wang Q, et al. The methodology and pharmacokinetics study of intraventricular administration of vancomycin in patients with intracranial infections after craniotomy. *J Crit Care*. 2015;30:218.e1–5.
16. Amod F, Moodley I, Peer AK, et al. Ventriculitis due to a hetero strain of vancomycin intermediate *Staphylococcus aureus* (hVISA): successful treatment with linezolid in combination with intraventricular vancomycin. *J Infect*. 2005;50:252–257.
17. Reesor C, Chow AW, Kureishi A, Jewesson PJ. Kinetics of intraventricular vancomycin in infections of cerebrospinal fluid shunts. *J Infect Dis*. 1988;158:1142–1143.
18. Nagl M, Neher C, Hager J, et al. Bactericidal activity of vancomycin in cerebrospinal fluid. *Antimicrob Agents Chemother*. 1999;43:1932–1934.
19. Luer MS, Hatton J. Vancomycin administration into the cerebrospinal fluid: a review. *Ann Pharmacother*. 1993;27:912–921.
20. Beenen LF, Touw DJ, Hekker TA, Haring DA. Pharmacokinetics of intraventricularly administered teicoplanin in Staphylococci ventriculitis. *Pharm World Sci*. 2000;22:127–9.

21. Nau R, Scholz P, Sharifi S, et al. Netilmicin cerebrospinal fluid concentrations after an intravenous infusion of 400 mg in patients without meningeal inflammation. *J Antimicrob Chemother.* 1993;32:893–896.

22. Briedis DJ, Robson HG. Cerebrospinal fluid penetration of amikacin. *Antimicrob Agents Chemother.* 1978;13:1042–1043.

23. Tangden T, Enblad P, Ullberg M, Sjolin J. Neurosurgical gram-negative bacillary ventriculitis and meningitis: a retrospective study evaluating the efficacy of intraventricular gentamicin therapy in 31 consecutive cases. *Clin Infect Dis.* 2011;52:1310–1316.

24. Mangi RJ, Holstein LL, Andriole VT. Treatment of gram-negative bacillary meningitis with intrathecal gentamicin. *Yale J Biol Med.* 1977;50:31–41.

25. Nevrekar S, Cunningham KC, Greathouse KM, Panos NG. Dual intraventricular plus systemic antibiotic therapy for the treatment of *Klebsiella pneumoniae* carbapenemase-producing *Klebsiella pneumoniae* ventriculitis. *Ann Pharmacother.* 2014;48:274–278.

26. McCracken GH, Nelson JD. Commentary: an appraisal of tobramycin usage in pediatrics. *J Pediatr.* 1976;88:315–317.

27. Kaiser AB, McGee ZA. Aminoglycoside therapy of gram-negative bacillary meningitis. *N Engl J Med.* 1975;293:1215–1220.

28. Manzella JP, Paul RL, Butler IL. CNS toxicity associated with intraventricular injection of cefazolin: report of three cases. *J Neurosurg.* 1988;68:970–971.

29. Markantonis SL, Markou N, Fousteri M, et al. Penetration of colistin into cerebrospinal fluid. *Antimicrob Agents Chemother.* 2009;53:4907–4910.

30. Kasiakou SK, Rafailidis PI, Liaropoulos K, Falagas ME. Cure of post-traumatic recurrent multiresistant gram-negative rod meningitis with intraventricular colistin. *J Infect.* 2005;50:348–352.

31. Ziaka M, Markantonis SL, Fousteri M, et al. Combined intravenous and intraventricular administration of colistin methanesulfonate in critically ill patients with central nervous system infection. *Antimicrob Agents Chemother.* 2013;57:1938–1940.

32. Butterfield JM, Mueller BA, Patel N, et al. Daptomycin pharmacokinetics and pharmacodynamics in a pooled sample of patients receiving thrice-weekly hemodialysis. *Antimicrob Agents Chemother.* 2013;57:864–872.

33. Mueller SW, Kiser TH, Anderson TA, Neumann RT. Intraventricular daptomycin and intravenous linezolid for the treatment of external ventricular-drain-associated ventriculitis due to vancomycin-resistant *Enterococcus faecium*. *Ann Pharmacother.* 2012;46:e35.

34. Friedman CA, Lovejoy FC, Smith AL. Chloramphenicol disposition in infants and children. *J Pediatr.* 1979;95:1071–1077.

35. Kramer AH, Mikolaenko I, Deis N, et al. Intraventricular hemorrhage volume predicts poor outcomes but not delayed ischemic neurological deficits among patients with ruptured cerebral aneurysms. *Neurosurgery.* 2010;67:1044–1053.

36. Akhtar A, Kamal AK. CLEAR: the intraventricular haemorrhage thrombolysis trial. *J Pak Med Assoc.* 2013;63:928.

37. Ziai WC, Tuhrim S, Lane K, et al. A multicenter, randomized, double-blinded, placebo-controlled phase III study of Clot Lysis Evaluation of Accelerated Resolution of Intraventricular Hemorrhage (CLEAR III). *Int J Stroke.* 2014;9:536–542.

38. Findlay JM, Weir BK, Stollery DE. Lysis of intraventricular hematoma with tissue plasminogen activator. Case report. *J Neurosurg.* 1991;74:803–807.

39. Findlay JM, Grace MG, Weir BK. Treatment of intraventricular hemorrhage with tissue plasminogen activator. *Neurosurgery.* 1993;32:941–947.

40. Naff N, Williams MA, Keyl PM, et al. Low-dose recombinant tissue-type plasminogen activator enhances clot resolution in brain hemorrhage: the intraventricular hemorrhage thrombolysis trial. *Stroke.* 2011;42:3009–3016.

41. Findlay JM, Jacka MJ. Cohort study of intraventricular thrombolysis with recombinant tissue plasminogen activator for aneurysmal intraventricular hemorrhage. *Neurosurgery.* 2004;55:532–538.

42. Naff NJ, Hanley DF, Keyl PM, et al. Intraventricular thrombolysis speeds blood clot resolution: results of a pilot, prospective, randomized, double-blind, controlled trial. *Neurosurgery.* 2004;54:577–584.

43. Lapointe M, Haines S. Fibrinolytic therapy for intraventricular hemorrhage in adults. *Cochrane Database Syst Rev.* 2002;(3):CD003692.

44. Morgan T, Awad I, Keyl P, et al. Preliminary report of the clot lysis evaluating accelerated resolution of intraventricular hemorrhage (CLEAR-IVH) clinical trial. *Acta Neurochir Suppl.* 2008;105:217–220.

45. Kramer AH, Roberts DJ, Holodinsky J, et al. Intraventricular tissue plasminogen activator in subarachnoid hemorrhage patients: a prospective, randomized, placebo-controlled pilot trial. *Neurocrit Care.* 2014;21:275–284.

46. Lee SB, Koh HC, Kim ON, et al. Intrathecal administration of sodium nitroprusside, a nitric oxide donor, increases blood pressure in anesthetized rats. *Neurosci Lett.* 1996; 203:53–56.

47. Thomas JE, Rosenwasser RH, Armonda RA, et al. Safety of intrathecal sodium nitroprusside for the treatment and prevention of refractory cerebral vasospasm and ischemia in humans. *Stroke.* 1999;30:1409–1416.

48. Agrawal A, Patir R, Kato Y, et al. Role of intraventricular sodium nitroprusside in vasospasm secondary to aneurysmal subarachnoid haemorrhage: a 5-year prospective study with review of the literature. *Minim Invasive Neurosurg.* 2009;52:5–8.

49. Goodson K, Lapointe M, Monroe T, Chalela JA. Intraventricular nicardipine for refractory cerebral vasospasm after subarachnoid hemorrhage. *Neurocrit Care.* 2008;8: 247–252.

50. Ehtisham A, Taylor S, Bayless L, et al. Use of intrathecal nicardipine for aneurysmal subarachnoid hemorrhage-induced cerebral vasospasm. *South Med J.* 2009;102:150–153.

51. Shibuya M, Suzuki Y, Enomoto H, et al. Effects of prophylactic intrathecal administrations of nicardipine on vasospasm in patients with severe aneurysmal subarachnoid haemorrhage. *Acta Neurochir (Wien).* 1994;131:19–25.

52. Barth M, Pena P, Seiz M, et al. Feasibility of intraventricular nicardipine prolonged release implants in patients following aneurysmal subarachnoid haemorrhage. *Br J Neurosurg.* 2011;25:677–683.

53. Kasuya H. Clinical trial of nicardipine prolonged-release implants for preventing cerebral vasospasm: multicenter cooperative study in Tokyo. *Acta Neurochir Suppl.* 2011; 110:165–167.

54. Schneider UC, Dreher S, Hoffmann KT, et al. The use of nicardipine prolonged release implants (NPRI) in microsurgical clipping after aneurysmal subarachnoid haemorrhage: comparison with endovascular treatment. *Acta Neurochir (Wien).* 2011;153:2119–2125.

55. Barker FG II, Ogilvy CS. Efficacy of prophylactic nimodipine for delayed ischemic deficit after subarachnoid hemorrhage: a metaanalysis. *J Neurosurg.* 1996;84:405–414.

56. Weyer GW, Nolan CP, Macdonald RL. Evidence-based cerebral vasospasm management. *Neurosurg Focus.* 2006;21:E8.

57. van den Bergh WM, Mees SM, Rinkel GJ. Intravenous magnesium versus nimodipine in the treatment of patients with aneurysmal subarachnoid hemorrhage: a randomized study. *Neurosurgery*. 2006;59:E1152.

58. Biondi A, Le Jean L, Puybasset L. Clinical experience of selective intra-arterial nimodipine treatment for cerebral vasospasm following subarachnoid hemorrhage. *Am J Neuroradiol*. 2006;27:474.

59. Auer LM, Ito Z, Suzuki A, Ohta H. Prevention of symptomatic vasospasm by topically applied nimodipine. *Acta Neurochir (Wien)*. 1982;63:297–302.

60. Auer LM, Oberbauer RW, Schalk HV. Human pial vascular reactions to intravenous nimodipine-infusion during EC-IC bypass surgery. *Stroke*. 1983;14:210–213.

61. Auer LM, Suzuki A, Yasui N, Ito Z. Intraoperative topical nimodipine after aneurysm clipping. *Neurochirurgia (Stuttg)*. 1984;27:36–38.

62. Hanggi D, Beseoglu K, Turowski B, Steiger HJ. Feasibility and safety of intrathecal nimodipine on posthaemorrhagic cerebral vasospasm refractory to medical and endovascular therapy. *Clin Neurol Neurosurg*. 2008;110:784–790.

63. Onofrio BM, Yaksh TL, Arnold PG. Continuous low-dose intrathecal morphine administration in the treatment of chronic pain of malignant origin. *Mayo Clin Proc*. 1981; 56:516–520.

64. Hassenbusch SJ, Paice JA, Patt RB, et al. Clinical realities and economic considerations: economics of intrathecal therapy. *J Pain Symptom Manage*. 1997;14:S36–S48.

65. Prager J, Deer T, Levy R, et al. Best practices for intrathecal drug delivery for pain. *Neuromodulation*. 2014;17:354–372.

66. Deer TR, Prager J, Levy R, et al. Polyanalgesic Consensus Conference. 2012: recommendations for the management of pain by intrathecal (intraspinal) drug delivery: report of an interdisciplinary expert panel. *Neuromodulation*. 2012;15:436–466.

67. Deer T, Winkelmuller W, Erdine S, et al. Intrathecal therapy for cancer and nonmalignant pain: patient selection and patient management. *Neuromodulation*. 1999;2:55–66.

68. Carvalho B, Drover DR, Ginosar Y, et al. Intrathecal fentanyl added to bupivacaine and morphine for cesarean delivery may induce a subtle acute opioid tolerance. *Int J Obstet Anesth*. 2012;21:29–34.

69. Goodchild CS, Nadeson R, Cohen E. Supraspinal and spinal cord opioid receptors are responsible for antinociception following intrathecal morphine injections. *Eur J Anaesthesiol*. 2004;21:179–185.

70. Duarte RV, Raphael JH, Southall JL, et al. Intrathecal granuloma formation as result of opioid delivery: systematic literature review of case reports and analysis against a control group. *Clin Neurol Neurosurg*. 2012;114:577–584.

71. Deer T, Chapple I, Classen A, et al. Intrathecal drug delivery for treatment of chronic low back pain: report from the National Outcomes Registry for Low Back Pain. *Pain Med*. 2004;5:6–13.

72. McGivern JG. Ziconotide: a review of its pharmacology and use in the treatment of pain. *Neuropsychiatr Dis Treat*. 2007;3:69–85.

73. Arroyo JC, Quindlen EA. Accumulation of vancomycin after intraventricular infusions. *South Med J*. 1983;76:1554–1555.

74. Taricco M, Pagliacci MC, Telaro E, Adone R. Pharmacological interventions for spasticity following spinal cord injury: results of a Cochrane systematic review. *Eura Medicophys*. 2006;42:5–15.

75. Cohen SP, Dragovich A. Intrathecal analgesia. *Anesthesiol Clin*. 2007;25:863–882, viii.

76. Harned ME, Salles SS, Grider JS. An introduction to trialing intrathecal baclofen in patients with hemiparetic spasticity: a description of 3 cases. *Pain Physician*. 2011; 14:483–489.

77. Ross JC, Cook AM, Stewart GL, Fahy BG. Acute intrathecal baclofen withdrawal: a brief review of treatment options. *Neurocrit Care*. 2011;14:103–108.

78. Greenberg MI, Hendrickson RG. Baclofen withdrawal following removal of an intrathecal baclofen pump despite oral baclofen replacement. *J Toxicol Clin Toxicol*. 2003; 41:83–85.

79. Bellinger A, Siriwetchadarak R, Rosenquist R, Greenlee JD. Prevention of intrathecal baclofen withdrawal syndrome: successful use of a temporary intrathecal catheter. *Reg Anesth Pain Med*. 2009;34:600–602.

80. Eroglu E, Gokcil Z, Bek S, et al. Long-term follow-up of patients with adult-onset subacute sclerosing panencephalitis. *J Neurol Sci*. 2008;275:113–116.

81. Solomon T, Hart CA, Vinjamuri S, et al. Treatment of subacute sclerosing panencephalitis with interferon-alpha, ribavirin, and inosiplex. *J Child Neurol*. 2002;17:703–705.

82. Kurai O, Nakajima S, Kuroki T, et al. Interferon-alpha/beta receptor in patients with HBV [in Japanese]. *Nihon Shokakibyo Gakkai Zasshi*. 1989;86:808.

83. Dastoli PA, Nicacio JM, Silva NS, et al. Cystic craniopharyngioma: intratumoral chemotherapy with alpha interferon. *Arq Neuropsiquiatr*. 2011;69:50–55.

84. Gascon GG, Yamani S, Cafege A, et al. Treatment of subacute sclerosing panencephalitis with alpha interferon. *Ann Neurol*. 1991;30:227–228.

85. Munts AG, van der Plas AA, Ferrari MD, et al. Efficacy and safety of a single intrathecal methylprednisolone bolus in chronic complex regional pain syndrome. *Eur J Pain*. 2010;14:523–528.

86. Rijsdijk M, van Wijck AJ, Meulenhoff PC, et al. No beneficial effect of intrathecal methylprednisolone acetate in postherpetic neuralgia patients. *Eur J Pain*. 2013;17:714–723.

87. Rijsdijk M, van Wijck AJ, Kalkman CJ, Yaksh TL. The effects of glucocorticoids on neuropathic pain: a review with emphasis on intrathecal methylprednisolone acetate delivery. *Anesth Analg*. 2014;118:1097–1112.

88. Kikuchi A, Kotani N, Sato T, et al. Comparative therapeutic evaluation of intrathecal versus epidural methylprednisolone for long-term analgesia in patients with intractable postherpetic neuralgia. *Reg Anesth Pain Med*. 1999;24:287–293.

89. Kotani N, Kushikata T, Hashimoto H, et al. Intrathecal methylprednisolone for intractable postherpetic neuralgia. *N Engl J Med*. 2000;343:1514–1519.

90. Kamin F, Rommer PS, Abu-Mugheisib M, et al. Effects of intrathecal triamincinolone-acetonide treatment in MS patients with therapy-resistant spasticity. *Spinal Cord*. 2015; 53:109–113.

INDEX

CPSIA information can be obtained
at www.ICGtesting.com
Printed in the USA
LVOW13s1349271217
560709LV00017B/20/P